India Migration Report 2022

India Migration Report 2022 is one of the first volumes to focus comprehensively on Indian health professionals' migration. The essays in the volume discuss the reasons, challenges, and opportunities that daunt and prompt health professionals to migrate within and outside India.

This volume:

- Explores the history of migration of health professionals, especially nurses from India;
- Focuses in economic and social drivers of migration among health professionals;
- Examines shifting patterns in migration as well as emergence of new destinations for migrants;
- Studies the economic and social impact of COVID-19 among migrant health professionals;
- Highlights the influence of remittances on rural economies in India.

Timely, data-driven and drawing on exhaustive fieldwork, the volume looks at Indian health professionals in North America, Middle East, Asia Pacific, and South Asia. It will be of interest to scholars and researchers of development studies, public health, public policy, economics, demography, sociology, and social anthropology, and migration and diaspora studies.

S. Irudaya Rajan is Chairman of the International Institute of Migration and Development (IIMAD), India, and Chair of the KNOMAD (the Global Knowledge Partnership on Migration and Development) thematic working group on internal migration and urbanization, World Bank. Earlier, he was Professor at the Centre for Development Studies, and Chair, Research Unit on International Migration (RUIM), funded by the erstwhile Ministry of Overseas Indian Affairs, Government of India (2006–2016). Dr Rajan is the Founding Editor-in-Chief of Migration and Development (Taylor and Francis), Refugee Survey Quarterly (Editorial Board member) and the editor of two Routledge series – India Migration Report and South Asia Migration Report. He has published extensively in national and international journals on demographic, social, economic, political, and psychological implications of international migration. He has also coordinated eight major large-scale migration surveys in Kerala since 1998 (with K.C. Zachariah), Goa (2008), Punjab (2009), Tamil Nadu (2015), and instrumental for Gujarat (2011).

India Migration Report

Editor: **S. Irudaya Rajan**, International Institute of Migration and Development (IIMAD), India

This annual series strives to bring together international networks of migration scholars and policymakers to document and discuss research on various facets of migration. It encourages interdisciplinary commentaries on diverse aspects of the migration experience and continues to focus on the economic, social, cultural, ethical, security, and policy ramifications of international movements of people.

India Migration Report 2016
Gulf Migration

India Migration Report 2017
Forced Migration

India Migration Report 2018
Migrants in Europe

India Migration Report 2019
Diaspora in Europe

India Migration Report 2020
Kerala Model of Migration Surveys

India Migration Report 2021
Migrants and Health

India Migration Report 2022
Health Professionals' Migration

India Migration Report 2023
Indians in Canada

For more information about this series, please visit: https://www.routledge
.com/India-Migration-Report/book-series/IMR

India Migration Report 2022
Health Professionals' Migration

Edited by S. Irudaya Rajan

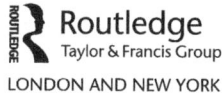

LONDON AND NEW YORK

First published 2023
by Routledge
4 Park Square, Milton Park, Abingdon, Oxon OX14 4RN

and by Routledge
605 Third Avenue, New York, NY 10158

Routledge is an imprint of the Taylor & Francis Group, an informa business

British Library Cataloguing-in-Publication Data
A catalogue record for this book is available from the British Library

Library of Congress Cataloging-in-Publication Data
A catalog record has been requested for this book

ISBN: 978-1-032-32457-9 (hbk)
ISBN: 978-1-032-32459-3 (pbk)
ISBN: 978-1-003-31512-4 (ebk)

DOI: 10.4324/9781003315124

Typeset in Sabon
by Deanta Global Publishing Services, Chennai, India

Contents

List of figures   viii
List of tables   xi
Notes on contributors   xvi
Preface   xviii
Acknowledgements   xxiv

1 The Women Who Paved the Way: At the Beginning of Indian
Nurses' Migration   1
MARIE PERCOT

2 Decision-Making of International Destination: A Case Study
of Indian Nurses in New Zealand   12
YUKO TSUJITA, HISAYA ODA AND S. IRUDAYA RAJAN

3 Analysing Health Professional Mobility from India to Canada   25
AYONA BHATTACHARJEE

4 Becoming a Migrant Healthcare Worker: Interrogating
Gender and Migration   43
SHRUTI GUPTA

5 Beyond the Caring Obligation: Indian Nurses Negotiating
Nursing Care and Migration   57
NEHA ADSUL AND ROHIT SHAH

6 Indian–EU Healthcare Workforce Migration in Data 2000–2019   87
GUNJAN SONDHI

7 An Analysis of Nurses' Intention Not to Migrate: Evidence
from Nurses in Tamil Nadu   108
HISAYA ODA, YUKO TSUJITA AND S. IRUDAYA RAJAN

 8 Health Worker Mobility from India: Trends and
    Opportunities for International Cooperation   121
    RUPA CHANDA AND SUDESHNA GHOSH

 9 The Transmutation of Care and Emotional Labour for a
    Technologically Advanced Workplace: A Case of Indian
    Nurse Migration   163
    NEHA ADSUL

10 India and the Global Provision of Health Professionals:
    Recent Developments and Potential Policy Responses   198
    MARGARET WALTON-ROBERTS AND S. IRUDAYA RAJAN

11 Aspirations of Health Professionals in India
    for Migration Abroad: A Pre-COVID and COVID-Time
    Comparison of Nurses   209
    BINOD KHADRIA AND SHEKHAR TOKAS

12 South–South Migration: Southern Interpretations of a
    Northern Discourse   230
    THEMRISE KHAN

13 Non-payment of Wages Among Gulf returnees in the First
    Wave of COVID-19   244
    S. IRUDAYA RAJAN AND C.S. AKHIL

14 Do Remittances Affect Labour Supply Decisions at a
    Household Level in India?   264
    AMAANI BASHIR

15 COVID-19 and International Migrants: Results from
    Post-Flood Migrant Survey in Kerala   289
    S. IRUDAYA RAJAN AND ROSHAN R. MENON

16 Internal Migrant Enumeration and Service Provision:
    A Municipal Governance Approach   305
    ANANTA KUKREJA AND ASMEETA DAS SHARMA

17 Shutdown Workers and Role of Agents in Tamil Nadu   320
    S. IRUDAYA RAJAN AND BERNARD D'SAMI

18 Understanding Economic Well-Being of the Elderly
Return Migrants in India 334
PINAK SARKAR AND HIMANSHU CHAURASIA

19 Emerging Relationship between Migration and Development
in West Bengal 349
JYOTI PARIMAL SARKAR

20 Migration, Remittances and Welfare: A Study of Ratnagiri
District of Rural Maharashtra 371
BHUPESH GOPAL CHINTAMANI

21 Drivers of Economic and Social Change: The Impact of Indian
Labour Migration to the Gulf 388
SHIBINU S.

Index 405

Figures

3.1   Stocks of India-trained physicians and nurses in major
      destination countries (2010–2018)   26
3.2   Annual inflow and share of foreign-trained HPs
      in Canada   28
3.3   Province-wise Physician density (per 100,000 population)
      by specialty and jurisdiction in Canada   31
3.4   Source country-wise share of foreign-trained physicians in
      Canada   33
3.5   Province-wise share of India-trained Physicians (as % of
      total IMGs in the province), 2018   34
3.6   Source country-wise share of foreign-trained nurses
      in Canada   35
3.7   Share of India-trained nursing workforce employed in direct
      care in Canada, during 2010–2019   36
6.1   Total Indian-born population in EU-27, 2010–2020   93
6.2   Percentage females as total Indian-born population in
      EU-27 by sex, 2020   94
6.3   Residence permits issued to Indians by reason,
      2015 and 2019   94
6.4   First permits issued to Indians, by reason and sex, 2019   95
6.5   First permits issued to Indians, by sex, 2017   95
6.6   Stock of Indian-trained doctors 2011–2018   96
6.7   Stock of Indian-trained nurses 2011–2019   97
6.8   Stock of Indian-trained doctors in Germany 2000–2018   97
6.9   Stock of Indian-trained nurses in Italy 2000–2019   98
6.10 Annual flow of Indian-trained nurses in Italy 2000–2019   100
6.11 Comparison of stocks and flow of Indian-trained nurses
      in Italy 2000–2019   101
6.12 Annual flow of Indian-trained doctors and nurses in
      Ireland 2010–2019   101

8.1	Share of foreign-born doctors in 27 OECD countries, 2015/16	125
8.2	Share of foreign-born nurses 2016	125
8.3	Growth in practising doctors between 2010/11 and 2015/16 attributed to foreign-born doctors in 15 OECD countries	126
8.4	Growth in practising nurses between 2010/11 and 2015/16 attributed to foreign-born nurses in 12 OECD countries	126
18.1	Quintile distribution of the NM and RM population cohorts in rural India	337
18.2	Quintile distribution of the NM and RM population cohorts in urban India	340
19.1	Classification of total migrant population in West Bengal by place of birth (POB): 1961–2011	353
19.2	Percentage of inter-district migrant population (place of birth) in districts of West Bengal: 1961–2011	354
19.3	Percentage of inter-state migrant population (place of birth) in districts of West Bengal: 1961–2011	354
19.4	Reasons for inter-district (ID) migration in West Bengal, 1981–2011	358
19.5	Reasons for inter-state (IS) migration in West Bengal, 1981–2011	358
19.6	Percentage of migrants based on landholding in West Bengal, 2007–08	359
19.7	Percentage of migrants in different educational levels in West Bengal, 2007–08	359
19.8	Migration rates for rural and urban in across MPCE Quintile Classes	361
19.9	Distribution of migrants and non-migrants in different economic status in rural and urban areas in West Bengal, 2007–08	362
19.10	Percentage of immigrants from Bangladesh in districts of West Bengal: 1981–2011	366
20.1	Marital status of migrants	377
20.2	Family status of migrants	378
20.3	Education status of migrants	379
20.4	Destination of migrants from sample households	379
20.5	Occupation structure of migrants	380
20.6	Expenditure pattern of the group of households on education, health, and food spending	384

21.1   Age composition of Gulf migrants by three districts   391
21.2   Religious distribution of Gulf migrants by districts   392
21.3   Educational .level of Gulf migrants by districts   393
21.4   Average monthly income of Gulf migrants during the
       pre- and post-migration phase by districts (in Rs.)   394

Tables

2.1	Foreign-Trained Nurses and the Country of Origin in New Zealand (Stock)	15
2.2	Survey Participants	18
3.1	Future Projections of the Number of HP-Related Job Openings and Job Seekers in Canada	29
3.2	Average Pass Rates Compared to Pass Rates of IENs During 2017 and 2018	37
4.1	Selected Healthcare Professions in the UAE by Nationality and Gender, Various Years	45
4.2	Average Salary of Healthcare Workers Interviewed (2017)	47
6.1	Annual Flow of Indian-Trained Doctors and Nurses in Ireland 2010–2019	102
7.1	Summary of the International Migration Experience of the Sample Nurses	111
7.2	Descriptive Statistics and Definitions of Explanatory Variables	113
7.3	Results of Logit Estimation (Odds Ratios)	114
7.4	Reasons for Non-Migration	115
7.5	Levels of Happiness of Nurses Who Did/Did Not Intend to Migrate	116
8.1	Share of Foreign-trained Doctors and Nurses in Selected OECD Countries, 2018 (Unless Otherwise Indicated)	124
8.2	Selected Bilateral Agreements on Health Worker Migration and Their Key Features	131
8.3	Stock of Foreign-trained Doctors in Selected OECD Countries (Numbers), 2014–19	133
8.4	Stock of Foreign-trained Nurses in Selected OECD Countries (Numbers), 2014–19	136
8.5	OECD Foreign-Trained Nurses: Share of Indian Nurses Among Total Foreign-Trained Nurses and Total Practising Nurses in Destination Countries, 2016	137

8.6	Registered Doctors and Nurses in the UK by Country of Primary Medical Qualification (Numbers), 2021	138
8.7	Number of Foreign-Born Health Workers, By Source Country and Occupational Category in OECD Countries, 2016	139
8.8	Partners' Scheduled Commitments in Health Worker Related Service Sectors/Subsectors in FTAs with India	145
8.9	India's Scheduled Mode 4 Commitments in Health Worker Related Sectors/Subsectors	148
10.1	Top Five Countries of Destination for India-Trained Doctors, 2014–19	201
10.2	Emigration of Nurses by State under Emigration Check Required (ECR), May 2015–November 2018	203
10.3	Indian State-Run Agencies through Which International Nurse Recruitment Is Allowed	204
11.1	Mobility Aspirations for Out-Migration of Nurses in India: 2002 and 2021	220
13.1	Return of Migrants to Kerala by Destination, 2021	248
13.2	Occupation of Return Migrants Prior to Return, 2021	249
13.3	Reason for Return Among Return Migrants in Kerala, 2021	250
13.4	Profile of Return Migrants Who Lost Job, 2021	250
13.5	Duration of Stay Among Return Migrants Who Lost Jobs, 2021	251
13.6	Occupation of the Return Migrants Who Lost Their Jobs, 2021	251
13.7	Nature of Job Loss Among Return Migrants, 2021	252
13.8	Occupational of the Return Migrants Who Were Asked to Resign, 2021	252
13.9	Duration of Stay and Non-payment of Wages, 2021	253
13.10	Breakdown of Non-payment of Dues and Benefits Reported by Return Migrants, 2021	254
14.1	General Ordinary Least Squares Regression	270
14.2	Structural Equation (Heckman Correction)	271
14.3	OLS vs. Heckman Correction	274
14.4	Heckman-Corrected IV	276
14.5	Average Model Cross Validation	277
14.6	Rural Ordinary Least Squares	279
14.7	Heckman Correction – Rural	281
14.8	Heckman Correction	282
14.9	Heckman-Corrected Rural IV	283
14.10	Average Rural Model Cross Validation	283

14.11   Multinomial Logistic Regression   284
15.1   District-wise Rainfall During the Period from 1 August to
        30 August 2018   291
15.2   District-wise Rainfall During the Period from 1 August to
        30 August 2019   292
15.3   Breakdown of Sampling Units   294
15.4   Households Affected by the Floods   295
15.5   Houses Damaged by the Floods   295
15.6   Insurance Status of Houses   296
15.7   Compensation Received from the Government Towards
        the Damage Caused   296
15.8   Damage Caused to Non-agricultural Land Due to Floods   296
15.9   Compensation Received From the Government Towards
        the Damage Caused to Non-agricultural Lands   297
15.10   Number of Days without Electricity after Floods   297
15.11   Number of Days without Water after Floods   298
15.12   Damage Caused to Agricultural Land Due to Floods   299
15.13   Compensation Received from the Government Towards
        the Damage Caused to Agricultural Land   299
15.14   Effect on Agricultural Crops Due to Floods   299
15.15   Impact of the Floods on Usual Economic Activities   299
15.16   Economic Activities Affected Due to the Floods and
        Reasons for Disruption   300
15.17   Impact of Floods on Businesses   300
15.18   Extent of Loss to Businesses Due to Floods   301
17.1   Destination of Returned Shutdown Workers, 2021   325
17.2   Characteristics of the Return Shutdown Workers, 2021   326
17.3   Occupation of the Return Shutdown Workers, 2021   327
17.4   Duration of Stay at the Countries of Destination by
        Return Shutdown migrants, 2021   327
17.5   Sponsorship of Return Flights as Reported by Return
        Shutdown Workers, 2021   327
17.6   Reason for Return Shutdown Migrants   328
17.7   Salaries Received by the Return Shutdown Migrants
        in the Destination, 2021   329
17.8   Future Plans of the Return Shutdown Migrants, 2021   329
18.1   Odds-Ratio Likelihood of Return Migration across the
        Major Indian States   337
18.2   Distribution of NM and RM Population Cohort for
        Illiterate and Literate Groups in Rural Area   338
18.3   Distribution of NM and RM Population Cohorts for
        Social Groups in Rural Area   339

18.4   Distribution of NM and RM Population Cohorts for
        Illiterate and Literate Groups in Urban Area   341
18.5   Distribution of NM and RM Population Cohorts for
        Social Groups in Urban Area   341
18.6   The RDI of Being Elderly RM Compared to Others RM
        in Rural India   345
18.7   The RDI of Being Elderly RM Compared to Others RM
        in Urban India   346
19.1   Identification of Levels of Development in Various Sectors 351
19.2   Sex-Wise Percentage of Migrant Population in Both Rural
        and Urban Areas of West Bengal (1961–2011)   352
19.3   Percentage of Inter-district Migrant Population
        (Place of Birth) in Districts of West Bengal (1961–2011)   356
19.4   Percentage of Inter-State Migrant Population
        (Place of Birth) in Districts of West Bengal (1961–2011)   357
19.5   Percentage Distribution of Migrants by Usual Principal
        Activity Status for Different Categories in West Bengal
        (2007–08)   360
19.6   Percentage of Migrants in Different Social Groups in
        West Bengal (2007–08)   360
19.7   (a): Coefficient of Correlation (r) between Inter-State
        Migration and Sectoral Indices of Development of
        Districts for 1971–2011   363
19.7   (b): Coefficient of Correlation (r) between Inter-state
        Male Migration and Sectoral Indices of Development of
        Districts for 1971–2011   363
19.8   (a): Coefficient of Correlation (r) between Inter-District
        Migration and Sectoral Indices of Development of
        Districts for 1971–2011   365
19.8   (b): Coefficient of Correlation (r) between Inter-District
        Male Migration and Sectoral Indices of Development of
        Districts for 1971–2011   365
19.9   Results of Regression Equation for Decennial Growth
        Rates in Population of Districts in West Bengal, 1961–2011 367
19.10   Coefficient of Correlation (r) between International
        Migration and Sectoral Indices of Development of
        Districts for 1971–2011   368
20.1   Sample Households Representation as per Social Groups   373
20.2   Sample Household Basic Characteristics in the
        Sample Groups   373
20.3   Descriptive Statistics of Sample Household   375
20.4   Age of Expatriates Before and After Migration   376

20.5   Mode of Transfer Information   381
21.1   Average Duration of Stay in Gulf by Gender   391
21.2   Main Occupation of Gulf Migrants before and
        after Migration   393
21.3   Utilization of the Loan Taken by the Gulf Migrant
        Households   395
21.4   Educational Level of Family Members in the Age Group
        20–49 by Households and Three Districts, 2016   396
21.5   Percentage Distribution of Older Person Households, 2016   397
21.6   Percentage Distribution of Households with Adult Male
        Members, 2016   397
21.7   Percentage Distribution of Type of Houses by the
        Households, 2016   398
21.8   Possession of Household Amenities by Type of
        Households, 2016   399
21.9   Standard of Living of Gulf Migrant and Non-migrant
        Households, 2016   400
21.10   Income Utilization Pattern by Type of Households, 2016   400

Contributors

Neha Adsul is Post-Doctoral Fellow, Centre for Policy Studies, Indian Institute of Technology, Mumbai.

C.S. Akhil is Research Fellow at the International Institute of Migration and Development, Kerala, India.

Amaani Bashir is Research Fellow at the National Institute of Public Finance and Policy, New Delhi, and an alumnus of the University of Warwick and School of Oriental and African Studies, United Kingdom.

Ayona Bhattacharjee is Assistant Professor, International Management Institute, New Delhi.

Rupa Chanda is RBI Chair Professor in Economics, Indian Institute of Management, Bangalore.

Himanshu Chaurasia is Scientist-B, National Institute for Research in Reproductive Health, Mumbai.

Bhupesh Gopal Chintamani is with Gokhale Institute of Politics and Economics, Pune, India.

Asmeeta Das Sharma is India Smart Cities Fellow, Ministry of Housing and Urban Affairs, Government of India affiliated to National Institute of Urban Affairs, New Delhi.

Bernard D'Sami is Senior Fellow, Loyola Institute of Social Science Training and Research (LISSTAR), Loyola College, Chennai, Tamil Nadu.

Sudeshna Ghosh is Research Associate, Indian Institute of Management, Bangalore.

Shruti Gupta is Doctoral Fellow, Faculty of Arts and Social Sciences, National University of Singapore.

Oda Hisaya is Professor, College of Policy Science, Department of Policy Science, Ritsumeikan University, Osaka, Japan.

S. Irudaya Rajan is Chairman, The International Institute of Migration and Development, Kerala.

Binod Khadria is Former Professor of Economics, Education and International Migration at Jawaharlal Nehru University, New Delhi.

Themrise Khan is an LSE DESTIN Alumnus and former Chevening Scholar (2000) and Honorary Visiting Professor at the International Institute of Migration and Development, India.

Ananta Kukreja is India Smart Cities Fellow, Ministry of Housing and Urban Affairs, Government of India affiliated to National Institute of Urban Affairs, New Delhi.

Roshan R. Menon is Research Fellow at the International Institute of Migration and Development, Kerala, India.

Marie Percot is Researcher with the French National Council for Scientific Research, Paris, France.

Jyoti Parimal Sarkar is Assistant Professor at SES's L.S.Raheja College of Arts and Commerce, Mumbai and Senior Research Fellow, The International Institute of Migration and Development, Kerala, India.

Pinak Sarkar is Assistant Professor, Centre for Development Practice & Research, Tata Institute of Social Sciences, Patna

Rohit Shah is Doctoral Fellow at Indian Institute of Technology, Mumbai and Monash Research Academy.

Shibinu, S, Head, Department of Economics, PSMO College, Tirurangadi, Kerala, India.

Gunjan Sondhi is Lecturer in Geography, Faculty of Arts and Social Sciences, School of Social Sciences and Global Studies, The Open University, United Kingdom.

Shekhar Tokas is Assistant Professor of Economics, Centre for New Initiatives and Research, SGT University, Gurugram, Delhi-NCR.

Yuko Tsujita is Researcher with Institute of Developing Economies of Japan External Trade Organization, Japan.

Margaret Walton-Roberts is Professor of Geography and Environmental Studies at Wilfrid Laurier University and the Balsillie School of International Affairs (BSIA), Waterloo Canada.

Preface

It is with great honour that I write this preface to introduce and present the *India Migration Report 2022* – the 13th report in the series. The theme of IMR 2022 is 'Health Professionals' Migration'. As I write this preface towards the beginning of 2022, the COVID-19 pandemic has taken 5.6 million lives and has lasted for almost two years. Now, most of the countries are in the third wave and it looks like there is no end to it till we complete the year 2022.

This timely collection of chapters from scholars on the migration of health professionals will be a great addition to the existing scholarship on migration. It is my hope that IMR 2022 will be studied and pondered over by researchers, policymakers, and the general public to understand the challenges and shortcomings in the current regime of migration of health professionals, so that we may solve some of the issues on migration that were brought to the surface by the pandemic.

Before I introduce the chapters of IMR 2022, I believe a recap of the previous India Migration Reports in their chronological order would be helpful. IMR 2010 looked at the various factors affecting migrants and migration in India. The report investigated gender-wise disparities and government policies pertaining to migration. While the first half of the report discussed the various impacts of migration on the country, the second half discussed the government's involvement in migration processes.

IMR 2011 studied internal migration in India and its different characteristics. The report also investigated the factors of caste and identity to gain a deeper understanding of the political and sociological impacts due to migration. In addition, IMR 2011 also critically examined the economic impact of migration. IMR 2012 investigated the effect of the Global Financial Crisis on migration. The report discussed how the Global Financial Crisis of 2008 affected Indian emigrants in different countries. The impact of the financial crisis in various Gulf countries and its consequences on migrants were particularly discussed in detail in this report.

IMR 2013 focused on the social, psychological, and human changes that migration imprints on members of the migrant households that are left behind, such as women, children, and the elderly. Issues such as the negotiation of children regarding parental migration, livelihood patterns of left out women, and the overall demographic implications on society that migration creates were also discussed. IMR 2014 looked at the Indian diaspora around the world and their contributions to the country. While the first half explored the features of the Indian diaspora and their contribution to development in their host and native countries, the second half examined the characteristics and nature of Indian diaspora in general.

IMR 2015 reported the experiences of internal migrants in India whilst also giving a focus on the role of gender in migration. The aspects of migration that are less researched such as marriage migration were discussed in the report. IMR 2015 also highlighted the relationship between the economy and changing gender dynamics brought about by migration. The IMR 2016 investigated Indian migration to the Middle East. It reviewed the current opportunities for and challenges faced by the existing and future migrants in Gulf countries. It also focused on different experiences of migrant workers and their living conditions in the Middle East.

IMR 2017 studied forced migration which is an ever-relevant phenomenon in India. The report detailed how various development projects such as industrialization and urban infrastructure construction in India have negatively affected the lives of marginalized communities and forced them to migrate to new locations. The report, in addition, analysed the outcome of this forced migration and the impact it has on the displaced people. IMR 2018 is a report on Indian migration to Europe. The report discussed the prospects and challenges of migrating to Europe while analysing different migration routes to Europe including skilled and unskilled labour migration and student migration. IMR 2018 also discussed the consequences of Brexit on migrants and how Indian migrant labourers are exploited in various parts of Europe.

IMR 2019 elaborated the lives and histories of the Indian diaspora in Europe. The report identified and described Indian communities in different parts of Europe and how they contribute to the economic development in India. The report also investigated the Indian diaspora's own subculture in these European countries, and how the social and political policies of these destination European countries affected their lives. IMR 2020 was an extensive report based on the wealth of data collected over two decades by the Kerala Migration Surveys. This report covered many topics on migration – from remittances and migration policy to return migration and gender. IMR 2020 is a classic example of the need for an all-India migration survey that can answer many questions on migration in India. The last IMR (2021) was a study on the health of migrants. The report brought to the fore the health characteristics of migrants before and during the COVID-19 pandemic. This IMR (2022) continues in this intellectual tradition to discuss a theme that is relevant, timely, and worthy of scholarly discussion – health professionals' migration.

In Chapter 1 of IMR 2022, Marie Percot traces the history of migration of nurses to the Middle East, beginning in the early 1980s. The chapter discusses the challenges that pioneer nurses from Kerala faced while migrating, and how they overcame the social stigma associated with young women travelling abroad alone. This chapter is the result of extensive fieldwork of the author among the first-generation nurse migrants between 2000 and 2011. The chapter also brings to the forefront the contribution of migrant nurses to their families and to the state of Kerala.

Yuko Tsujita, Hisaya Oda, and S. Irudaya Rajan explore the migration of Indian nurses to New Zealand in Chapter 2. Based on a larger study conducted among Indian nurses in Auckland, this chapter illuminates factors that make countries like New Zealand attractive for migrant Indian nurses. In this chapter, the authors' critical examination of the qualifications required to work as a nurse in New Zealand will also be a great source of information for prospective migrant nurses.

In Chapter 3, Ayona Bhattacharjee presents the results of an exploratory research project on the mobility of health professionals (HPs) to Canada, with a special focus on Indian health professionals. The chapter seeks to plug the gaps in research on migration of HPs to Canada when compared to countries like the United States or the United Kingdom. Bringing the uncertainty surrounding migration due the pandemic to the limelight, the author argues for a joint effort by the Indian and Canadian authorities to improve the mobility of Indian HPs.

Shruti Gupta highlights the gendered experiences of migrant healthcare workers in Asia, with a special reference to the migration of women healthcare workers from India to the United Arab Emirates (UAE) in Chapter 4. Based on semi-structured interviews with women migrant HPs, the author explores the interplay between gender and the migration of Indian healthcare professionals to UAE, the creation of the demand for and supply of workers, the channels of migration, and the policies governing migration and professionalisation. In this chapter, the author also emphasises the lack of data on women migrant health workers, and the complex immigration policies and licensing regimes imposed in this regard.

In Chapter 5, Neha Adsul and Rohit Shah discuss what skilled nursing care consists of and its contribution to the well-being of the patients. Based on in-depth interviews conducted among nurses working in different hospitals in India, the chapter reveals the various economic and social dimensions of being a nurse and the need for enhanced support for nurses.

Gunjan Sondhi provides country-wise data on the mobility of healthcare workers between India and EU during the period 2018–2019 in Chapter 6. Through this, the chapter aims to support evidence-based policy-making to ensure the safe migration and decent working conditions for the migrant healthcare professionals. The chapter also throws light into the question on the limitations of OECD datasets and emphasises the need for further research on the migration of healthcare professionals in the India–EU corridor.

In Chapter 7, Hisaya Oda, Yuko Tsujita, and Irudaya Rajan discuss the numerous factors that contribute towards the decision of non-migrating nurses. Based on a survey conducted among the alumni of two prominent nursing schools in Tamil Nadu, the chapter underscores the massive salary gap between nurses working in the public and private sectors. The authors conclude that as long as private employment salary falls remarkably short of government salary, nurses in the private sector will continue to seek opportunities abroad.

Rupa Chanda and Sudeshna Ghosh explore the salient features of India's health worker migration to the rest of the world, and the management of this migration through bilateral and other arrangements in Chapter 8. While highlighting factors that enhance the mobility of health workers, the authors recommend policies that provide opportunity as well as safeguard the rights of migrant health workers,

In Chapter 9, Neha Adsul investigates the role of techno-social structures, including social networks and training institutions in decision-making to migrate among nurses. Based on interviews conducted among nurses in 2016–2017, the author observes that market demands penetrating the training regime of nurses, advances in science and technology creating a competent workforce, overseas network of nursing professionals, etc., are some factors driving migration among nurses in India.

Margaret Walton-Roberts and S. Irudaya Rajan examine India's role in the global provision of HPs by exploring international migration patterns and processes, considering established and emerging patterns of migration and presenting relevant Indian policy responses in Chapter 10. The chapter underscores the frailties in the Indian healthcare sector as a major reason for the migration of the Indian healthcare professionals and encourages the formulation of policies that protect the interests of healthcare professionals both at home and overseas.

In Chapter 11, Binod Khadria and Shekhar Tokas explore the imposition of travel restrictions in the wake of the COVID-19 pandemic and its impact on the mobility aspirations of health workers in general and nurses in particular. Based on surveys conducted among two samples of nurses separated by almost two decades, the authors conclude that while better living and working conditions were the primary motives for migration prior to the disruptions caused by the pandemic, personal safety as well as safety of the family members emerged as a major factor hampering migration in a world made chaotic by the pandemic.

Themrise Khan explores the phenomenon of migration and mobility within the global south, based on the experiences of the author as a southern practitioner and researcher on migration and development and as a migrant herself from the traditional north–south migration corridor in Chapter 12. The author identifies major perception deficits in the northern literature on south–south migration and calls for creating a counter-narrative or self-narrative on south–south migration.

In Chapter 13, S. Irudaya Rajan and C.S. Akhil investigate the nature and scale of wage-theft among returnee migrants from Gulf countries in

Kerala, in the wake of the pandemic based on the recent return migrants survey in Kerala. The authors observe that wage-theft is more prevalent among the low-skilled workers, and the lack of access to legal recourse and the absence of effective labour protection laws are the major hurdles in addressing the grievances of migrant labourers facing the threat of wage-theft.

Amaani Bashir examines the impact of remittances on labour supply decisions of households dependent on migration in India, especially in the rural setting in Chapter 14. The author posits that the remittance impact is more pronounced in the rural sector which displays a higher elasticity to remittances. This chapter also further proves the micro-foundations of the literature surrounding remittances, inducing a Dutch disease effect by positing that remittances have a persistently negative and significant impact on the decision to work in Indian households.

In Chapter 15, S. Irudaya Rajan and Roshan R. Menon assess the impact of floods in Kerala in 2018 and 2019. Based on a large-scale survey conducted by the senior author, the chapter analyses the impact of the floods on agriculture, economic activity, business/commerce, self-employment, etc., and the cascading disruptions that followed.

Ananta Kukreja and Asmeeta Das Sharma employ phenomenological research to investigate the condition of migrant workers in the city and the practical gaps in migration governance with a special reference to the city of Surat in Gujarat in Chapter 16. The authors posit data collection on the state of migrant labourers by the Urban Local Bodies (ULB) as a major step towards initiating welfare measures for the migrant labourers – one that can prevent the mass exodus of migrant labour in instances of sudden uncertainty.

In Chapter 17, S. Irudaya Rajan and Bernard D'Sami examine the impact of travel restrictions on the 'shutdown' migrant workers from Tamil Nadu, who had been making a living in the GCC countries. Based on a survey conducted during the return migrant survey in 2021 among 'shutdown' workers in Tamil Nadu, the authors shine a light onto this unexplored phenomenon and deliver recommendations to streamline the recruitment process so as to prevent the exploitation of migrant workers.

Pinak Sarkar and Himanshu Chaurasia compare the economic well-being of elderly return migrants with all return migrants and non-migrants in Chapter 18. Based on the National Sample Survey (64th round), the authors find that elderly return migrants are in a relatively better economic position compared to all-age return migrants and non-migrants across various states and migrant groups.

In Chapter 19, Jyoti Parimal Sarkar explores the trends associated with migration to the Indian state of West Bengal over the past few decades. The author aims to establish possible linkages between migration and diversified development in West Bengal and by observing concentration of the migrant population in the industrially and agriculturally advanced districts, lack of land ownership, and poor educational background in the rural areas, etc., the author posits the validation of modernisation theory of migration.

Bhupesh Gopal Chintamani examines basic characteristics of emigrants, their age, education, occupation, destination, and mode of transfers in Maharashtra in Chapter 20. To determine the pace of development among the recipients, the study has interviewed two categories of respondents, namely migrant and non-migrant households, with a structured question-naire and the analysis validated a positive association between inward remit-tances on the economic welfare and subsistence of the recipient households.

Emigration and remittances have been praised as a source of funding for household and community transformation. Due to its historical linkage to overseas migration, Kerala has been one of the most significant source regions for Indian temporary workers, mainly to the Gulf. In Chapter 21, Shibinu examines/empirical findings of the socio-economic discourses of Gulf migration on the emigrants, their households, and the region from which they emigrated, and how they differ from the non-migrant households.

The India Migration Report 2023 will focus on Indians in Canada while the India Migration Report 2024 will examine Indians in the United States.

S. Irudaya Rajan

Acknowledgements

Over the last 13 years, the India Migration Report (IMR) series have received overwhelming support and global recognition from readers that include development practitioners, policymakers, and researchers as well as activists, and the IMR series have emerged as prime reference works in the field of migration. I take this opportunity to thank all the contributors who have helped to make every report in the series a must-read. In particular, I take this occasion to thank all the contributors for the IMR 2022, for providing stimulating and thought-provoking articles on the health of migrants, in both the origin and destination, both at the time of migration and during the health crisis unleashed by the COVID pandemic.

The IMR series was in my dream since 2006, conceived formally in 2008 and commenced in 2010, with the first IMR made possible with the support and guidance of the erstwhile Ministry of Overseas Indian Affairs (MOIA), Government of India, which established the first Research Unit on International Migration (RUIM) from 2006 to 2016, at the Centre for Development Studies, where I worked as the Chair Professor. I express my gratitude to all the secretaries of the MOIA, especially to S. Krishna Kumar, K. Mohandas and Dr A. Didar Singh, without whose help this series would not have begun and become what it is today.

The 13th IMR is the second IMR being organized after my departure from the Centre for Development Studies in April 2020 to the newly established think-tank, the International Institute of Migration and Development (IIMAD) (www.iiimad.org). I would like to take this opportunity to thank the board members, in particular, K.C. Zachariah and U.S. Misrha and the research team – Sunitha, Sreeja, Migdad, Anand, Nelgyn, Anjana, Arya, Lathika, Nikhil, Aneeta, and Ashwin – of the IIMAD for their hard work and enthusiastic support in putting the series together.

I am eternally grateful for the emotional support, patience, and understanding I have received from my wife Hema and our three children – Rahul, Rohit, and Mary Catherine – without which none of this would have been possible.

Last but not least, I would like to put on record my appreciation for the hard work of the editorial and sales team at Routledge for bringing out this report on time.

S. Irudaya Rajan

1 The Women Who Paved the Way

At the Beginning of Indian Nurses' Migration

Marie Percot

Introduction

It has been nearly half a century since the Indian nurses started to migrate abroad, beginning with the Gulf countries. Despite the pitfalls, possible exploitation or disappointment, for the young generation of migrant nurses, the expectations are rather well measured and strategies broadly mastered (Percot, 2006; Percot and Rajan, 2007; Nair and Rajan, 2017; Walton-Roberts et al., 2017; Walton-Roberts and Rajan, 2013, 2020). The migration culture that today women have acquired was slowly built on the experience of older ones who, as pioneers, had to struggle hard both in the receiving country and in their home country. This chapter deals with the first generation of nurses who paved the way for a well-established robust network of migration, which is existent even today.

This study is based on fieldworks stretched over a long period of time, conducted in India and in the Gulf between 2000 and 2011. In addition to the notes taken during the fieldwork, this chapter also relies on telephonic conversations with the participants, which took place prior to the writing of the chapter.

The chapter deals with the circumstances surrounding the departure from the place of origin and arrival at the host community. The second section deals with the way they were perceived at home, in Kerala, as the first female migrants. The concluding section traces how these pioneers contributed to the development of the migratory network.

Learning Migration, Learning About the Gulf

It is at the end of the 1970s that the nurses from India were first recruited in order to work in the Gulf. These countries were just beginning to develop their infrastructure, including the healthcare system. (Al Khayat, 1981; Qutub, 1983) As the salaries offered were not attractive enough for the nurses from the West, nurses from countries like the Philippines and India found a favourable option. Although India and the Philippines had a strong and reliable network for training nurses, the job opportunities and salary

DOI: 10.4324/9781003315124-1

were not so promising to keep them in their homeland. The first hospitals in the Gulf were mainly government institutions, and the recruitment in India was executed directly by their agents who conducted interviews and selection in big cities such as Delhi and Mumbai. Later, a few Indian recruiting agencies were also operating on their behalf, but they were limited to the same places and were offering fewer positions. For the potential migrants, it was at that time almost free of cost, which means there were no recruitment fees and a paid flight to destination, in a move to encourage candidates to apply. The first women who took the chance were around 35–40 years old, having years of experience as nurses. Although some had stopped working after attaining motherhood, all of them were married. Almost all of them too were Malayali Christians. They were among the very first women from India to migrate abroad alone.

Maryama who left for Kuwait in 1977 at the age of 36 and had spent 14 years over there explained:

> We were living in Delhi where my husband was working in an airplane company. He came to know that special planes were reserved in his company to transport nurses to the Gulf from Bombay. We thought about this opportunity and I started to check newspapers for information about it, but could not find anything. Then a cousin of mine who is also a nurse and lives in Bombay told me that recruiters were offering good proposals there. That is how we decided that I should try. The recruitment took place in hotel. There were some twenty candidates, all from Kerala. Almost all of us were recruited. We eventually left on the same day in order to work in the same hospital.

They stated that they had indeed very little information about their destination. They had been told that the remuneration was high, 10–15 times higher than what was paid then in India and that it would be paid on time. It was also said that the conditions of living were safe. However, since not much was known, it was a risk for those who decided to accept the challenge.

Lethika who had arrived in Muscat in 1980 said:

> There were already Malayali men working abroad, but they were not so many. It's not like how it is today when everybody knows much about the Gulf. Even those who haven't been there, they are able to figure out how it looks like. In the 80's, it was different. When I left for Muscat, I had no picture in my mind. It was like living a big adventure. It is fortunate that I left with other nurses, but all of us were rather afraid. [The recruiters] had said "Don't worry, everything is organized. We will wait for you at the airport, we will take you directly to the hostel and the hostel is in the hospital compound". They insisted that we will never be left alone. Still, it was my first real trip, my first time without the family. Had I not been so motivated by the prospect of helping my

family, I would not have climbed the first step of the plane. You had to be brave to take the plunge at that time.

After having taken the difficult decision to leave and once they had arrived at their destination, most remembered the beginning of their stay as a real shock. At first, it was the underdevelopment of most places that surprised them. They underlined for instance that *Kuwait City was not even like a small town of Kerala.* "Muscat was almost a village with very few tarred roads. There were some buildings here and there and nothing in the middle" or "My hospital [in Abu Dhabi] was in the middle of the desert with nothing around but camels and the people rearing them".

As nurses, they were also surprised by patients who still had a very limited experience of modern hospitals or medicine:

> You can't imagine how it was. Only rich people there knew what a hospital is because they used to go to Bombay if they needed to. But the others were afraid of everything in the hospital and, of course, they were not able to speak a single word of English. I remember a woman who was delivering and needed an episiotomy [a common operation to facilitate a difficult delivery]. She was crying aloud but she refused to be touched and so the baby died.

This account was given by Mary, who arrived in Dubai in 1978 and stayed there for 25 years. The educated and professionally qualified Indian nurses who arrived in the Gulf developed clearly a disdain for their destination country and for its people that they have certainly contributed to propagate at home. Here is a statement which was repeated in the 2000s as well and it is something that is being told very often almost verbatim:

> These people are totally uneducated; they are not even able to do things by themselves. It's the foreigners who are doing everything. These Arabs, they have just been lucky to have oil, otherwise they would still be walking behind their camels!

But Pax, for instance, also added: "They were rude, with no respect. You know, as if foreigners were lower than them". Considering themselves coming from a lot more refined civilization and as a lot more educated, it has been all the more difficult for those women to bear being treated with scorn by the local people.

So, it was hard dealing with patients and it was not so easy either to deal with the physicians. For the first nurses, the level of proficiency in English was not very high. In addition, physicians coming from very different places had a variety of English accents. Communication was indeed a bit uncertain, increasing the fear of misunderstanding an order and making mistakes. Many described a long period of stress before being able to quietly collaborate with all the medical staff. To overcome such difficulties, nurses needed to develop a strong solidarity as Radhika stated:

> We were helping each other a lot. Working more with such or such physician, we were getting used to work with him, so we would advise a colleague who was not used to him of what to do according to his habits. If one of us was stuck because she has not understood, we would find a trick to have the order repeated. At that time, we were really considering each other as sisters.

As a matter of fact, the pioneers were not only working but also living together. No family life was then possible in the Gulf and no nurse had independent housing. All of them were residing in hostels located in the hospital's compounds. As it is still mostly the norm today in hostels, nurses from the same community shared a common ward. Indian nurses were thus sharing rooms, cooking and eating, and spending free time together. It must be remembered that in the 1980s there was still no internet. Calling home was very expensive, watching an Indian TV channel impossible. To get news from home, nurses had to wait for letters which came very late. This isolation from the family was certainly the most difficult aspect of their migration, particularly as mothers. All of them remember the suffering inflicted by being separated from their children.

Maryama remarked:

> You can't compare with today's situation. Now, even if your children are far away, you can speak to and see them every day on WhatsApp. You can decide with their father or their keepers what do in case a problem arises. You can see for yourself if they are ok or not. At that time, you just had a few lines every ten or fifteen days. You were always wondering if those lines were even true or if they had not written them just to make you feel good. Even pictures were expensive and more complicated, so they were not so commonly sent. It means that, for a full year, you were just terribly missing your family and children. I remember thinking that my youngest one may not even recognize me when I go back for the next holidays.

The 1980s witnessed a spurt in the number of Indians migrating to the Gulf countries, and among them Malayalees were the most prominent group. As a fallout of the presence of Indian migrants, shops, movie theatres, religious associations, etc., were established. Yet hospitals and hostels continued for some years to be the only horizon migrant nurses had. Although most of them described the leisure time they spent within the hospital campus boring, they did not venture out to the so-called Indian neighbourhoods, as they thought it would not augur well for their status as women. The stigma attached to female migrants was prevalent in Kerala and there were chances of them being suspected of prostitution (cf. section "From Loose Women to Useful Women"). Apart from a certain fear of venturing in unknown spaces, not to be seen outside of the hospital by fellow countrymen was considered as the best strategy not to be branded as *loose women* at a personal as well as at a collective level. As Mary said: "If only one of us would have behaved badly, it would have given a bad name to all of us". It is not before a familial migration was established (by the very end of the 1980s or beginning of the 1990s) that nurses started to go in the public space for shopping, attending religious, or cultural events. In this new environment, they were not directly recognizable anymore as women having migrated alone, i.e., without a male "guardian" somewhere around.

From Loose Women to Useful Women

In Kerala, in the context of strong patriarchy (Devika, 2006) when, at least in the social milieu they were coming from (low middle class), the standard for women was broadly to be housewives, the first nurses to go abroad were really breaking a norm. The economic gain was certainly strong enough to incite their close parenthood to let them attempting the adventure, but the first nurses had certainly to pay a high price because of not only their difficult life abroad but also the social stigma they had to endure for long at home (George, 2005; Naïr, 2012; Percot, 2006).

As Naïr (2012) stated, nurses in India had always been suffering from a low status: because of their close contact with men, their night shifts were rendering these women suspects of immoral behavior; the low salaries they were receiving were not helping to enhance their situation. Nevertheless, they were still under a potential social control by family or neighborhood. It was not the case anymore for those who went abroad. A remark that a taxi driver once made to me illustrates the feeling that was still prevailing: "One really wonders what they are doing once they are off duty ... because they are on their own there, so it is easy for them to earn more by wandering in the streets, if you understand what I mean". George (2005: 146) insists on this bad name of being loose women that sticks to nurses, particularly for migrant nurses. Osella and Osella (2000: 44) note that the blame could even be extended to the full Christian community, from which a vast majority of nurses are coming, for being greedy enough not only to push women to work outside their home, but even to be ready to "send them to the Arabs as nurses".

As most of these early migrants told me, they were proud to be good earners for their family, having the feeling to help a lot for the future of their children, but they had, as Maryama expressed it, to "keep a very low profile" when they were back home, showing even more respect for the social norms regarding married women. Lethika with whom I had discussions very recently about that time, remembered:

When I was coming home, I could see the suspicion in my neighbors' eyes. I knew there were gossips. For the two months I was staying, I think I never went out without husband or mother-in law. At home too, it was not holidaying. I was doing more than my duty, cooking all day long, massaging mother or father's feet; you get it, the perfect daughter-in-law! I had the support of my husband for going abroad, but he too was relieved that I behaved so traditionally once back home. For him, it was like, you know, "See, she has not changed at all". It took years before things started to change a bit.

Several early migrants remarked that up to the 1990s, it would have been hardly imaginable for a non-married young nurse to migrate because the stigma was strong enough to really hamper her chances to find a husband. According to them, the first single women to go were coming from families who were facing a very difficult economic situation. It was the case of Rosa, who left for Abu Dhabi in 1985 when she was 23. Her father had a lot of debts and she – as she put it – "sacrificed herself in order to save the family". She has since pursued a particularly brilliant career, still in Abu Dhabi, but was only able to get married when she was 36, namely very late according to Malayali social norms; in the meantime, after paying her father's debts, she had saved a lot, meaning a potential interesting dowry, and the stigma attached to migrant nurses had also started to wane.

Two factors played a role:

At first, people in Kerala could see that there was really a financial gain for migrant nurses' families, enough to push more families to eventually accept the migration of a daughter, wife, or daughter-in-law; Rosa remembered having witnessed this trend in her own neighborhood in Kottayam:

People in the neighborhood were mostly like us, very simple Christian families. Not very poor, not very rich. Many girls had studied nursing [...] By the mid-80s, we were around 10 nurses to work in the Gulf. After some time, it was possible for the neighbors to see the economic change in our families. They had also seen that we were like normal women when we were coming back. If there was a nurse in their family, they became less afraid to be criticized for having her going like us. It was like "Why should she continue to work for a few rupees, if she can earn plenty there?" You know, nursing was not so well considered anyway, so it is better at least to have the nurse of the family earning money. Money can change a mentality!

Then, and maybe, more importantly, the many other Malayali migrants who had in the meantime reached the Gulf – some with their family – were able to give a less phantasmatic picture of the life of migrant nurses. Wives of migrants could, for instance, share activities with nurses like in the very common prayer groups or in the cultural events organized by the numerous associations which had rapidly blossomed in most of the Gulf cities. However, Pax remember that it was not so easy to be fully admitted:

> The first time I joined a prayer group in St Pierre and Paul Church [in Muscat], I was with three of my colleagues. There were 6 to 8 other women who had just joined their husbands, housewives. I can't say they were hostile, but they were not very friendly either. You could see they had some sort of prejudice. Once we started to better know each other the atmosphere got warmer, but it took time. It took even more time before they started to invite us at home, but then we became friends.

Moreover, many nurses were eventually able to have their husband coming to the Gulf.[1] It can thus be argued that, in a way, the "normal" social control over nurses as women was reestablished. Yet, like many women who are living or have lived in the Gulf acknowledge, those norms in migration were, little by little, distancing themselves from the ones of the home country (Emirbayer & Mische 1998: 984), with a bit more freedom and autonomy (Percot, 2007),[2] but they were however evolving with the consent and voluntary participation of the men with whom women were sharing migration. Having accepted as the new normal the way Malayali men and women were acting or interacting in the Gulf, the male migrants, once back home, were also attesting to the "good behavior" of the female migrants, including nurses. The large dissemination of knowledge about Gulf's life into the Malayali society, the culture of migration which developed during the following decades, contributed largely to the trivialization of nurses' migration. With more and more nurses migrating, the phenomenon became in a way very banal. It did not totally erase the stigma attached to them, but it drastically reduced it; enough at least, in their own social milieu, to consider them as good potential spouses as it could be verified in marriage classifieds, for instance, where the mention "nurse working abroad wanted" could be seen more and more. Marrying a nurse had become an easy – if not the only – gateway to international migration, particularly for men with few qualifications. To quote Lindstrom & López Ramírez (2010: 55), "Pioneers do not just provide an example of new behavior; they also facilitate the adoption of this behavior by others".

The pioneers had eventually proved they were "decent" women, facilitating the path for the newcomers, whether it is for other nurses or for men of their community.

Paving the Way

Bakewell et al. (2012: 18) wrote:

> The innovative orientation towards the future might make pioneer migrants interested in facilitating further migration of their group

members, so that the new experiences, change and betterment that stem from migration as a livelihood strategy might be shared by more community members and put in motion more intense processes of social change and transformation.

Pioneer nurses have contributed to a migration system by showing both the economic benefit for their family and changing the gaze on women migrating alone. And they were indeed very active in helping other women to follow their path. One can spot there three different motivations: at first, the oddity of their migration would furthermore decrease with a higher number of women doing the same; then, there was a real commitment to help families – and more especially women – of their community by pushing them to grab a good opportunity of earning well[3]; at last, more practically, migrant nurses were considering as a good thing to have fellow citizens as colleagues whether it is at work or as roommates in the hostels.

Rosa explained all of this clearly:

> When you help somebody to migrate, when you find for her a position in a good hospital with a good contract, people are thankful. Generally, they will remember it […] As soon as we were aware of recruitment somewhere, we would inform nurses we knew at home; we would give them information about the hospital which was recruiting, about the place and everything. It was also better for the newcomers to already know people on the spot. Of course, it was to help, it was a generous move, but it was also good for us, because it is easier to live and work with people like you.

In the meantime, the structuring of nurses' recruitment industry had been accomplished. Fewer recruitments were done directly by Gulf hospitals; brokers had seized this market, and they were now based throughout India, at least in all big metropolises and all Kerala's cities. At the same time, nurses training had also become a blossoming private market, a shift from the previously mainly government schools. A very large proportion of trainees[4] were aiming at migrating as soon as possible, meaning after the two years of the required experience. The migration opportunities had even pushed many young men to enter into this profession (Walton-Roberts 2019). To become a migrant nurse was now a big investment with the cost of school and the recruitment fees which could not be avoided anymore.

In the first years of this migratory network development, when the brokerage system was still not as complex as it is today, migrant nurses had often been in a position to directly help to the recruitment of fellow nurses in India.[5] It became not so directly possible later, but the advices they continued to give were however still helpful to avoid as much as possible the pitfalls of the recruitment process. At a time where agencies were sprouting up everywhere, resorting to fellow nurses who had already gone through this process was a security that most candidates to migration to the Gulf used. Information about reasonable fees, about the reliability of such or such agency, about the type of contract that should be proposed, etc., were (and still are) exchanged extensively through borders.

I have met very few nurses having emigrated after 1985 who had not been in close contact before their departure with women who were already in the destination country as migrants. They had contacted them at each stage of their migratory process. Jenny, who left Kerala in 2001, is an example:

> When I was about to finish the two years of compulsory service at the hospital in Kottayam[6], I was looking for a good place to migrate. There were plenty of recruitment agencies in the city; they were advertising for many places, UAE, Kuwait, Saudi Arabia, etc. I knew very well three nurses in the Gulf. Two were in UAE and one was in Oman. When Mary, a neighbor I knew since childhood and who was working in Dubai, came on holiday I asked her what to do. She told me that Dubai was a better place, that life was nice there. She told me which hospitals were good and which places in UAE were not so interesting like Al Ain. She also managed to get valuable information about the best agencies. Eventually, I was able to join her. The second day after my arrival, she came to see me at the hostel [...] She was the one to explain to me everything there. She was like a big sister to me.

Older migrant nurses had indeed also an important role in making the newcomers feeling safer on arrival. They were helping them in terms of communication (with other staff and patients), in adjusting to the hostel life, and later – when a life outside the hospital's compound had developed – they were also helping in the city discovering (introducing the newcomers to the community's activities or to the spaces of interest like worshipping, shopping places, etc.). As older women and as older migrants, their experience of the Gulf was obviously very beneficial to the new generation, this time mostly consisting of very young women whose life experience was still mostly confined within their parents' home and just a few years of training or hospital work.

Conclusion

The first generation of Indian nurses to the Gulf had to face many challenges in their destination as well as in their home country. They were Indian pioneers in female migration, with all the stigma which were attached to such a move; they were also among the pioneers of Indian migration to the Gulf at a time when a potential support from the diaspora was almost nonexistent. They had bravely managed to somehow resist the difficulties they were facing. They contributed to a change in the way migrant nurses were considered in Kerala, at least in their community, opening an easier path for newcomers.

They have also practically contributed to the arrival of these new migrants by helping them since the moment the latter decided to migrate. The solidarity older nurses were displaying towards fresher migrants – and that was well known in nursing circles – had certainly facilitated many migratory decisions and the way new migrants would be able to cope in their early months abroad. There are certainly a number of structural factors underlying the development of this migratory niche; among them one can quote the increasing number of staff needed in the Gulf, the poor working status of nurses in India and the lack of attractive job opportunities, the appearance of a nursing school market dedicated to training for migration, etc. Yet, the role of pioneer nurses as agents in this migratory phenomenon cannot be underplayed.

Over time, new difficulties appeared for prospective migrant nurses: in India itself, the rising cost of private nursing schools as well as recruitment fees, the more frequent scams by a blossoming and not sufficiently controlled recruitment sector; in the Gulf, for instance, the frequent recruitment in private hospitals or nursing homes for which conditions of work as well as salaries could be unsatisfactory (particularly compared to government hospitals, only ones to recruit at the beginning). The new generation had to also face their own challenges. However, with the development of a strong diaspora and its growth, they are spared nowadays from the loneliness their first colleagues had to bear, from the courage they had to show, as first women and as first Indians to live and work in the Gulf.

Notes

1 Most men arrived with a touristic visa which was quickly transformed into a working visa, thanks the job found through the network the nurses had been able to establish in the Malayali community in the Gulf's city they were living in. Venier (2011) remarks that having a nurse as a spouse was also a way to establish a small business for men having joined them in the Gulf (thanks to loans that were accessible to nurses working in governmental hospitals).

2 Women remark in particular that, freed from the constant gaze of the joint family or of the close neighborhood, they can behave differently in such things as going out with friends, dressing differently. They also often stress the different type of relation they are able to establish with their husband.

3 The feedback at home in term of gratitude, if not even prestige, from relatives or neighbors for such a help cannot be ruled either as a motivation.

4 According to the surveys, I have done during the 2000s in private as well as governmental schools shown that up to 90% of trainees had chosen to study nursing in order to migrate, at least for a few years (Percot, 2006).

5 Being informed of potential recruitment in their hospital, they could find out through the hospital's administration how, when and where the – at that time direct – recruitment would take place in India. The information was quickly passed on to nurses they knew at home.

6 Nursing trainees are bond to work for two years after their degree for the hospital linked to their school. It is a way for hospitals to partly alleviate the shortage of nurses most institutions face in India, but also a way to have a very cheap labor since young nurses' salaries are particularly low.

References

Al Khayat, H. (1981). *Urban revolution in the Arab Gulf states, geography and the third world.* Kuala Lumpur: University of Malaysia, 226 p.

Bakewell, O, de Haas, H, & Kubal, A. (2012). Migration systems, pioneer migrants, and the role of Agency. *Journal of Critical Realism*, 11: 413–437.

Devika, J. (2006). Negotiating women's social space: Public debates on gender in early modern Kerala, India. *Inter-Asia Cultural Studies*, 7(1): 43–61.

Emirbayer, M., & Mische, A. (1998). What is agency? *American Journal of Sociology*, 103: 962–1023.

George, S. (2005). *When women come first: Gender and class in transnational migration.* Berkeley, CA: University of California Press, 296 p.

Lindstrom, D. P., & López Ramírez, A. (2010). Pioneers and followers: Migrant selectivity and the development of U.S. migration streams in Latin America. *Annual American Academy of Political and Social Sciences*, 630: 53–77.

Nair, S. (2012). *Moving with the times: Gender, status and migration of nurses in India.* New Delhi: Routledge.

Nair, S., & Rajan, S. I. (2017). Nursing education in India: Changing facets and emerging trends. *Economic and Political Weekly*, 52(24): 38–42.

Osella, F., & Osella, C. (2000). *Social mobility in Kerala, modernity and identity in conflict.* London: Pluto Press, 320 p.

Percot, M. (2006). Indian nurses in the Gulf: Two generations of female migration. *South Asia Research*, 26(1): 41–62.

Percot, M. (2007). Migration of Indian nurses to the Gulf countries: A step toward more autonomy. *Autrepart*, 3: 135–145.

Percot, M., & Rajan, S. I. (2007). Female emigration from India: Case study of nurses. *Economic and Political Weekly*, 42(4): 318–325.

Qutub, I. Y. (1983). Urbanization in contemporary Arab Gulf states. *Ekistics*, 50(300): 170–182.

Venier, P. (2011). Development of entrepreneurial initiatives in the UAE among Kerala emigrants. In S. I. Rajan & M. Percot (Eds.), *Dynamics of Indian migration: Historical and current perspectives* (pp. 164–194). New Delhi: Routledge.

Walton-Roberts, M. (2019). Asymmetrical therapeutic mobilities: Masculine advantage in nurse migration from India. *Mobilities*, 14(1): 20–37.

Walton-Roberts, M., & Rajan, S. I. (2013). Nurse emigration from Kerala: 'Brain circulation' or 'trap'. In S. I. Rajan (Ed.), *India migration report* (pp. 206–223). New Delhi: Routledge.

Walton-Roberts, M., & Rajan, S. I. (2020). Global demand for medical professionals drives Indian abroad despite acute domestic health-care worker shortages. *Migration Information Source*. January 23, 2020. https://www.migrationpolicy.org/article/global-demand-medical-professionals-drives-indians-abroad.

Walton-Roberts, M., Runnels, V., Rajan, S. I., Sood, A., Nair, S., Thomas, P., Packer, C., Mackenzie, A., Murphy, G. T., Labonté, R., & Bourgeault, I. L. (2017). Causes, consequences, and policy responses to the migration of health workers: Key findings from India. *Human Resources for Health*, 15(1): 28.

2 Decision-Making of International Destination

A Case Study of Indian Nurses in New Zealand

Yuko Tsujita, Hisaya Oda and
S. Irudaya Rajan

Introduction

Many developed countries face a shortage of nurses, primarily due to the progressively ageing population, shortage of 'home-grown' nurses, and the inability of families to take care of dependents under the current demographic, economic, and social transformation. The recruitment of internationally educated nurses addresses staff shortages in many countries. As of 2015–2016, on average, 15.8% of nurses in Organisation for Economic Cooperation and Development (OECD) countries were born abroad (OECD, 2020). India sends the second-highest number of nurses to OECD countries after the Philippines (*ibid.*). In 2015–2016, 87,871 Indian-trained nurses were working in OECD countries (*ibid.*), and an estimated 640,000 were working abroad, including the Gulf countries (a primary destination for Indian-trained nurses) (Rajan and Nair, 2013).

A traditional push-pull factor analysis of migration found that nurses migrate overseas primarily for higher salaries, better working resources and conditions, more training opportunities, transparent promotion, exposure to new advanced knowledge and technology, skill enhancement, and higher occupational status among others (e.g., Kingma, 2006; Kline, 2003). They are also compelled by push factors, such as lower wages, poor working conditions, and lack of training opportunities, among others, in the country of origin. Consideration of the specific context and background of international migration is needed in both source and destination countries.

Regarding nurses migrating from India, those working in private hospitals are more likely to migrate abroad than their counterparts in public hospitals are (Oda et al., 2018). This is mainly because the salary, benefits, and working conditions in private hospitals are inferior to those in the public sector.

A key decision for nurses while considering international migration is the destination. This decision-making might be once or more. It is increasingly apparent that the nurse migration trajectory is not always a single-tracked journey from one country to another. International nurse migration can be

DOI: 10.4324/9781003315124-2

repeated involving multiple overseas destinations after spending substantial time in each destination during their career (Carlos, 2013). However, decision-making on destinations by nurses is currently under-researched.

This chapter investigates why certain countries may be favoured over others by Indian nurses through semi-structured interviews of nurses in New Zealand. The remainder of this chapter describes the background of a destination country; explains data collection, reports and findings; and discusses the findings before concluding the chapter.

Background: Foreign-Trained Nurses in New Zealand

Shortage of Nurses

In 2017, the number of practicing nurses per 1,000 people was 10.2 in New Zealand, higher than 8.8 in the OECD countries.[1] However, the demand for the nursing workforce has been increasing. A primary reason has been the ageing population. The proportion of the population aged over 65 years was 9.9% in 1981, 14.3% in 2013, and is projected to be 26.7% by 2063 (New Zealand Census).[2] Moreover, the population grew at a rate of 1.44% annually in 2019, higher than the 1.18% in 1991 and 0.57% in 2000 (Stats NZ website)[3] because of the influx of migrants. Therefore, it is predicted that 25,000 additional nurses will be required by 2030 (Hancock, 2019). However, the supply of home-grown nurses did not meet the growing demand. There are three main reasons for this.[4] First, the number of new graduates passing the Nursing Council's state exam increased from 1,321 in 2010 to 1,817 in 2013 (Ministry of Health, 2014). However, the new potential workforce does not always gain employment nor stay in the country. Second, the workforce experiences attrition and ageing. The Ministry of Health (2016) reported that the average age of nurses was 46.3 years, and 45.2% of nurses were over 50 years old. A large part of the current workforce will reach retirement age within the next 10–15 years. Third, many nurses from New Zealand have migrated to Australia. The Trans-Tasman Mutual Recognition Arrangement (MRA) enables nurses from New Zealand to work in Australia and vice versa. Although they do not have the same nursing curriculum and have a separate registration system in both countries, more nurses migrate from New Zealand to Australia than the other way around. In 2018, the number of Australian nurses in New Zealand was 698, and the corresponding figure of New Zealand nurses in Australia was 6,767.[5] These factors have led to the recruitment of more nurses from overseas.

Recruiting Foreign-Trained Nurses

The Ministry of Health (2014) reports that 'Locally trained doctors and nurses are leaving to work overseas, and there is a heavy reliance on highly mobile locums and overseas-trained health professionals to fill the vacancies' (pp. 2–3). New overseas registrations have nearly equalled or exceeded the number of locally trained new registrations every year (Walker and Clendon, 2015). Accordingly, some schemes have been introduced to address the recruitment, retention, and distribution challenges of home-grown nurses from a mid-term to long-term perspective. However, they are not efficiently utilised by nurses.

Regardless, immigration policy has addressed the shortage of registered nurses and has listed their requirements in skill shortage lists. Although the categories or names of the lists have changed over time, a wide range of registered nurses, including those specialised in mental health, aged care, clinical care, emergency, medical, and perioperative care, have been listed as priority occupations for immigrants since the early 2000s (North, 2007) until February 2017. Once all registered nurse categories were removed in 2017,[6] the current lists consisted of the Long-term Skill Shortage List (LTSSL),[7] Regional Skill Shortage List, and Construction and Infrastructure Skill Shortage List. These lists had only registered nurses (aged care) after the aged care association actively lobbied to add registered nurses (Jackson, 2019).

If their expertise is in the skill shortages list (currently aged care), foreign-trained nurses can gain bonus points when it comes to the assessment of obtaining various visas, including work visa, resident visa, and others. Meanwhile, employers do not have to go through the formal labour recruitment processes to prove that they cannot find locals for the job. Even if registered nurses are not listed in the skill shortage category, it is still possible for employers to hire foreign-trained nurses after employers have made genuine but unsuccessful efforts to recruit a suitable citizen or resident.

As a nurse-receiving country, New Zealand has a high proportion of foreign-trained nurses, 26.2% (OECD, 2020). Table 2.1 shows that the number of foreign-trained nurses (stock) increased from 8,931 in 2008 to 13,115 in 2018. Besides, the countries of origin have changed during this period. In 2008, 4,169 (46.7% of foreign-trained nurses) nurses came from the United Kingdom, followed by 672 (7.5%) from Australia, and 645 (7.2%) from South Africa. In 2018, 4,282 nurses (32.6%) were from the Philippines, followed by 3,380 (25.8%) from the United Kingdom, and 2,369 (18.1%) from India. More foreign-trained nurses are from Asian countries, especially the Philippines and India.

Some Characteristics of Asian Nurses

There are three main characteristics of Asian nurses, including Indian nurses. First, foreign-trained nurses are significantly younger than home-trained nurses are (Walker and Clendon, 2015; the Nursing Council of New Zealand, 2020). Age is related to the willingness to work abroad and higher points given based on age, as per the immigration policies, by receiving countries. We found that younger nurses from India are more likely to go abroad (Oda et al., 2018). In New Zealand, the younger the nurses are, the

Table 2.1 Foreign-Trained Nurses and the Country of Origin in New Zealand (Stock)

Country	2008	2009	2010	2011	2012	2013	2014	2015	2016	2017	2018
Australia	672	648	657	740	675	639	636	652	698	652	698
China	71	70	118	125	130	134	143	99	145	142	147
Fiji	-	-	-	452	441	436	424	421	434	409	402
India	563	666	882	1200	1457	1526	1697	2076	2373	2330	2369
Philippines	-	-	-	1694	2009	2234	2498	2975	3684	3924	4282
South Africa	645	672	695	712	649	656	627	607	595	558	571
United Kingdom	4169	4301	4303	4036	3925	3831	3759	3695	3545	3415	3380
Others	2811	2941	3460	1573	1478	1429	1386	1447	1420	1250	1266
Total	8931	9298	10115	10532	10764	10885	11170	11972	12894	12680	13115

Source: OECD Health Stat: https://stats.oecd.org/Index.aspx?ThemeTreeId=9# (accessed on 2 February 2021).

more points they earn to work, reside, and achieve permanent residency. Second, foreign-trained nurses are concentrated in Auckland, including 36.7% of the overall nursing workforce in the city, far higher than in other regions (the national average is 26.6%) (Nursing Council of New Zealand, 2020).[8] Third, Asian-trained migrant nurses typically work in the aged care sector (Walker and Clendon, 2015; Nursing Council of New Zealand, 2020). In New Zealand, aged care services are largely privatised, while the District Health Boards, which the government fully funds, provide health and medical services. Nurses in aged care are paid approximately NZD5 per hour less than those working in the public sector are (Wallance, 2019). That is why home-trained nurses prefer not to work in the aged care sector.

Pathway to Become a Registered Nurse

In New Zealand, those who complete a three-year BSc programme leading to registration as a nurse are required to pass the Nursing Council State Final Examination. In the case of foreign-trained nurses, according to the New Zealand Nursing Council website,[9] the process of registration is different for those registered in Australia and those registered in any other country. Registered nurses in the former category are also registered in New Zealand through Trans-Tasmanian MRA. However, the latter category of nurses is first required to send documents to the Credentials Verification Services for the Nursing Council of New Zealand at Commission on Graduates of Foreign Nursing Schools (CGFNS) International Inc. The documents include ID documents, employment history, nursing education history, licence validation, and language proficiency.[10] Once the CGFNS completes the verification process, the Nursing Council decides on each person's registration. Foreign-trained nurses from Asian countries are often required to take a bridging course called the Competency Assessment Programme (CAP).

CAP, stipulated by the Health Practitioners Competence Assurance Act 2003, is a bridging course for foreign-trained nurses, and local nurses who have been away from practice for more than five years. The CAP is offered by the Nursing Council's accredited providers, which included 20 institutions as of August 2019. The course consists of theory and clinical practice over 5–12 weeks. During the course, the registered nurse candidates are continuously assessed. Those who complete the CAP course are officially recognised as registered nurses. Institutions tend to prefer international students, as they pay a higher fee (price range from NZD6720 to NZD15000) than local nurses do. Admission to the CAP course for international students is competitive. Some nurses opt for the one-year-graduate diploma course combined with CAP, as the validity of the English proficiency test expires if they wait to be admitted to the short-term CAP course. During the fieldwork, we came across an Indian-migrant nurse who was studying nursing in a one-year-graduate diploma course after she was admitted to a CAP course starting one year later.

Data Collection

This chapter is a part of a larger study conducted in and around Christchurch, New Zealand. We conducted face-to-face semi-structured interviews in September 2019 and February 2020 with nurses born, educated, and worked as registered nurses in India, and were currently working as registered nurses in New Zealand. Since the register of those who meet the criteria is not available to us, snowball sampling was employed whereby respondents introduced us to their colleagues and friends. The semi-structured questions included personal background, educational experience, clinical experience in India, job history, migration to New Zealand, the process of becoming a registered nurse, and current problems faced in the destination country among others. The number of survey participants in this analysis was confined to 15 registered nurses in New Zealand. Nurses were usually interviewed at their homes except three whom we met at a café in their neighbourhood. The interviews were in English, took approximately 60 min on average, and were audio-recorded and transcribed. Some profiles of the participants are shown in Table 2.2.

Most of the sample nurses were Christians from the state of Kerala. Their current workplace was public hospitals, community nursing, or rest homes. All of them had arrived in New Zealand after 2008, indicating that Indian migrants increased only recently (Table 2.1). Interestingly, one-third of the participants (five nurses) came to New Zealand after working in another foreign country. At the time of the arrival, all the participants had Indian nationality, i.e., Indian passport. All participants, except for one nurse who had worked in Ireland, had completed a CAP course or a similar bridging course in Australia before searching for a job in New Zealand.

Findings

Requirements in Destination Countries

International destinations in developed countries for Indian nurses are mainly English-speaking countries. Why did the nurses choose New Zealand among their potential destinations? Only two nurses, whose spouses worked in New Zealand, were decisive about their preferred destination (Participants 12 and 15). The others did not know anybody in New Zealand when they arrived there for the first time.

The important factor turned out to be English proficiency. At the time of the survey, New Zealand allowed foreign-trained nurses to combine all the English test scores taken over 12 months. The requirement at the time of the survey to apply for nursing registration was a minimum score of 7 in the International English Language Testing System (IELTS) or B in the Occupation English Test (OET) for every band, that is, reading, listening, writing, and speaking. If a person could not achieve the minimum score in any band in either the IELTS or OET, they could attempt the exam until

Table 2.2 Survey Participants

No.	State of Origin	Sex	Marital Status	Religion	Workplace	Nursing Education in India	Completed Year of Nursing Education in India	Year Arrived at NZ	Experience Abroad
1	Kerala	F	Married	Christian	Hospital	BSc	2010	2012	
2	Kerala	F	Married	Christian	Hospital	BSc	2007	2009	
3	Kerala	F	Married	Christian	Rest home	BSc	2007	2012	
4	Kerala	F	Divorced	Christian	Rest home	BSc	2009	2016	Saudi Arabia
5	Kerala	F	Married	Christian	Community nursing	BSc	2006	2012	
6	Kerala	M	Married	Christian	Community nursing	BSc	2008	2012	
7	Kerala	F	Married	Christian	Hospital	BSc	2004	2011	Maldives
8	Uttarakhand	F	Married	Sikh	Rest home	GNM	2009	2012	
9	Kerala	F	Married	Christian	Hospital	BSc	2009	2013	
10	Kerala	F	Married	Christian	Community nursing	GNM	2006	2008	
11	Kerala	F	Married	Christian	Rest home	BSc	2012	2015	
12	Kerala	F	Married	Christian	Hospital	BSc	2010	2015	Saudi Arabia
13	Kerala	F	Married	Christian	Hospital	GNM	2006	2014	Qatar
14	Kerala	F	Married	Christian	Hospital	BSc	2012	2018	
15	Kerala	M	Married	Muslim	Hospital	BSc	2013	2019	Ireland

Note: In India, GNM is currently three-year-General Nursing & Midwifery, while BSc nursing is a four-year course. Care homes are commonly referred to as rest homes in New Zealand.
Source: Authors' survey.

they fulfilled the requirement for the next year. This flexibility was not available in other English-speaking countries such as Australia, the United Kingdom, and Ireland at their time of arrival. Thus, many of the sampled nurses came to New Zealand due to their English proficiency scores. For example,

> I wanted to go to Australia but could not obtain the minimum score in one test, so I came to New Zealand
>
> (Participant 4)

> My English score only matched the New Zealand requirements when I investigated the requirements of other English-speaking countries
>
> (Participant 14)

Migration Cost

The cost of migration plays an important role in making decisions on destinations. From the semi-structured interviews, we found that the migration cost to New Zealand, except for English tests, is high. It is approximately INR 800,000 to INR 1,000,000 (approx. US$10,800 to US$13,500). As per our on-going survey, this amount is similar for those migrating to Australia. As per our previous survey, this is at least ten times more expensive than the migration cost to the Gulf countries from India. As most of the sampled nurses earned only a few thousand Indian rupees per month in private hospitals in India before they arrived in New Zealand, the question arises about how they financed their migration cost.

Some of the sampled nurses who had worked in other countries such as Saudi Arabia, Qatar, or Ireland, before arriving in New Zealand, were able to finance the migration costs to New Zealand on their own. However, the rest of the sampled nurses had to borrow some money as either an education loan or other loans from their family and relatives. Going to New Zealand as a nurse is a life-long opportunity for family members that enable them to settle down in a developed country legally. Thus, it becomes the household's strategy. As the cost of migration is much higher than in destinations such as Gulf countries, these nurses are possibly from relatively well-off families.

Family

Migration does not always mean moving from one place to another. It can be repeating processes such that nurses move from one place to another or move back and forth. Some sampled nurses came to New Zealand via overseas destinations. A sample nurse told us the reason she left a Gulf country, her previous country of destination.

It was a good job and a well-paid job. However, when we think about the future of our life and the kids, we cannot live there forever. It will be hard for my kids so that one of the main reasons for us to move.

(Participant 13)

Even when migrants move from India (via a third country) to New Zealand, they can still move back. New Zealand and Australia have an MRA, whereby registered nurses in New Zealand can work in Australia. It has been reported that a large number of foreign-trained nurses have been found in New Zealand, particularly because they can move directly to Australia under this MRA (Walker 2008; New Zealand Nurse Organization, 2017). In our semi-structured interviews, most of the participants mentioned 'Australia' as the first preferred destination before arriving in New Zealand, except for participants who came after their marriage, as their spouses had already settled in the country (Participants 12 and 15). Another example is a nurse (Participant 13) who took a bridge course in Melbourne, Australia because her relatives lived there. However, she moved to New Zealand as she could not find a job in Australia.

When we asked the nurses if they intended to migrate to Australia or elsewhere, the results were mixed. They were likely to remain in New Zealand because of 'children's schooling', 'purchase of home', and others. Those considering migrating to Australia described their reasons as follows:

A lot of friends have already left for Australia. In Australia, nurses are better paid, and the cost of living is lower than here. In particular, the rent is very expensive, and the houses are smaller than those in Australia.

(Participant 7)

It is not only better paid in Australia, but also closer to India, and more flight options are available. We cannot go home easily from here at the time of an emergency back home.

(Participant 10)

Importantly, 4 out of 29 Indian-migrant nurses in our parallel survey in Australia had previously worked in New Zealand. One nurse said,

My husband is educated but could not find a job in Auckland. That is the main reason why we came to Australia.

(Australia Participant 4)

Many female nurses' husbands were engaged in unskilled jobs or were self-employed, as it is not easy for them to find a reasonable job in New Zealand. Some nurses confessed that they were professionally satisfied in the public hospitals of smaller towns in New Zealand. However, due to the employment opportunities for their husband, they came to Christchurch, a larger town (Participants 4, 12, and 13).

Discussion

This chapter discusses how nurses decide their migration destination. One of the important factors that affect their decision-making is the regulatory framework in destination countries. Nurse-receiving countries tend to ease the qualification standards for foreign-trained nurses when they suffer from a shortage of nurses, while they tighten the requirements when they have relatively enough resources. Work experience, language proficiency, and educational background are the common criteria that nurse-receiving countries adjust from time to time. Accordingly, New Zealand also changes the standard qualifications for registered nurses from abroad from time to time. Correspondingly, nurses try to find a destination that meets their qualifications. If migrant nurses do not meet the minimum criteria set by the receiving countries, they face a greater hurdle to become registered nurses. For example, New Zealand previously allowed India's three-year diploma in nursing to register; however, the rule has changed to requiring a BSc nursing degree. One nurse said,

> Since my brother settled in Australia, I was planning to go there, but it was difficult to find a nursing job in 2012, so I came to New Zealand without knowing that India's nursing diploma qualification was not qualified to join the CAP course anymore. I ended up doing a BSc in nursing in this country.
>
> (Participant 8)

Although it is beyond the scope of this chapter, we also came across some caregivers in New Zealand who had completed the diploma in nursing course and had a nursing licence in India. They were unaware that their educational qualification did not meet the minimum criteria to become a registered nurse in New Zealand, and they came to New Zealand to study any health-related course. They were last known to be working as caregivers and struggling to find a way to become a registered nurse.

Cost plays an important role in their decision of the destination. Indian nurses who come to New Zealand without loans or family help are mainly confined to those who worked in other foreign countries. As the remuneration of nurses, particularly those in private hospitals, remains low in India, they cannot often afford to move to other countries depending on their own savings. Therefore, they depend on bank loans or family members to help finance their journey. As nurses can work and reside in a destination country that enables family members to settle down, like New Zealand, it may be the family that influences nurses' decision-making on their destination. This chapter found that whether the sampled nurses are willing to move to anywhere else, particularly Australia under the MRA, their decision to migrate is based on economic reasons and their family.

The New Economics of Labour Migration posits migration as a family strategy to overcome resource constraints and avoid risks (Stark and Bloom, 1985). While some nurses go abroad as part of a family strategy, others encounter more considerable hurdles in migrating overseas due to their family's objection (Tsujita and Komazawa, 2020). Our findings suggest that the family or household is an important factor when and to where nurses consider migration.

Conclusions

This chapter discusses the factors that affect nurses' migration decision-making regarding their destination, using semi-structured interviews with registered nurses in New Zealand. Our findings suggest that the receiving country's transmutative requirements that nurses must comply with, international migration costs that nurses incur, and family affect their decision on international migration and its destination.

The implication drawn from this chapter is to provide nurses with accurate information on the overseas labour market, so that nurses can avoid facing greater hurdles in the journey to becoming a registered nurse in a destination country even after spending large sums of money to migrate. A three-year diploma in nursing does not meet the minimum criteria in many nurse-receiving countries. Although India recently oriented towards BSc nursing, diploma students still outnumber BSc students in the country. Those who are willing to migrate should be aware of this. Moreover, the Indian nurses' underlying reason for emigrating is the low remuneration of nursing jobs, particularly in the private sector. Worse, in recent years, contract-based public sector jobs have increased in many parts of the country. India needs better nursing jobs in both the private and public sectors.

Notes

1 OECD website: https://www.oecd-ilibrary.org/sites/98e2d5de-en/index.html ?itemId=/content/component/98e2d5de-en (accessed on 2 February 2021).
2 http://archive.stats.govt.nz/Census/2013-census/profile-and-summary-reports/ quickstats-65-plus/population-overview.aspx (accessed on 24 February 2020).
3 https://www.stats.govt.nz/topics/population (accessed on 24 February 2020).
4 Local New Zealander nurses work up to 40 hours per week. We found that nurses could decide how many hours per week they work. This may contribute to the fact that a greater number of nurses are required.
5 OECD health stat: https://stats.oecd.org/Index.aspx?ThemeTreeId=9# (accessed on 5 February 2021).
6 New Zealand Nurses Organisation (NZNO), the largest nurse labour union, and professional organisation for nurses, midwives, and caregivers, along with other national nursing organisations, recommended that all nursing categories should be removed from the list (NZNO, 2017 p. 2). They mentioned that long-term

health work planning is required rather than relying on the recruitment of nurses from overseas (*ibid.* p. 4).

7 Long-term skill shortage list, generally reviewed every six months, identifies occupations where there is a sustained and ongoing shortage of highly skilled workers, both globally and throughout New Zealand: https://skillshortages .immigration.govt.nz/ (accessed on 23 February 2020).

8 The government currently discourages foreign-trained nurses to work in Auckland. Our interviews with Indian migrant nurses found that, to avoid the concentration in Auckland, those who worked outside Auckland could earn higher points to obtain permanent residency and those who studied a nursing bridge course outside Auckland were given longer years of post-study visa.

9 https://www.nursingcouncil.org.nz/Public/Nursing/How_to_become_a_nurse/ NCNZ/nursing-section/How_to_become_a_nurse.aspx (accessed on 23 February and 4 March 2020).

10 Language proficiency is waived for those who were registered in the United Kingdom, Ireland, Canada, or the United States.

References

Carlos, M. R. D. (2013). The stepwise international migration of Filipino nurses and its policy implications for their retention in Japan, Working Paper Series, Studies on Multicultural Societies No. 23, Afrasian Research Centre, Ryukoku University.

Hancock, F. (2019). Where are all the extra nurses? *Newsroom*, 26 February 2019. Retrieved from (https://www.newsroom.co.nz/2019/02/26/462930/still -understaffed-say-nurses-1500-nursing-gaps) on 22 February 2020.

Irudaya Rajan, S. and S. Nair. (2013). Assessment of existing services for skilled migrant workers: India project site, ILO Promoting Decent work across borders: A pilot project for migrant health professional and skilled workers. Draft Report submitted to International Labour Organization.

Jackson, P. (2019). 'Immigration adds registered nurses to skills list' the Northland Age, 16 May 2019. Retrieved from (age/news/article.cfm?c_id=1503402&objectid =12231405) on 1 February 2021.

Kinga, M. (2006). *Nurses on the move: Migration and the global health care economy.* Ithaca, NY: Cornell University Press.

Kline, D. (2003). Push and pull factors in international nurse migration. *Journal of Nursing Scholarship*, 35(2), 107–111.

Ministry of Health. (2014). *The role of health workforce New Zealand.* Wellington: Ministry of Health.

Ministry of Health. (2016). *Health of the health workforce 2015: A report by health workforce New Zealand.* Wellington: Ministry of Health.

New Zealand Nurses Organization. (2017). Internationally qualified nurses: Immigration and other issues. Wellington: New Zealand Nurses Organization.

North, N. (2007). International nurse migration: Impacts on New Zealand. *Policy, Politics, & Nursing Practice*, 8(3), 220–228. https://doi.org/10.1177 /1527154407308410

Nursing Council of New Zealand. (2020). The New Zealand nursing workforce: A profile of nurse practitioners, registered nurses and enrolled nurses 2018–2019. Wellington: Nursing Council of New Zealand.

Oda, H., Y. Tsujita and S. I. Rajan. (2018). An analysis of factors influencing the international migration of Indian nurses. *Journal of International Migration and Integration*, 19(3), 607–624.

OECD. (2020). *Contribution of migrant doctors and nurses to tackling COVID-19 crisis in OECD countries. OECD Policy Responses to Coronavirus (COVID-19).* Paris: OECD Publishing.

Stark, O. and D. Bloom. (1985). The new economics of labor migration. *American Economic Review*, 75(2), 173–178.

Tsujita, Y. and O. Komazawa. (2020). Human resources for the health and long-term care of older persons in Asia. Chiba, Japan: Economic Research Institute for ASEAN and East Asia, Jakarta, Indonesia and Institute of Developing Economics-Japan External Trade Organization.

Walker, L. (2008). A mixed picture: The experiences of overseas trained nurses in New Zealand. *Labour, Employment and Work in New Zealand*, November 2008. https://doi.org/10.26686/lew.v0i0.2221.

Walker, L. and J. Clendon. (2015). New Zealand's migrant Asian nurses: Recent trends, future plans. *Labour, Employment and Work in New Zealand*, February 2015.

Wallace, S. (2019). There's no excuse for the way we undervalue aged-care nurses. *Stuff*, 12 July 2019. Retrieved from (https://www.stuff.co.nz/national/health/114125275/theres-no-excuse-for-the-way-we-undervalue-agedcare-nurses) on 7 March 2020.

3 Analysing Health Professional Mobility from India to Canada

Ayona Bhattacharjee

Introduction

> During the COVID-19 pandemic, many of the OECD countries already reliant on migrant health workers have further recognised them as key assets and implemented additional policy measures to ease their entry and the recognition of their professional qualification.
>
> (Scarpetta et al., 2020)

The COVID-19 pandemic has made the world realize how crucial it is to optimally allocate human resources for health (HRH) in order to enhance public health preparedness. To meet the sudden upsurge in healthcare demand, many countries had to adopt measures to mobilize health professionals (HPs),[1] including initiatives facilitating the arrival and qualification recognition of foreign-trained HPs.[2] For instance, doctors, nurses, and paramedics in the United Kingdom (UK), with visas due to expire before October 2020 got automatic extension of their visas for one year; France allowed non-licensed foreign-trained HPs to work as support staff in non-medical occupations; Italy adopted a decree that enabled temporary licensing of foreign-trained HPs. The pandemic has thus re-emphasized the importance of HPs, irrespective of the healthcare system and shown that cross-country HP mobility barriers are more malleable than what they are made out to be (Dempster & Smith, 2020).

HRH shortages plaguing healthcare delivery is not new. For a long time, the prospect of retirement of the 'baby-boom' generation of HPs has been threatening HRH availability in many countries (Merçay et al., 2016). To address HRH shortages, policymakers have usually increased the number of medical colleges, adding to the pool of graduating students, or relied on the immigration of foreign-born/foreign-trained HPs (OECD, 2019a and 2019b).[3] Drawing from the literature on migration of professionals, there are push and pull factors for HP migration too.[4] The commonly cited push factors include poor remuneration, poor working conditions, limited training and education opportunities, unclear or poor career prospects. The pull

DOI: 10.4324/9781003315124-3

factors are usually attributed to the shortage of personnel in destination countries, better remuneration, better working conditions, career advancement opportunities and better quality of life. Additionally, HP mobility is responsive to demographic shifts, disease burden, and population health conditions. Cross-country HP mobility calls for special attention as it involves ethical and equity concerns.[5]

Decades back, Jeffrey (1976) mentioned the prospects of Indian doctor emigration as domestic employment opportunities were likely to deteriorate over time. Considering more recent data, we do observe that Indian HPs contribute significantly to the HP stocks in several developed countries. Figure 3.1 summarizes the stock of Indian HPs, namely physicians and nurses, practising in top four destination countries over the last decade. The United States (US) and the UK have reported the highest stocks of Indian physicians and nurses, respectively. The other common destination countries have been Canada and Australia. The high year-on-year stock numbers in these countries reflect high annual flow of Indian HPs to each of these destination countries.

The existing literature has mostly looked at the US or UK as important destination countries for Indian HPs. However, in a detailed analysis, presented more than a decade back, Dumont et al. (2008) highlighted how the composition of source countries for foreign HPs in Canada had been changing with rising shares of physicians from South Africa and India, replacing the high shares of HPs from the UK and Ireland. This chapter contributes by exploring Canada as a destination country for Indian HPs.

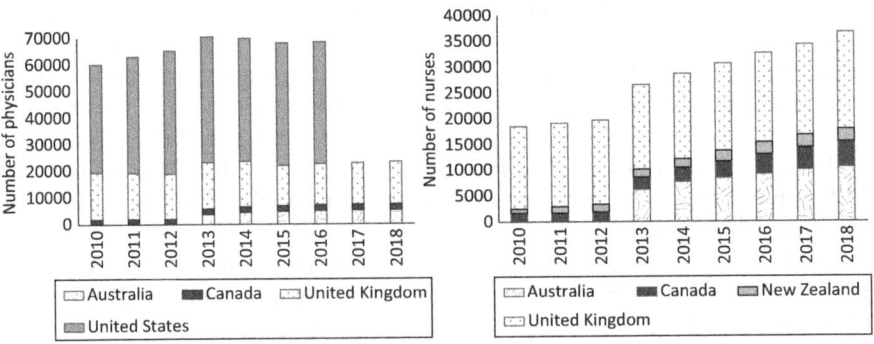

Figure 3.1 Stocks of India-trained physicians and nurses in major destination countries (2010–2018).

Source: Health Workforce Migration Database, from OECDSTAT, accessed on 15 July 2020. Note: The data are on the number of physicians and nurses trained in India, registered and working in the destination countries during the respective year of reporting. Data for physician stock are missing for: US during 2017–2018; Australia, during 2010–2012. Data for stock of nurses are missing for: Australia during 2010–2012. For the US, only nurse inflow data are available, not the stock data.

Canada suits the framework of study as it is not only a major destination country for Indian migrants, but over the years it has altered immigration regulations concerning HPs. The current pandemic is unlikely to have any adverse effect on the future employment of HPs, domestic or foreign-trained, as prior experiences with 1990 and 2008–2009 recessions have shown the Canadian health and social sector employment to be resilient to unforeseen shocks (Merçay et al., 2016). Recent evidence suggests that some Canadian provinces have facilitated qualification recognition of foreign-trained physicians to mobilize additional workers during the pandemic.[6] This strengthens the proof of Canada's flexibility in accommodating international HP mobility as and when the need arises.

The rest of the chapter is organized as follows: The second section discusses the overall structure of the Canadian health system with subsections on physicians and nursing professionals, discussing the distribution, demographics, and shares of foreign-trained HPs. The third section elaborates on the specifics of immigrant HPs in Canada with a focus on the share trained in India. The fourth section discusses the few international and cross-provincial collaborations that Canada has had regarding HP mobility. The fifth section concludes with future implications of HP mobility.

The Canadian Health System

A crucial element of healthcare policies in Canada has been the issue of HRH optimization. The decade of the 1990s started with a perception of surplus health workforce in Canada, calling for curtailment of the number of HPs (Evans & McGrail, 2008). The Advisory Committee on Health Delivery and Human Resources (ACHDHR), established in 2002, outlined key objectives for conducting human resource planning and enhancing health workforce planning capacity (Marchildon, 2013). A 10-year plan to strengthen health care was introduced in 2004, whereby the government committed to reforming HRH, wait times, primary health care, etc.[7] As the Canadian health system has specified roles and responsibilities segregated at the federal, provincial, and territorial levels, provincial governments can actively establish enrolment targets at the medical institutions and affect their HRH distribution. Such targets are determined by population health requirements, demographics, technology and the organization of health services. These targets determine enrolment levels for domestic health workforce (Sweetman, et al., 2015) and have implications for cross-border HP mobility.

Figure 3.2 presents the stock and flow of foreign-trained HPs in Canada over the last two decades. The inflow of foreign-trained physicians has shown a steady increase while the inflow of nurses has fluctuated with a slight increase in recent years. Relative to that of the physicians, there is a widening gap between the number of domestic and foreign-trained nurses

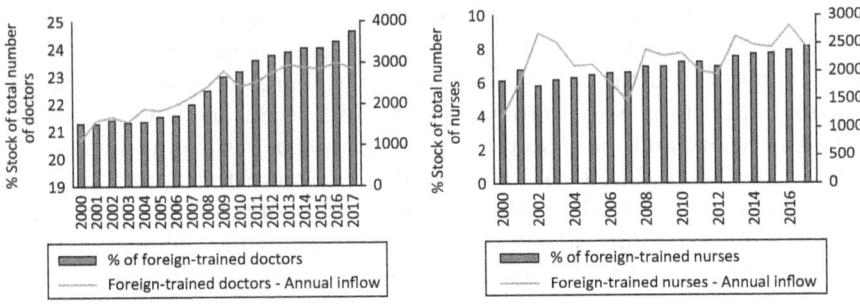

Figure 3.2 Annual inflow and share of foreign-trained HPs in Canada.

Source: OECDSTAT Health Workforce Migration Database, accessed on 3 July 2020. The percentage of foreign-trained doctors (nurses) is the number of foreign-trained physicians (nurses) as a share of total number of physicians (nurses) in a particular year. The secondary axis in either case represents the number of foreign-trained physicians and nurses.

in Canada. Data as of 2017 show that around 25% and 9% of the total number of physicians and nurses in Canada are foreign-trained.

Employment and Social Development Canada (ESDC) uses models of the Canadian Occupational Projection System (COPS) and the National Occupational Classification to predict the number of occupation-wise job openings at the national level. The projections conducted under pre-COVID scenario suggest that labour shortages are imminent in health care. Table 3.1 summarizes the projections of some of the HP-related job openings in Canada. These predictions show that there will be a sharp rise in the demand for nurses and physicians. Combining this information with the proposed number of domestic HP availability clearly implies an emerging situation of shortage.

Traditionally, economic migrants, identified by their respective "occupations in demand", have constituted the largest immigration stream in Canada. Earlier, without enough occupational points, or a job offer, it was difficult to migrate to Canada under this category. An immigration reform introduced in Canada in 2002 shifted the selection criteria for migrants from occupational to educational characteristics. This reform enabled HPs to receive priority as their profession entailed high levels of education. In the same year, the federal government introduced the Immigration and Refugee Protection Act (IRPA), which assigned points to the applicants, based on their measures of education, language, and age. The latest development in the immigration regulations has been the introduction of the "Express Entry" system in 2015.

While easing the entry of migrant HPs may be a short-term cost-efficient solution for HRH optimization, it raises concerns about obtaining resources that are neither accredited to Canadian standards nor have any stake in

Table 3.1 Future Projections of the Number of HP-Related Job Openings and Job Seekers in Canada

	2021	2022	2023	2024	2025	2026	2027	2028
Nurse aides, orderlies, patient service associates, and other assisting occupations in support of health services	349,900	358,700	367,700	376,700	385,900	394,900	404,300	413,900
Registered nurses and registered psychiatric nurses	346,400	356,200	366,200	376,200	386,300	396,300	406,600	417,100
General practitioners and family physicians	84,100	86,900	89,600	92,400	95,100	97,800	100,600	103,400
Licensed practical nurses	84,000	85,300	86,700	88,000	89,400	90,800	92,200	93,700
Specialist physicians	54,400	56,100	57,900	59,700	61,500	63,200	65,000	66,800
Nursing coordinators and supervisors	38,100	39,300	40,500	41,800	43,000	44,200	45,500	46,700
Paramedical occupations	29,200	29,600	30,000	30,300	30,700	31,100	31,500	31,900

Source: COPS – 2019 to 2028 projections available at https://open.canada.ca/data/en/dataset/e80851b8-de68-43bd-a85c-c72e1b3a3890, accessed on 20 July 2020.

its health system. Thus, while keeping the systems open to foreign-trained HPs, restrictions in different forms have been imposed to ensure quality. The Canadian provinces recommend immigrant HPs to have their medical degrees from schools identified by the World Directory of Medical Schools. The foreign HPs are further required to clear language tests and licensure examinations.

Physicians in Canada

The decade of the 1980s witnessed concerns regarding the growing number of physicians in Canada. The issue was addressed by reducing the number of medical school admissions and training positions in Canada (Tyrrell & Dauphinee, 1999). The early 1990s brought in specific policies on physician supply following the Barer–Stoddart (1991) report, which recommended reducing medical school enrolment and the number of provincially funded postgraduate training positions. The objective was to ensure that the needs of the graduating medical students were met. This accentuated the fall in the number of physicians, nurses, and other public healthcare workers. By 2006, there was again perception of a growing shortage in physician availability in Canada and measures were adopted to address the same.

More recently, during 2014–2018, the population in Canada increased by 4.6% while the number of physicians grew by 12.5%, with Manitoba and British Columbia reporting the largest increase in physician population. Manitoba reported the largest per capita increase among all jurisdictions during that period (CIHI, 2018). Nova Scotia and Quebec reported the smallest increase.[8] In 2018, there were 89,911 physicians in Canada, representing a 3.8% increase over 2017. This accounted for a density of 241 physicians per 100,000 population, constituted by 122 family medicine physicians and 119 specialists (CIHI, 2018). In 2018, among the provinces, Newfoundland and Labrador reported the highest number of family physicians per 100,000 population while Nova Scotia reported the highest number of specialists per 100,000 population (Figure 3.3). Medical regulatory authorities of provinces are responsible for setting the licensing criteria and thus the availability of physicians in their provinces.[9]

Gender and age of HPs play important roles in determining physician availability. The share of female physicians in Canada has steadily increased from 31% of total physicians in 2000 to 43.2% in the year 2018. The share of female physicians aged between 55 and 74 years has contributed the most to the growth in female physician workforce. The corresponding decline in relative share of male physicians is attributable to the decline in male physicians aged between 45 and 64 years.[10]The average age of physicians in 2018 was 50 years, with the highest average age reported in Prince Edward Island (52.5 years) and the lowest in Newfoundland and Labrador (48.7 years) (CIHI, 2018).

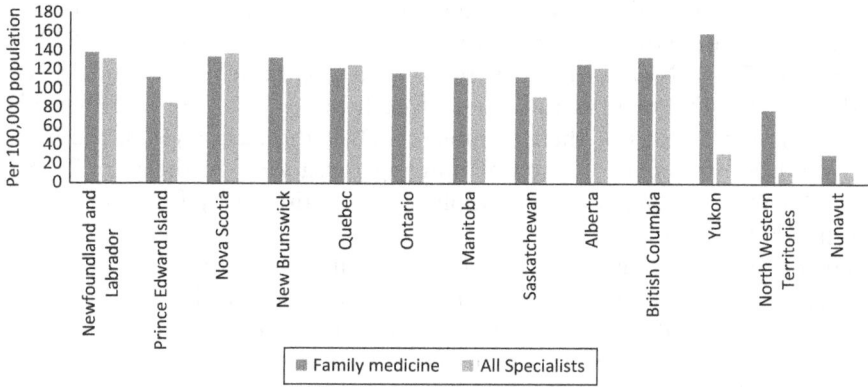

Figure 3.3 Province-wise Physician density (per 100,000 population) by specialty and jurisdiction in Canada.

Source: Supply, Distribution, and Migration of Physicians in Canada, Canadian Institute for Health Information (CIHI, 2018), accessed on 25 June 2020. The bar chart shows the province-wise physician (family medicine and specialist) density in Canada.

Physician mobility in the context of Canada is not just restricted to foreign countries of origin but also across the provinces and the Canadian students studying abroad. Canadian Resident Matching Service (CaRMS) reports that most of the Canadian citizens studying undergraduate medicine abroad were in Caribbean-based schools and without enough prospects.[11] With limited opportunities at their disposal, the Canadian medical students studying abroad prefer coming back for practice. On their return, they compete with the foreign HPs aspiring to work in Canada (Monavvari et al., 2015). Cross-provincial HP mobility in Canada is relatively less pronounced. In 2018, the highest cross-provincial migration of physicians happened between Ontario, Alberta, and British Columbia; minimal flows were reported across Yukon and North Western Territories (CIHI 2018).

Nurses in Canada

Canada's nursing workforce is categorized as nurse practitioners (NPs), registered nurses (RNs), registered psychiatric nurses (RPNs), and licensed practical nurses (LPNs). Each province has its own legislation and a separate body governing nursing practice. NPs practise autonomously and are licensed by jurisdictional nursing regulators. RNs work both autonomously and in collaboration to facilitate healthcare delivery. RPNs focus on mental illnesses, developmental health, and addictions. They are regulated in Manitoba, Saskatchewan, Alberta and British Columbia, and Yukon. LPNs are regulated in all the 13 provinces. The total supply of RNs in Canada was 439,975 in 2019 with 300,669 RNs, 127,097 LPNs, 6,159 NPs, and 6,050 RPNs. While almost all provinces experienced an increase in nurses per 100,000 population, Manitoba reported a decrease in RNs and RPNs during 2017–18. New Brunswick reported a decline in RPNs and LPNs (CIHI, 2019). The regulatory bodies of each province are responsible for overseeing the actions of their members.[12] Over the past 5 years, the NPs had the largest increase among all nursing categories. In the year 2019, around 8.9% of Canada's RNs supply was constituted by foreign-trained nurses (CIHI, 2019).

Historically, nursing has been a female-dominated profession. In 2019, at least 90% of the NPs, RNs, and LPNs were females, while 81% of RPNs were females (CIHI, 2019). Over time, the number of male RNs (15.4% during 2015–2019) has been growing faster than the number of female RNs in Canada (3.9%. during 2015–2019). A major part of the increase in nursing professionals has been contributed by the younger generation. Among RNs, the share of nurses less than 34 years old has been rising while the share of those above 65 has been gradually declining. Among the NPs, the highest share is constituted by the 35–39 years old followed by 30–34 years old. The share of those aged 40–49 years has steadily declined. Among the LPNs, the highest share is constituted by those below 30 years of age and rising shares are constituted by those aged 30–39 years. Among the RPNs, a significant increase has been in the share of those less than 34 years.

Nursing employment in Canada is reported to be growing after a period of healthcare restructuring and hospital downsizing. The late 1990s witnessed labour strife due to dissatisfaction of the nursing professionals with their working conditions and stagnant remuneration (Marchildon, 2013). Gradually, the governments and health organizations tried recruiting nurses, thereby improving the staffing levels, work conditions, and remuneration (CIHI, 2011). Canadian Nursing Association reports that under ceteris paribus conditions, Canada may fall short of 60,000 full-time equivalent RNs by 2022.[13] This ballpark measure only provides a lower limit of the potential shortage, which is likely to affect public policies concerning the domestic capacity and foreign-trained nurses.

Foreign-Trained HPs in Canada and India's Role

International Medical Graduates in Canada

Historically, Canada has shown reliance on International Medical Graduates (IMGs). The share of IMGs has remained relatively stable since 2014, ranging between 25.6% in 2014 and 26.4% in 2018. The corresponding shares of family physicians increased from 28.6% in 2014 to 29.9% in 2018; the share of specialists hovered around 22.5% to 22.7% during 2014–2018 (CIHI, 2018). Figure 3.4 shows the overall share of the eight major source countries of IMGs in Canada, contributing between 35% and 50% since the

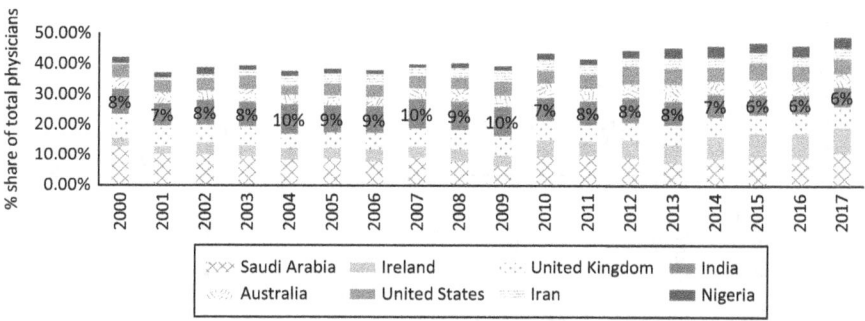

Figure 3.4 Source country-wise share of foreign-trained physicians in Canada.

Source: OECDSTAT, accessed on 25 June 2020. Only eight major source countries of IMGs are reported, which are – Australia, Iran, Ireland, India, Nigeria, Saudi Arabia, UK, and US.

year 2000. In 2018, the IMGs from South Africa, India, and the UK made up 28.7% of all internationally trained physicians (CIHI, 2018). India's share in annual stock of IMGs in Canada has mostly been less than 10% each year.

Disaggregated data at the provincial level provides information on the share of foreign-trained family physicians and specialists. During 2014–18, Saskatchewan, Newfoundland, and Labrador report the largest shares of IMGs while Quebec and Prince Edward Island report the smallest shares. Manitoba and Alberta report high shares of foreign-trained family physicians while North Western Territories and New Brunswick report high shares of foreign-trained specialists. South Africa is the most important source of graduation for foreign-trained family physicians, while India is the most important source country for foreign-trained specialists (CIHI, 2018).

In 2018, a majority of India-trained family physicians practising in Canada were reported in New Brunswick and Ontario (Figure 3.5). Similarly, in the case of specialists, a majority were in Newfoundland and Labrador and Manitoba. In absolute numbers, India-trained physicians outnumbered IMGs from other countries in Newfoundland and Labrador, New Brunswick, and Ontario but hardly had any presence in Prince Edward Island and the territories.

Let us consider the case of Ontario, the province which not only has the maximum number of IMGs but also the highest number of India-trained physicians, as of 2018. Ontario has adopted measures to increase physician supply, improve retention, and enhance the distribution of physicians in the province. The Ministry of Health and Long-Term Care does not promote or actively recruit foreign-trained HPs (WHO, 2018). To practice medicine independently in Ontario, IMGs must hold an Independent Practice Certificate of Registration issued by the College of Physicians and Surgeons

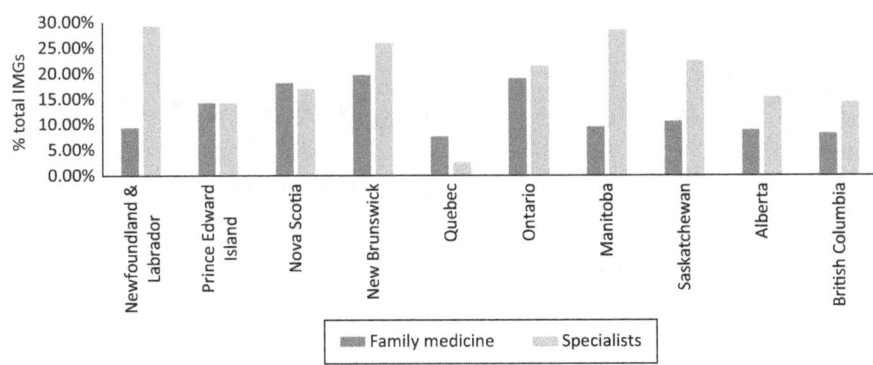

Figure 3.5 Province-wise share of India-trained Physicians (as % of total IMGs in the province), 2018.

Source: Supply, Distribution, and Migration of Physicians in Canada, Canadian Institute for Health Information, (CIHI, 2018), accessed on 25 June 2020. Yukon, Northwest Territories, and Nunavut are not represented as zero Indian-trained physicians were reported in those provinces in 2018.

of Ontario (CPSO). To qualify for the certificate, the applicant must have a recognized medical degree; qualify in the Medical Council of Canada Qualifying Examination (MCCQE); obtain certification of the Royal College of Physicians and Surgeons of Canada (RCPSC) or the College of Family Physicians of Canada (CFPC); complete one-year postgraduate training or active medical practice with relevant clinical experience in Canada; Canadian citizenship or permanent resident status.[14] An IMG can live and practice in Canada after obtaining Royal College certification.[15] Like any other IMG in Canada, the primary requirement for a physician trained in India is also to get a valid medical licence for the province where one wishes to practice. The mandatory licensure examinations serve as entry barriers. Records from 2017 show that while 95% and 97% of Canadian physicians qualified the MCCQE Part I and Part II, respectively; the corresponding success rates for IMGs were only 62% and 74%, respectively.[16]

Internationally Educated Nurses in Canada

The major source countries for foreign-trained nurses in Canada have been Philippines, India, UK, and US. The shares of these countries for each year are represented in Figure 3.6. Though the Philippines has contributed the highest number of trained nurses in Canada every year, India has reported a steadily rising share of 4% to 14% during 2000–2017.

The wide variation across provinces and territories in terms of the supply of domestic versus foreign-trained nursing graduates is worth mentioning.

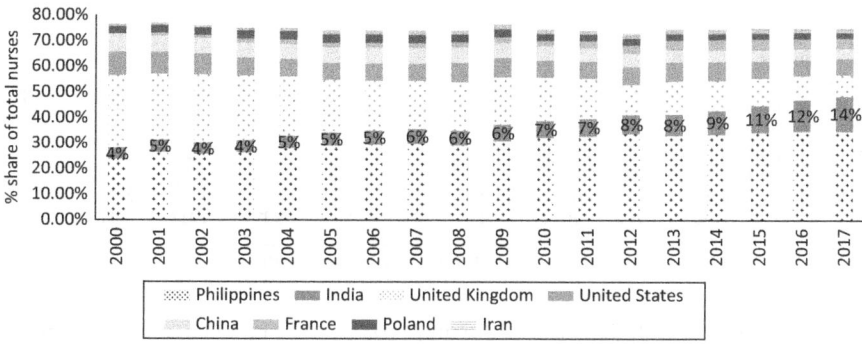

Figure 3.6 Source country-wise share of foreign-trained nurses in Canada.

Source: OECDSTAT, accessed on 25 June 2020. Only eight major source countries of IENs are reported, which are – China, France, India, Iran, Philippines, Poland, UK, and US.

In the year 2019, Manitoba, Alberta, and Ontario reported the highest shares of immigrant nursing professionals.[17]

A common concern regarding migrant professionals is their inability to get absorbed in professions for which they have been trained. To assess the same for the Internationally Educated Nurses (IENs) in Canada, we compute the ratio of regulated nursing workforce employed in direct care to the total supply by provinces/territories. Available data spanning 2010–2019 show that around 90% of NPs, around 85% of RNs and RPNs, and around 86% of LPNs on average have been employed in direct care (CIHI, 2020). This shows the likelihood of migrant NPs getting absorbed in direct care is relatively high. This has implications for the career prospects of IENs in Canada.

Figure 3.7 shows the varying composition of India-trained nursing professionals as percentage of IENs in Canada each year. While the overall share of India-trained nurses has been increasing, the highest increase has been in the share of LPNs. In 2010, the shares of LPNs and RNs were of similar magnitude. As of 2019, the share of LPNs compared to that of RNs is almost 43% higher. In absolute terms, there were 3105 RNs (out of 17,124) and 2069 LPNs (out of 6533), from India in Canada, in the year 2019. US and UK-trained NPs have outnumbered other IENs since 2010. Philippines and India have taken over the US and UK as the major source countries for RNs and especially for LPNs. India hardly has any contribution to the pool of RPNs. The major source country for RPNs has been the UK.

To illustrate the process of practising as a nurse in a province, let us take the example of Ontario, with consistently the highest share of IENs every year. An IEN must establish Canadian citizenship or permanent residence or hold authorization under the *IRPA* to engage in the practice of nursing

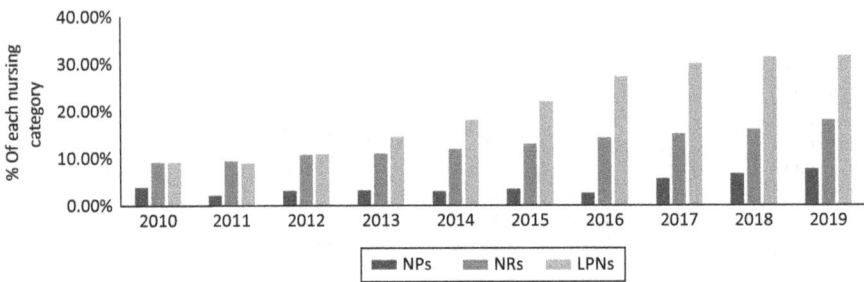

Figure 3.7 Share of India-trained nursing workforce employed in direct care in Canada, during 2010–2019.

Source: Canadian Institute for Health Information. Nursing in Canada, 2019 – Data Tables. Ottawa, ON: CIHI; 2020, accessed on 25 June 2020. Note: The shares have been calculated as India's share in the corresponding three IEN categories each year.

in Ontario. Becoming an RN or RPN in Ontario further requires opening an account with the National Nursing Assessment Service (NNAS). Exams such as the National Council Licensure Examination (NCLEX-RN) for RN and Canadian Practical Nurse Registration Examination (CPNRE) for RPN must be cleared by the applicant. Pass results for the licensure examinations over the last two years show that the average pass rates for foreign applicants were lower than average pass rates (see Table 3.2). The applicant must complete a jurisprudence exam to prove knowledge of the regulations, college by-laws, and practice standards that govern the nursing profession in Ontario.

Like the IMGs, the IENs must also go through an expensive and time-consuming process of licensing to prove their medical knowledge suitable for practising in Canada.

International Collaborations Concerning HP Mobility in Canada

Earlier, the Canadian Medical Association (CMA) viewed foreign HPs as a significant "planning component for sustainable Canadian physician workforce" (CMA & CCCPR, 2008). However, the multiple steps involved in HP mobility, such as the recognition of medical degree, licensure examinations, language tests, residency permits, etc., are time consuming, complicated entry barriers with financial implications for the applicants. As the above discussions reveal, Canada has reported an increasing share of IMGs and IENs in its HRH pool despite entry barriers for foreign-trained HPs. Unlike the migration of other professional categories covered in different agreements, Canada has mostly excluded health and social services from its

Table 3.2 Average Pass Rates Compared to Pass Rates of IENs During 2017 and 2018

	2017		2018		2017		2018	
	Average Pass Rate for RN	*Foreign-Trained RN Exam Writers*	*Average RPN pass rate*	*Foreign-Trained RPN Exam Writers*	*Average RPN Pass Rate*	*Foreign-Trained RPN Exam Writers*	*Average RPN Pass Rate*	*Foreign-Trained Exam Writers*
First attempt	83.5	51.1	85.2	53.6	86.4	71.8	83	65.1
Second attempt	33.3	38.8	26.3	34.8	63.2	56.2	58.3	48.3
Third attempt	50	39.3	50	32	62.6	63.3	57.3	51.4

Source: Nursing Registration Exams Report, 2018, available at http://www.cno.org/globalassets/2-howweprotectthepublic/statistical-reports/nursing-registration-exams-report-2018.pdf, accessed on 1 August 2020.

commitments. The Regional Trade Agreements (RTAs) signed with Chile, Colombia, Honduras, Panama, Peru or the North American Free Trade Agreement (NAFTA), or the bilateral agreements cover several migration-related commitments but healthcare. A multilateral agreement exists between Canada, US, Australia, Ireland, and UK for recognized training and certification of IMGs.

More than the trade agreements, Canada has Memorandum of Understanding (MoUs) facilitating international cooperation and coordination for HP mobility. Such agreements include a bilateral MoU between Philippines and Manitoba for physicians, nurses, and midwives; a bilateral MoU between Philippines and Saskatchewan for occupations such as the regulated health professions; a bilateral MoU between France and Quebec; a bilateral Memorandum of Agreement (MoA) between Philippines and Alberta concerning cooperation in Human Resource Deployment and Development (WHO, 2018). Within Canada, an interprovincial MoU exists between the government recruitment agencies in Saskatchewan, Alberta, British Columbia, and Manitoba covering family physicians and specialists for shared ethical recruitment practices in recruitment of IMGs.

Some specific policies and laws governing foreign-trained HPs at the provincial levels have been adopted to facilitate their inclusion. For instance, Ontario offers different career options to IMGs with varying qualification levels. The ministry funds postgraduate training positions and assessments to provide IMGs an opportunity for obtaining the additional qualifications they need to be eligible for independent practice in Ontario. The ministry is funding Touchstone Institute to provide standardized evaluation and training services. It delivers the Internationally Educated Nurses Competency Assessment Program (IENCAP) to assess the competence of RNs. It includes a clinical examination and an examination to evaluate knowledge, judgement, language, and comprehension related to nursing practice in Ontario. Health Force Ontario Marketing and Recruitment Agency (HFO MRA) offers a range of services to support IMGs in exploring and assessing their options with respect to alternative careers. The HIRE IEHP project, administered by HFO MRA and the University of Toronto, is aimed at integrating foreign HPs into the Canadian workplace. In Newfoundland and Labrador, funding has been provided to support foreign HP integration into practice and into the community (WHO, 2018).

Despite the rising share of Indian HPs in several Canadian provinces, no HP mobility agreement exists concerning the same. Overall, India is the second most important source country of IMGs in Canada. In terms of nursing professionals, India is second only to the Philippines as the major source country for Canada. As of 2019, India was reported as the second most important contributor of RNs and LPNs in Canada. India-trained HPs have comparative advantage in the global market, but they face the same entry barriers as any HP from other countries without collaborations/agreements with Canada. The extent of collaboration is only limited to health research institutes without direct implications for HP mobility. In 2015, Canadian and Indian Prime Ministers noted the opportunities inherent in India's goals of skill development. MoUs were signed between the National Skill Development Council of India and Canadian institutes and Sector Skills Councils in different fields including healthcare. The lack of any bilateral agreement regarding HP mobility between India and Canada leaves behind a potential demand–supply imbalance with trade policy implications.

Conclusion

Over the last decade, health systems around the world have been undergoing technological transformation. The aftermath of COVID-19 pandemic is only likely to catalyse these transformations. It will be worth watching out for a new paradigm of healthcare delivery with newer ways of optimizing healthcare resources. The pandemic has ushered in uncertainties in various aspects, including uncertainties about how the countries will settle for the new normal in healthcare delivery. The only certainty in this whole event is that the importance of HPs will not wane. Given the economic repercussions of the pandemic, a downside could be the adoption of austerity measures affecting the level and structure of HP remuneration in a publicly financed health system like Canada's. A secondary effect could be the need for strengthening the availability of domestic HRH with adverse effects on allowing foreign HPs. Nonetheless, it is essential for the individual countries to assess their trade-offs of engaging in cross-border HP mobility to alleviate HRH shortages and be prepared to confront adverse health shocks in the future.

The global nature of the current pandemic will undoubtedly leave behind a need for collective action to formulate long-term solutions for future health workforce shortages. Greater involvement of both the source and destination countries will be essential. It might be worthwhile for countries to diversify and strengthen their ties with partner countries with which they have significant migration flows of professionals. India–Canada HP mobility is a case in point for the same. A joint effort would accordingly be essential to improve global health conditions with spillover effects on domestic health outcomes. Such global cooperation will not only improve population health conditions but also make us better prepared for any future domestic or global health challenge.

Notes

1 Around 30 health professions are regulated under legislation in Canada. This chapter focuses on HP sub-categories of Medical Doctors/physicians and Nursing Professionals only, while acknowledging that other categories of health professionals also play a vital role in healthcare delivery but leaves the latter for future research.

2 These measures include facilitating renewal of working authorization, recruitment, temporary licensing, and fast-track processing of foreign qualifications recognition in the health sector. (OECD, 2020) http://www.oecd.org/coronavirus/policy-responses/beyond-containment-health-systems-responses-to-covid-19-in-the-oecd-6ab740c0/, accessed on 20 July 2020).

3 The definition of the foreign-trained HPs varies according to the data source or the corresponding country. For example, in Canada, foreign HPs are identified based on the country where their medical school or the nursing school was located, not necessarily the place where postgraduate training occurred (WHO, 2014).

4 See Chanda (2002); Buchan & Sochalski (2004); Blouin, Drager, & Smith (2005); Smith, Chanda, & Tangcharoensathien (2009); Tjadens, Weilandt, & Eckert (2012); Buchan, Wismar, Glinos, & Bremner (2014), Bhattacharjee (2018), and others for discussions on these factors.

5 The WHO Global Code of Practice on International Recruitment of Health Personnel (2010) aims at promoting practices for the ethical international recruitment of health personnel and facilitate the strengthening of health systems (WHO, 2010).

6 For instance, in Ontario, foreign-trained physicians who have passed their exams to practise in Canada or have graduated in the past two years were allowed to apply for a supervised 30-day medical licence to help fight COVID-19 (OECD, 2020).

7 Source: https://www.canada.ca/en/health-canada/services/health-care-system/reports-publications/health-care-system/canada.html, accessed on 27ʳJuly 2020.

8 Source: https://www.cihi.ca/en/canadas-doctor-supply-continues-to-grow-faster-than-the-population, accessed on 20 July 2020.

9 Examples of these authorities are: College of Physicians and Surgeons of British Columbia, College of Physicians and Surgeons of Alberta, College of Physicians and Surgeons of Saskatchewan, College of Physicians and Surgeons of Manitoba, College of Physicians and Surgeons of Ontario, Collège des médecins du Québec, College of Physicians and Surgeons of New Brunswick, College of Physicians and Surgeons of Nova Scotia, College of Physicians and Surgeons of Prince Edward Island, College of Physicians and Surgeons of Newfoundland & Labrador, Yukon Medical Council, Health and Social Services Government of the Northwest Territories, and Department of Health and Social Services Government of Nunavut.

10 Source: OECDSTAT, Dataset: Health Care Resources, accessed on 29 June 2020.

11 Source: Canadian Resident Matching Service. Canadian students studying medicine abroad. Ottawa, ON: Canadian Resident Matching Service; 2010. Available from: www.carms.ca/pdfs/2010_CSA_Report/CaRMS_2010_CSA_Report.pdf.

12 The regulatory authorities for RNs are: British Columbia College of Nursing Professionals, College and Association of Registered Nurses of Alberta, Saskatchewan Registered Nurses Association, College of Registered Nurses of Manitoba, College of Nurses of Ontario, Ordre des infirmières et infirmiers du Québec, Nurses Association of New Brunswick, Nova Scotia College of Nursing, College of Registered Nurses of Newfoundland and Labrador, Registered Nurses Association of the Northwest Territories and Nunavut, Registered Nurses Association of the Northwest Territories and Nunavut, Yukon Registered Nurses Association.

13 Source: https://www.cna-aiic.ca/-/media/cna/page-content/pdf-en/rn_highlights_e.pdf?la=en&hash=22B42E6B470963D8EDEAC3DCCBD026EDA1F6468D, accessed on 2 August 2020.

14 Source: https://www.cpso.on.ca/Physicians/Registration/Requirements, accessed on 1 August 2020.
15 Source: http://www.royalcollege.ca/rcsite/credentials-exams/assessment-international-medical-graduates-e#ac3, accessed on 20 July 2020.
16 Source: Medical Council of Canada 2017-18 Annual Report: https://mcc.ca/media/MCC-ANNUAL-REPORT-2017-2018.pdf, accessed on 30 July 2020.
17 Source: Data on "Supply and workforce" from CIHI Nursing Data Tables 2019.

Bibliography

Barer, M. L., & Stoddart, G. L. (1991). *Toward integrated medical resource policies for Canada*. Report prepared for the Federal/Provincial/Territorial Conference of Deputy Ministers of Health.

Bhattacharjee, A. (2018). Migration of Indian health professionals to the European Union: An analysis of policies and patterns. In S. I. Rajan ed. *In India migration report 2018: Migrants in Europe* (pp. 108–127). India: Routledge India.

Blouin, C., Drager, N., & Smith, R. (2005). *International trade in health services and the GATS: Current issues and debates*. World Bank Publications. https://doi.org/10.1596/978-0-8213-6211-2.

Buchan, J., & Sochalski, J. (2004). The migration of nurses: Trends and policies. *Bulletin of the World Health Organization, 82*(8), 587–594.

Buchan, J., Wismar, M., Glinos, I., & Bremner, J. (2014). *Health professional mobility in a changing Europe: New dynamics, mobile individuals and diverse responses*. Geneva: World Health Organisation (WHO).

Chanda, R. (2002). Trade in health services. *Bulletin of the World Health Organization, 80*, 158–163.

CIHI. (2011). *Canada's health care providers, 2000 to 2009: A reference guide*. Ottawa, ON: Canadian Institute for Health Information.

CIHI. (2018). *Physicians in Canada*. Ottawa, ON: Canadian Institute for Health Information.

CIHI. (2019). *Canadian institute for health information: Nursing in Canada, 2019 —A lens on supply and workforce*. Ottawa, ON: Canadian Institute for Health Information.

CIHI. (2020). *Nursing in Canada, 2019 — Data tables*. Ottawa, ON: Canadian Institute for Health Information.

CMA, & CCCPR. (2008). *International medical graduates in Canada*, January 16. Ottawa, ON: Canadian Medical Association and Canadian Collaborative Centre for Physician Resources. (http://www.cma.ca/multimedia/CMA/Content_Images/Policy_Advocacy/) on accessed 20 June 2012.

Dempster, H., & Smith, R. (2020). *Migrant health workers are on the covid-19 frontline: We need more of them*. Center For Global Development. Available at: https://www. cgdev. org/blog/migrant-health-workers-are-covid-19-frontline-we-need-more-them.

Dumont, J. C., Zurn, P., Church, J., & LeThi, C. (2008). *International mobility of health professionals and health workforce management in Canada: Myths and realities*. OECD Health Working Paper No. 40. Available at https://www.oecd.org/els/health-systems/41590427.pdf.

Evans, R. G., & McGrail, K. M. (2008). Richard III, Barer–Stoddart and the daughter of time. *Healthcare Policy, 3*(3), 18.

Jeffery, R. (1976). Migration of doctors from India. *Economic and Political Weekly*, *11*(13), 502–507.

Marchildon, G. (2013). Canada: Health system review. *Health Systems*, *15*(1), 1–179.

Merçay, C., Dumont, J. C., & Lafortune, G. (2016). *Health workforce policies in OECD countries-right jobs, right skills, right places*. OECD Publishing.

Monavvari, A. A., Peters, C., & Feldman, P. (2015). International medical graduates: Past, present, and future. *Canadian Family Physician*, *61*(3), 205–208.

OECD. (2016). *Health Workforce Policies in OECD Countries: Right Jobs, Right Skills, Right Places*. Paris: OECD Health Policy Studies, OECD Publishing. https://www.oecd.org/publications/health-workforce-policies-in-oecd-countries -9789264239517-en.

OECD. (2019a). *Recent trends in international migration of doctors, nurses and medical students*. Paris: OECD Publishing. https://doi.org/10.1787/5571ef48-en.

OECD. (2019b). *Recruiting immigrant workers: Canada 2019, recruiting immigrant workers*. Paris: OECD Publishing. https://doi.org/10.1787/4abab00d-en.

OECD. (2020). *Beyond containment: Health systems responses to COVID-19 in the OECD*. Paris: OECD Publishing.

Scarpetta, S., Dumont, J. C., & Socha-Dietrich, K. (2020). *Contribution of migrant doctors and nurses to tackling COVID-19 crisis in OECD countries*. Paris: OECD Publishing.

Siyam, A., & Dal Poz, M. R. (2014). *Migration of health workers: The WHO code of practice and the global economic crisis*. Geneva: World Health Organisation.

Smith, R. D., Chanda, R., & Tangcharoensathien, V. (2009). Trade in health-related services. *The Lancet*, *373* (9663), 593–601.

Sweetman, A., McDonald, J. T., & Hawthorne, L. (2015). Occupational regulation and foreign qualification recognition: An overview. *Canadian Public Policy*, *41*(Supplement 1), S1–S13.

Tjadens, F., Weilandt, C., & Eckert, J. (2012). Mobility of health professionals: Health systems, work conditions, patterns of health workers' mobility and implications for policy makers. WIAD – Scientific Institute of the Medical Association of German Doctor.

Tyrrell, L., & Dauphinee, D. (1999). *Task force on physician supply in Canada*. Canadian Medical Forum Task Force on Physician Supply in Canada. Available at: http://www.physicianhr.ca/reports/PhysicianSupplyInCanada-Final1999.pdf.

Wang, L., Rosenberg, M., & Lo, L. (2008). Ethnicity and utilization of family physicians: A case study of Mainland Chinese immigrants in Toronto, Canada. *Social Science & Medicine*, *67*(9), 1410–1422.

WHO. (2010). *User's guide to the WHO global code of practice on the international recruitment of health personnel*. Geneva: World Health Organisation.

WHO. (2018). *National reporting instrument*. Canada: World Health Organisation.

4 Becoming a Migrant Healthcare Worker

Interrogating Gender and Migration

Shruti Gupta

Introduction

The historical mobility of Indians for employment coupled with the increasing feminisation of migration has created particular migratory flows within which the migration of healthcare workers, particularly nurses, has been significant. As per the World Migration Report (2020), India has the largest absolute number of migrants living abroad. While men dominated the earlier migration streams, there has been an increasing demand for migrant women, particularly, in the services industry. Within these flows, the presence of skilled women working as doctors, nurses and technicians has increased. However, research on their migratory experiences and economic participation remains scarce, particularly for gendered migration between countries within Asia.

This chapter traces the process of becoming a migrant healthcare worker through the case study of Indian women in the United Arab Emirates (UAE) – the creation of the demand for and supply of workers, the channels of migration, and policies governing migration and professionalisation. It illustrates that the becoming of a woman migrant healthcare worker lies at the intersection of varied scales and is deeply intertwined with economic, social, political and cultural factors. This argument is developed in three sections. The first section highlights the interlinking of care needs across borders through the theoretical framework of global care chains. It asserts that the commodification of care work has resulted in an increasingly stratified workforce along the axes of gender, race and class, and this influences and impacts the particular experiences of migrant healthcare workers. The second section shows how these care chains are configured by immigration policies on both sides of the border. Unintended gendering of immigration channels and policies impacts women's freedom of mobility, access to employment opportunities and benefits of family reunification both implicitly and explicitly. The third and final section focuses on the close relationship between licensing and accreditation procedures and gendered access to economic, cultural and social capital. The findings are based on semi-structured interviews conducted in 2017 with 26 Indian women employed in the

DOI: 10.4324/9781003315124-4

healthcare sector across institutional settings in the UAE. It forms part of a larger project in which over 150 Indian migrant women across income categories were interviewed, along with migrant agents and returned migrants in India. For the purpose of this chapter, data from the larger dataset were also drawn upon to understand the process of becoming a migrant healthcare worker more holistically. Overall, the chapter aims to highlight the gendered experiences of migrant healthcare workers in Asia and, in doing so, contribute to academic, policy and developmental discourses on the topic.

The Interplay of Care, Migration and Gender

The work of healthcare professionals is rooted in practices of caregiving and care-receiving, which are socially constructed and culturally situated. Conventionally, women were expected to perform care work out of love and obligation for family members. These were unpaid services, shouldered exclusively by women. However, with the increase in social differentiation, several of these activities moved out of the private realm of the home to the public arena. These came to be managed and performed by live-in caregivers and by professionally trained skilled workers in state and market-governed institutions. Many of these care arrangements today are dependent on the migration of healthcare workers, which has created global care chains that link care regimes of different countries such as India and the UAE. Hochschild (2015) theorised global care chains as a "series of personal links between people across the globe based on the paid or unpaid work of caring". While global care chains have been poignant in integrating gender within migratory care work, this conceptualisation remains limited in its analytical scope. Yeates (2009) argues for an expansion of the literature on global care chains to include a range of commodified forms of social reproduction and paid carework through the study of healthcare workers, in particular, nurses. In doing so, skilled women working in institutional settings can provide an alternative understanding of gender, care regimes and migration from that of domestic workers. The broadening of the global care chain's literature to include healthcare professionals makes visible the issue of gender, the complexities of gendered migration and its interconnections with political, social and economic factors that determine care regimes.

I find that the extension of the global care chains literature to the healthcare sector in the UAE illustrates the high reliance on migrant workers and its gendered composition. As per Younies et al. (2008), 82 percent of healthcare workers in the UAE are migrants. Table 4.1 draws data from the four health authorities in the UAE – the Health Authority of Abu Dhabi (HAAD) for Abu Dhabi, the Dubai Health Authority (DHA) and Dubai Healthcare Authority (DHCA) for Dubai, and the Ministry of Health and Prevention (MOHAP) for the other five Emirates – Sharjah, Ajman, Ras Al Khaimah, Umm Al Quwain and Fujairah, and it primarily focuses on professions that research participants are engaged in. The table shows the overwhelming

Table 4.1 Selected Healthcare Professions in the UAE by Nationality and Gender, Various Years

Profession	Nationality	Gender	MOHAP (2017)	Dubai (2019)[1]	HAAD (2017)
Doctors	Citizen	Male	36	221	314
		Female	242	455	732
		Total	278	676	1046
	Non-citizen	Male	859	5371	5503
		Female	550	3560	2895
		Total	1409	8931	8398
Dentists	Citizen	Male	19	46	39
		Female	171	147	120
		Total	190	193	159
	Non-citizen	Male	31	1139	990
		Female	39	1215	771
		Total	70	2354	1761
Nurses[2]	Citizen	Male	1	2	7
		Female	306	74	181
		Total	307	76	188
	Non-citizen	Male	289	2781	6610
		Female	2209	15262	20770
		Total	2498	18043	27380
Assistant nurses	Citizen	Male	0		
		Female	2		
		Total	2		
	Non-citizen	Male	170		
		Female	584		
		Total	754	0	
Technicians	Citizen	Male	19	41	
		Female	743	332	
		Total	762	373	
	Non-citizen	Male	724	3906	
		Female	749	9493	
		Total	1473	13399	

HAAD, Health Authority of Abu Dhabi; MOHAP, Ministry of Health and Prevention; UAE, United Arab Emirates.

Source: Annual Statistical Book, 2017. Ministry of Health and Prevention, UAE; Annual Health Statistic Book, 2019. Dubai Health Authority; Abu Dhabi Health Statistics 2017. Department of Health, Abu Dhabi.

presence of migrants and, in particular, migrant women in the sector across professions. Table 4.1 also adds a layer of complexity to the overall sectoral composition by highlighting the stratification of the workforce along the axes of race, class and gender. I draw on Roberts" (1997) division of domestic carework into spiritual and menial to explain the composition of the sector. She asserts that spiritual or relational carework is a highly complex activity which makes the standardisation, mechanisation and capitalisation of the work difficult. Such work in the healthcare sector is performed by specialists such as doctors and dentists. Menial or non-relational carework performed by nurses, assistant nurses, midwives and technicians is arduous, routine and unpleasant. This ideological split between the different domains of carework pushes the burden of relational carework onto women and the performance of non-relational carework to migrant women of colour and women in the lower socio-economic strata. Segregation of occupations based on nationality and gender shows that the number of nationals and men reduces as we move down the income and skill ladder. Foremost, Emirati men are engaged as doctors and dentists as these professions are associated with skills and expertise which are deemed appropriate for men to acquire and practise through their economic, social and cultural capital. Further, in the UAE, professions like nursing have a poor social image and are considered to be women's work (El-Jardali et al., 2008) due to which there is an overrepresentation of women.

In the healthcare sector, hierarchy was institutionalised through the colonial model of nursing education which favoured British women as nurses while women of other races worked as nurse assistants (Percot and Rajan, 2007). This ideological differentiation and hierarchy have manifested in a higher number of Emirati women working as doctors and dentists in comparison with those working as nurses. In 2013, only 3 percent of the nurses in the UAE were Emiratis (D'Souza, 2013). As per data published by the Ministry of Health in 2007, 63 percent of nurses are from South and Southeast Asian countries, primarily, India, Pakistan and the Philippines and 28 percent are from Arab countries such as Palestine, Jordan, Oman, Syria, Egypt, Sudan and Somalia (El-Jardali et al., 2008). Based on fieldwork, it was seen that even among migrant women, those of marginalised socio-economic positions are employed as assistant nurses and technicians. In addition to the manner in which carework in the healthcare sector is perceived, these professional hierarchies can also be attributed to the high cost of medical and nursing education, economic capital required for overseas accreditation and certifications and social capital required for professionalisation – issues discussed in detail in the next sections.

The overrepresentation of women and migrants in the healthcare sector, particularly, in non-relational work leads to an undervaluation of carework. Table 4.2 provides an overview of average salaries received by participants interviewed and these varied based on institutional settings and seniority. The table illustrates large variations in income, especially among nurses. Further, as per El-Jardali et al. (2008), the remuneration received by Emirati nurses while higher than that received by migrant nurses is lower than that of other professions. In recognition of the low engagement of nationals as nurses, the MOHAP has since made concerted efforts to increase their presence in the profession. In 2013, in Ministry facilities, 8 percent of nurses were Emirati, which was to be increased to 10–16 percent. In Table 4.1, the target has been achieved, as 11 percent of nurses were nationals in 2017. Similar to the overall labour force composition, the majority of national

Table 4.2 Average Salary of Healthcare Workers Interviewed (2017)

Profession	Type of Institute	Average Monthly Salary (AED)
Physicians	Private hospital	8,500 and above
Nurses	Private hospital	5,500–7,000
Nurses	Private clinic	3,500
Nurses	School	3,750
Assistant nurses	Private hospital	3,500
Cleaning and sanitation	Private hospital	3,500

Source: Fieldwork, 2017.

healthcare workers are employed in the public sector which can ensure competitive salaries, flexible working hours and other incentives such as scholarships, trainings and paid-time off. Thus, the economic value of carework is deeply intertwined with its racial, classed and gendered composition.

The shortage of healthcare workers in rich countries such as the UAE, increasing demand for health services and the presence of trained workers in developing countries such as India defines who is cared for, by whom and how (Kofman & Raghuram, 2009). The Gulf in particular became an extremely popular migrant destination for healthcare workers from India as the immigration procedures are faster and relatively cheaper than those in Western countries. As per estimates, there are approximately 40,000–50,000 Indian nurses in Gulf countries with 90 percent of them from Kerala (Percot & Rajan, 2007). Higher salaries in these countries than those in private hospitals in India and a favourable rate of exchange between the two currencies have been a key motivating factor for migration. For example, a young nurse from Kerala in a private clinic in Dubai earned nearly four times higher in the UAE: approximately Emirate Dirham (AED) 3,500 per month in the UAE in comparison with INR 16,000 per month in India. Temporary migration stretching over several years enables individuals and families to not only provide for those in India but also to invest in property, save and purchase consumer durables through remittances.

In addition to care imbalances between countries and economic factors, migration of healthcare professionals is also linked to socio-economic relations across scales. Nursing in India was rooted in social stigma as it carried caste connotations, dictated by the rules of ritual purity and pollution. However, the possibility of economic mobility and migration changed the perception of nursing over the last 20 years. Percot and Rajan (2007) show that nurses no longer come from poor families. My findings indicate an even greater shift towards the de-stigmatisation of the profession, as the nurses I interviewed came primarily from lower-middle or middle-class backgrounds. A majority of the participants' fathers and/or husbands worked in administrative positions in private organisations or government departments. Further, it was seen that nurses were considered positively in the matrimonial market for men working overseas. 82 percent of nurses interviewed migrated overseas for the first time after marriage. Their spouses were already in the UAE and they entered the country on a visit or residence visa, depending on the husband's income level. Similarly, the doctors interviewed also migrated after marriage. In addition to the improving status of nursing in India, the finding also shows that nurses might be preferable because of their income earning capacity. Nurses earn higher than other skilled migrant women in the UAE such as teachers and those in administrative positions in private organisations. Given the high cost of living in the UAE, healthcare workers can combine their sexual and reproductive labour with economic labour (Kaur, 2010). Thus, nursing is now seen as a vehicle to gain economic and social mobility for the family and to secure better matrimonial prospects for the woman (Percot, 2006).

Despite the interdependence between India and the UAE for healthcare workers, there are no bilateral agreements on the management of migrants in the sector. Varied institutions undertake recruitment based on periodic requirements. For example, Aster group of hospitals with the help of the Indian consulate in Dubai and the UAE government flew in 88 Indian nurses in May 2020 to fulfil the shortages in their field hospitals during the COVID-19 pandemic (Saseendran, 2020). Poor healthcare workforce planning by both countries, social stigma against nursing, and incomplete, outdated data has furthered the care imbalance and the undervaluation of the profession. An intersectional approach through the lens of global care chains captures these overarching problems and highlights the particular experiences and positionalities of migrant healthcare workers.

Gendered Immigration Policies

From the minute women decide to migrate, their experiences are differentiated from those of men. Immigration policies for women and their subsequent integration upon migration are different from those that govern men. Gendered immigration policies erase women's role as economic agents, devalue their skills and impact their migratory outcomes. In this section, I highlight how the mobility of healthcare workers is tightly regulated and how their identities are determined based on their gender before and after migration.

The Emigration Act 1983 bifurcates the status of Indian citizenship into Emigration Check Required (ECR) and Emigration Check Not Required (ECNR) (Kodoth & Varghese, 2012). Prospective migrants with an education qualification below matriculation are classified into the ECR category. In response to growing reports of exploitation and harassment of Indian nurses in the Gulf, in 2015, the Indian government-imposed restrictions on the mobility of nurses migrating to 18 countries, one of them being the UAE, by placing them in the ECR category. Following the notification, nurses can be recruited either through registered recruitment agencies in India or through registered foreign recruiters on the eMigrate system operated by the Ministry of External Affairs. As per data gathered by Walton-Roberts and Rajan (2020), the number of ECR nurses fell after the regulation from 4,858 in 2016 to 4,123 in 2017 but has increased since to 5,562 in 2018. However, through my fieldwork in 2017, I found that none of the nurses interviewed migrated through the ECR channel. A majority of the married nurses migrated on their husband's visa while others migrated through a visit visa. Those entering the UAE on a visit visa were sponsored by their husbands, siblings or cousins in the UAE and were aware of the restrictions imposed on their immigration. Many recited the script they had practised in response to the questioning by immigration officials in India and they carried sufficient documentary proof of their visa sponsor's credentials in the UAE. After arriving in the UAE, they endeavoured to clear the licensing examinations and looked for jobs before the expiration of their three-month visit visa.

At its most fundamental level, the ECR categorisation of nurses, majority of whom are women, points towards a gendered conceptualisation of citizenship and mobility. Migrant women, particularly domestic workers and nurses, are viewed as symbols of national honour whose exploitation abroad becomes unacceptable to the state irrespective of the lack of protection accorded to them at home (Pattadath & Moors, 2012). Threat of abuse and exploitation overseas has resulted in the denial of the right to migrate and the right to work. At the policy level, it remains uncertain if ECR regulations have reduced the exploitation of migrant nurses. As per an interview conducted with a recruitment agency in New Delhi, the database of registered recruitment agencies made publicly available by the Ministry of External Affairs is used by unregistered agencies to pose as registered agents. These agents use details available online to print fake licences to dupe prospective migrations who have no way of verifying the validity of the licence[3]. Further, a recruitment agency official explained that the ECR procedure is susceptible to corruption:

> The emigration procedure involves a lot of bribing. Every agency has a middleman who liaisons with the Ministry of External Affairs. We transfer the requisite amount to him and he handles the immigration clearance for workers in the ECR category.

These restrictive immigration procedures also increase the economic burden for migrant women. Women migrating on visit visas have to bear the cost of their visas and a return flight ticket, which is usually borne by the employer if recruited directly. Further, many do not find employment before their visit visa runs out, paying extra for a visa extension or exiting and returning to the UAE for renewal purposes. In addition, women migrating through the alternative route of family migration are categorised in familial terms – mothers, sisters and daughters. They face similar conditions and barriers as women migrating as labour migrants but their gender-specific experiences and their contribution in the labour market are not recognised.

Consequently, skilled women such as healthcare workers are not recognised as economic agents, they are incorrectly included in migration data and research on their migration experiences remains limited.

Additionally, migrants' immigration and subsequent legal status must be understood as the triangular relation between sending states, receiving states and the socio-economic position of individual migrants (Baubock, 2017). In the UAE, an employer bases the governance of migrants on the *Kafala* system wherein the worker is sponsored for a predetermined contract period. While the sponsorship rules and immigration criteria are similar for all migrants, the rules for family reunification are differentiated based on migrants' class positionality determined by their place in the occupational structure and their gender. Male migrants can sponsor their families if they earn a minimum salary of AED 4,000 or AED 3,000 plus accommodation. Earlier, men belonging to only certain professions were allowed to sponsor their families. The new regulation marks a radical shift in immigration policies allowing for greater inclusion and belonging for migrants. However, for women, the occupation criteria and income threshold still apply. In Abu Dhabi and Dubai, a woman can apply to sponsor her family if she is an engineer, teacher, doctor, nurse or in any other profession related to the medical sector and if her monthly salary is more than AED 10,000 or AED 8,000 plus accommodation. In Dubai, women not employed in one of these professional categories can also apply to sponsor their families if their income is more than AED 10,000. The website with residency rules does not provide information for women sponsoring families in Emirates other than Abu Dhabi and Dubai. As previously shown, all healthcare professionals interviewed fall below the required income threshold. While online news reports claim that the rules have been changed recently to bring parity between men and women (Nagraj, 2019), these still do not reflect on official government websites. Removing the occupational criteria and lowering of the income threshold for women will have positive impacts on women's migratory experiences and their sense of belonging as migrant workers.

The UAE does not provide the option of naturalisation and permanent residency. The residency status of migrants is intricately tied to their employment contract, generally ranging between a period of one to three years and in the case of healthcare workers, linked to the renewal of their professional licence. Thus, migrants live simultaneously across multiple borders involving "the active consideration of the present in terms of the past, the future in terms of the present, and so on" (Bailey et al., 2002). However, I found that legal statuses accorded through visas are actively resisted by migrants and continuously in flux. High-income workers and professionals in particular enjoy easy visa and contract renewal, allowing for long-term residency. Healthcare workers interviewed had stayed for an average of 10 years at the time of the study, with the longest duration being 19 years. A large number of participants[4] reported that they would like to stay in the country for as long as possible and would move back only if their visas were cancelled. Greater professional and personal comfort, saving opportunities and preserving of the family unit by being with the husband were the main motivators to continue living in the UAE. Additionally, visa rules are altered based on the economic and social needs of the destination countries. Dubai changed its visa regulations in 2019 and 2020 to allow long-term residency for certain groups of migrants. Within this scheme, selected healthcare professionals were given a 10-year golden residency visa in recognition of their services in fighting the COVID-19 pandemic. Additionally, 80,000 frontline workers were identified to be given social benefits such as mental health services, discounts and educational scholarships for their children as gratitude for their service and sacrifice during the pandemic (Abubaker, 2020).

Thus, migrant women contend with gendered immigration policies on both ends of the transnational field forcing them to bear greater uncertainties and pressures than their male counterparts. Despite these strong controls over their mobility and identities, women negotiate with patriarchal constructs and gendered ideologies when undertaking migration and work. In doing so, they create spaces of exception wherein they claim inclusion and belonging. At the level of the state, they acquire acceptance through their remittances in the home country and their labour and skills in the destination country. At an individual level, they facilitate belonging through the acquisition of economic and social capital across borders.

Qualifications and Licensing Procedures

The entry of skilled workers into the labour market after the migration is heavily reliant on the verification of their educational qualifications and professional experience. Without bilateral agreements and mutual certification recognitions, the rigid structures of accreditation and verification can adversely impact migrants' labour market participation and have varying outcomes for men and women. Alongside government agencies and professional associations, institutions such as employers, universities and families also determine the value of qualifications and prior work experience.

In order to practice in the UAE, all healthcare professionals are required to obtain a licence from one of the four healthcare authorities. The pre-screening entails the verification of education credentials (high school and professional qualifications) and licence in home or previous country and submission of an experience certificate (minimum two years). Each authority has its own fee structure and might require additional documents. Indian candidates are also required to undertake a licensing exam. While these licensing and accreditation requirements seem gender neutral on the surface, I find that experiences vary for men and women. This is because most women occupy marginal positions within labour markets due to their differentiated access to economic and social capital. Additionally, women's engagement in paid employment must be understood within the context of their unpaid reproductive labour within the household.

As there are four healthcare authorities in the UAE, the selection of the licensing exam for many might be a difficult decision as migrant women have limited knowledge of local labour markets and might be out of professional networks (Iredale, 2005). Further, many take decisions based on their husband's job. For example, a homemaker interviewed applied for the DHA exam as her husband's job was based in Dubai. Due to high living expenses, the family moved to Sharjah pushing her out of the labour market as she could not balance childcare, household responsibilities, the long commute and an 8-hour shift as a nurse. Further, to be eligible for the licensure exam, doctors and nurses must have two years of work experience and there must not be a gap greater than two years in their work record. She currently does not have the economic capital to take another exam[5] and fears her professional qualifications will be devalued as she approaches two years out of the job market. Thus, women's ability to gain accreditation and enter the labour market is also dependent on the negotiations undertaken within the household (Iredale, 2005). High costs of accreditation exams[6] is an added burden which forces women to prioritise the needs of their children and partner over their own career aspirations (Hawthrone, 2000).

The licensure procedure is an embodiment of not only the skills of the professional but also their race, class and gender. The licensing criteria in the UAE are not uniform across nationalities as those with qualifications and credentials from Western countries (Canada, South Africa, USA, Ireland, Australia, New Zealand and Britain) and select Gulf Cooperation Council (GCC) countries are exempt from the licensing exams. In addition, I found that education qualifications and work experiences even among Indian migrants have varying credibility. For example, several women working as cleaning staff in private organisations have nursing diplomas with over five years of work experience as nurses in India. However, due to the perceived value of their credentials and the cost of licensure, the majority did not attempt to convert their credentials upon migration. Further, the certification procedure to gain equivalency is often discretionary. In the UAE, primary source verification (PSV) is undertaken directly after submitting documents through online portals. While the integrated PSV system eases the process for applicants, there is no guarantee that those who have the required qualifications will be certified. A participant working as a conductor and cleaner in a school illustrated how women, particularly, those of marginal socio-economic positions face deskilling, reduced earnings and potential unemployment due to licensing requirements on migration:

> First, I worked as a lab technician for six months in a private clinic. I had problems at the time of document verification and could not work as a lab technician anymore. I was forced to migrate because of my financial situation; my husband is an alcoholic who troubles me and my

son was unwell. So, I paid AED 9,000 to an agent who got me a cleaning job at a school.

While reskilling and upskilling are essential for healthcare workers to perform their professional duties, these requirements are difficult to comply with for women of lower socio-economic status. This was seen in 2019 when a bachelor's degree was mandated as the minimum prerequisite for registered nurses, irrespective of their years of experience. Following the notification, approximately 200 Indian nurses with diplomas lost their jobs while several others were demoted to assistant nurses (Gokulan, 2019). As per a local newspaper, the bridging courses offered by the UAE universities which cost between AED 60,000 to AED 70,000 are unaffordable for many nurses (Gokulan, 2019). Additionally, the UAE only recognises nursing diplomas issued by the Kerala Nursing Council, therefore, many who might be able to afford the bridge courses are ineligible.

It must be noted that the immigration policies and licensing procedures in the UAE are simpler, cheaper and more accessible than the point-based immigration systems in Western countries, particularly, Australia, Canada and New Zealand. This makes the UAE an attractive migration destination for skilled professionals. Further, migration to the UAE allows for the accumulation of economic and social capital to migrate to more developed countries, allowing for access to better opportunities and naturalisation (El-Jardali et al., 2008). While on the surface and by intent, the UAE's licensing requirements are gender neutral, a closer examination supported by empirical evidence shows that these policies can have varying outcomes due to the complex intersection of gender, race and class. Immigration policies along with labour market regulations are structured upon unequal gender relations which result in unemployment, deskilling and devaluation of women workers. The impact of these unequal policies is acute for healthcare workers due to the strict regulation of the sector resulting inmigrants' reliance on their educational qualifications and economic and social capital to make their skills internationally recognisable (Kofman & Raghuram, 2006). Thus, policies governing migration such as immigration, licensing and accreditation must not only be gender neutral but gender-sensitive to accommodate the particular needs of women (Iredale, 2005).

Conclusion

The chapter studies the process of becoming a migrant woman healthcare worker through the case study of Indian women in the UAE. It highlights that migration and employment are determined by a myriad of actors, institutions and factors, influencing one another in multiple ways. In doing so, the research endeavours to highlight and contribute to the gaps in literature on three fronts: intra-Asia migration, gendered migration of skilled women and information and data on migration. Recognising and filling these gaps can have vital implications for developmental and policy discussions.

Over the past years, migration research has begun to acknowledge the limited focus on flows between countries in the Global South, including intra-Asia migration. Data indicate that flows between the South are nearly as large as those between countries in the Global North and the Global South (Chanda, 2012). In particular, a distinctive feature of Asian migration is its intraregional and sub-regional nature, of which certain corridors such as the India–UAE corridor have substantial flows. The India Migration Report series has been significant in recognising and plugging this gap, and this chapter aims to further the endeavour by focusing on the particular social and cultural relations and economic and political contexts of inter-Asia migration.

Further, the narrative on migration has privileged the mobility of men and their experiences in the productive sphere. In studying women's migration, an overwhelming amount of research has focused on migrant domestic workers. While women's dominance in the domestic work sector is reflected in the quantum of research on the subject, it has erased women's engagement in other forms of productive and reproductive labour. Thus, the study of healthcare workers enables an expanded understanding and rethinking of the multiple ways women intersect with the labour market, their differentiated migration experiences and their identity as not only women but also as classed and racialised actors. In the Asian context in particular, as countries such as the UAE transition to a more knowledge-based economy and as countries invest more in public health, the reliance on unskilled men will decrease and skilled women's prominence within these flows will increase.

Finally, there is limited availability of data on the mobility of women and in particular healthcare workers. As seen through this study, data have been compiled from incomplete and fragmented datasets gathered from national records, newspaper articles, research papers and reports. The characterisation of migrant women in familial terms furthers data inaccuracies. Limited information and data make the monitoring of migration, resource allocation and formation of social policy difficult and lacking.

Notes

1 The statistics for Dubai provides details for healthcare workers in both DHA and DHCA.
2 The categorisation of nurses differs for each source. DHA does not provide figures for assistant nurses, whereas HAAD includes midwives in the nursing figures.
3 The list is regularly updated by the Ministry of External Affairs and can be accessed at:https://emigrate.gov.in/ext/openPDF?strFile=RA_LIST_REPORT.pdf.
4 When asked about the primary reason to leave the UAE in the future, the leading reason selected by participants was divided equally between cancellation/expiration of visa and education of children. In addition, a number of participants

anticipated moving back to India due to family obligations, particularly caregiving responsibilities towards ageing parents. I found corporal and cognitive agencies as central to women's migratory decisions; forged at the intersection of varied scales and undertaken through active thinking, strategising and imaginings (Silvey, 2004).

5 In 2014, the health authorities signed an agreement for the unification of licences, making it easier for professionals to work anywhere in the country. However, for many, such as the participant in question, the additional fee is a financial strain on the family income. Further, in the participant's case in particular, as she does not have the required six months of work experience using her licence, she would need to take another exam to work in Sharjah.

6 The accreditation cost varies per authority and qualification. For example, in the case of nurses, the minimum cost for the MOHAP licence is AED 1,000 (INR 20,000), AED 3,060 (INR 61,300) for DHA and AED 900 (INR 18,000) for HAAD. Charges increase for any additional document verification and processes required. Also, the cost for licensure is substantially higher for physicians and doctors across authorities.

References

Abubaker, R. (2020, September). UAE Press: Frontline workers recognised and rewarded in the UAE. WAM, Emirates News Agency. http://wam.ae/en/details /1395302868448 retrieved 3 January 2021.

Bailey, A. J., Wright, R. A., Mountz, A., & Miyares, I. M. (2002). (Re)producing salvadoran transnational geographies. *Annals of the Association of American Geographers*, 92(1), 125–144. https://doi.org/10.1111/1467-8306.00283

Baubock, R. (2017). Political boundaries and democratic membership. In A. Shachar, R. Bauböck, I. Bloemraad, & M. Vink (Eds.), *The Oxford handbook of citizenship* (pp. 60–78). New York: Oxford University Press.

Chanda, R. (2012). *Migration between South and Southeast Asia: Overview of trends and issues* (ISAS Working Paper No. 140). Institute of South Asian Studies.

D'Souza, C. (2013, March). Emirati nurses make up just 3% in UAE. *Gulf News*. https://gulfnews.com/uae/health/emirati-nurses-make-up-just-3-in-uae-1 .1161080 retrieved 21 December 2020.

El-Jardali, F., Jamal, D., Jaafar, M., & Rahal, Z. (2008). *Analysis of health professionals migration: A two-country case study for the United Arab Emirates and Lebanon*. Beirut: Faculty of Health Sciences, American University of Beirut.

Gokulan, D. (2019, October). Qualification issues of Indian nurses in UAE to be resolved soon: Muraleedharan. *Khaleej Times*. https://www.khaleejtimes.com /uae/dubai/qualification-issues-of-indian-nurses-in-uae-to-be-resolved-soon -muraleedharan retrieved 28 December 2020.

Hawthrone, L. (2000). *The international transfer of skills to Australia: The 'NESB' factor in labour market disadvantage for migrant nurses and engineers* [Unpublished Ph.D. Thesis]. Monash University.

Hochschild, A. R. (2015). Global care chains and emotional surplus value. In D. Engster & T. Metz (Eds.), *Justice, politics, and the family* (1st ed., pp. 249–261). Routledge, New York: New Press, Distributed by W.W. Norton.

Iredale, R. (2005). Gender, immigration policies and accreditation: Valuing the skills of professional women migrants. *Geoforum*, 36(2), 155–166. https://doi.org/10 .1016/j.geoforum.2004.04.002

Kaur, R. (2010). Bengali bridal diaspora: Marriage as a livelihood strategy. *Economic & Political Weekly, 45*(5), 16–18.

Kodoth, P., & Varghese, V. J. (2012). Protecting women or endangering the emigration process: Emigrant women domestic workers, gender and state policy. *Economic and Political Weekly, 47*(43), 56–66.

Kofman, E., & Raghuram, P. (2006). Gender and global labour migrations: Incorporating skilled workers. *Antipode, 38*(2), 282–303. https://doi.org/10.1111/j.1467-8330.2006.00580.x

Kofman, E., & Raghuram, P. (2009). *The implications of migration for gender and care regimes in the South* (Social Policy and Development Programme Paper No. 41). United Nations Research Institute for Social Development.

Nagraj, A. (2019, July 14). New family sponsorship law for expats in the UAE takes effect. *Gulf Business.* https://gulfbusiness.com/new-family-sponsorship-law-for-expats-in-the-uae-takes-effect/ retrieved 16 November 2020.

Pattadath, B., & Moors, A. (2012). Moving between Kerala and Dubai. In B. Kalir & M. Sur (Eds.), *Transnational flows and permissive polities* (pp. 151–168). Amsterdam University Press; JSTOR. http://www.jstor.org/stable/j.ctt45kfk8.12

Percot, M. (2006). Indian Nurses in the Gulf: Two Generations of Female Migration. *South Asia Research, 26*(1), 41–62. https://doi.org/10.1177/0262728006063198

Percot, M., & Rajan, S. I. (2007). Female emigration from India: Case study of nurses. *Economic & Political Weekly, 42*(4), 318–325.

Roberts, E. D. (1997). Spiritual and menial housework. *Yale J.L. & Feminism, 9*(51), 51–78.

Saseendran, S. (2020, August). Indian nurses on COVID-19 duty in UAE fly back home with valuable lessons, cherished memories. *Gulf News.* https://gulfnews.com/uae/indian-nurses-on-covid-19-duty-in-uae-fly-back-home-with-valuable-lessons-cherished-memories-1.73025932 retrieved 23 December 2020.

Silvey, R. (2004). Power, difference and mobility: Feminist advances in migration studies. *Progress in Human Geography, 28*(4), 490–506. https://doi.org/10.1191/0309132504ph490oa

Walton-Roberts, M., & Rajan, S. I. (2020, January 21). *Global demand for medical professionals drives Indians abroad despite acute domestic health-care worker shortages.* Migrationpolicy.Org. https://www.migrationpolicy.org/article/global-demand-medical-professionals-drives-indians-abroad retrieved 21 December 2020.

World Migration Report 2020. (2020). International Organization for Migration. https://publications.iom.int/system/files/pdf/wmr_2020.pdf

Yeates, N. (2009). Production for export: The role of the state in the development and operation of global care chains. *Population, Space and Place, 15*(2), 175–187. https://doi.org/10.1002/psp.546

Younies, H., Barhem, B., & Younis, M. Z. (2008). Ranking of priorities in employees' reward and recognition schemes: From the perspective of UAE health care employees. *The International Journal of Health Planning and Management, 23*(4), 357–371. https://doi.org/10.1002/hpm.912

5 Beyond the Caring Obligation
Indian Nurses Negotiating Nursing Care and Migration

Neha Adsul and Rohit Shah

Introduction

"Caring" a Very Emotional and Material Activity

Nurses have always contended to balance the dichotomy between their desire to care and the right to control and define this activity. This can largely be attributed to a societal order, which undermines the value of "care." Over time, this balance between the desire to care and the rights to it seems to have changed, but the obligation to care remains at the core of this profession. "Caring in nursing" concerns with virtue having its roots running deep into an ethical and empathetic imperative to help others (Noddings, 1984).

When we become seriously ill, and its management goes beyond the capacity of our circle of family and friends, we look for more intensive professional care, such as from a nursing professional or a healthcare worker trained to provide such care. Being responsive to such obligations of care based upon people's expectations forms the backbone of nursing as a profession. Concurrently, this makes "caring" a very emotional and material activity. This duality makes "caring" very difficult to define and control, which reiterates it across the globe as an unbounded act, yet undervalued as part of a profession.

In the Indian context, to understand this existent asymmetry, the status of nursing as a profession needs to be examined through the lens of intersectionality (Crenshaw, 1989; Sen and Iyer, 2012; Springer, Hankivsky and Bates, 2012; Young et al., 2020). The principal reason for this is that it helps overcome the binaries associated with nursing as a gendered profession. It would help understand a complex social order which has been historically intertwined with notions of caste, religion, and gender and how it helped evolve such a profession. In its absence, it would be a myopic and limited examination if the principal questions of who the individuals are who uptake nursing as a profession and what draws them to it are not delved into.

Bearing in mind that caring encounters are considered fundamental to nursing, this research articulates an understanding of the importance of caring work in nursing. This chapter is one of the few studies which brings to

DOI: 10.4324/9781003315124-5

the forefront what nurses in India do: of what skilled nursing care consists of and how it contributes to the well-being of the patients. The central idea which remains to be communicated to policymakers is that when something is not easily measurable, it often goes unnoticed and remains neglected in value, and it is essential to account for it.

The interpretivist in-depth interviews belonging to a range of nurses from different generations bring in a temporal effect while laying the understanding of "what it means to care in nursing", understanding the ethos of nursing, and the reasons for choosing nursing as a career. These get intertwined with contemporary nurses talking about their prime objective of emigrating to developed nations. Their reasons make sense when looked at from an empathetic understanding of the nurses' context.

The chapter intends to bring attention to the neglected aspects of nursing care arising from the damaging stereotypes and how a new generation of Indian nurses face the dilemma of negotiating care, professional status, and emigration. This remains important to subvert the prolonged de-valuation of the "care" work in nursing, which would add to recognising the worth of this profession. It would avert the already strained Indian health system from suboptimal compromised care to patients and retain the "status quo" in the nursing profession.

The Indian Nurse Labour Market

A study by Rao, Shahrawat, and Bhatnagar (2016), based on a nationally representative household survey by the National Sample Survey Office (2011/2012), estimated the density of qualified nurses and midwives as 3.16 per 10,000 population in India, which is much below the World Health Organization's (WHO) suggested minimal threshold of at least 44.5 health workers per 10,000 population by 2030 (WHO and SEARO, 2019).

On the contrary, India remains one of the largest exporters of all health professionals, and the emigration of nurses is also significant, with estimates ranging from 20% to 50% of Indian nursing program graduates intending to seek overseas opportunities (Thomas, 2006; Walton-Roberts, Margaret in Rajan, 2010, pp. 196–216; Roberts and Rajan, 2013; 2020; Roberts et al., 2017). Irrespective of nursing availability as directly correlating with the health status of the country's population, nursing continues to grapple to get its due recognition as an important profession in India. The fear of losing out nurses through an exodus continues to engulf an already compromised Indian health system. This evident polarity remains an issue of major concern as India continues to battle with the challenge of dealing with a mismatch between health prerequisites and the lack of a healthy human workforce while concurrently experiencing a dual burden of disease and persistent nursing shortage (Gill, 2016).

The "Nursing" versus the "Clinical" Gaze: Does Caring Matter?

The late eighteenth and nineteenth centuries had witnessed a fundamental change in western medicine, which was evident through how medical practitioners comprehended the body's working in health and disease. The spaces in which medical knowledge evolved impinged the social relations of medicine and the doctor–patient and doctor–nurse relationships. The final products of these processes were the creation of modern medicine.

Jewson (1976) provides a framework in which he describes the historical shifts in how a patient is treated from being a whole person to a set of organs to a collection of cells. He describes a shift from "bed-side medicine" to "hospital-medicine", which resulted in changes in the power relations between doctors–patients and doctors over other health professionals.

Concurrently he maintains that there prevailed a system of medicine known as the "bed-side medicine." This system viewed the sick in a holistic framework seeking to locate the patient's condition in a wider context as sickness being caused by several social, environmental, or lifestyle factors. It was the medical practitioner's job to understand the patient's personality and circumstances and then use various techniques to restore the body to balance. It was a world where patients and practitioners shared the same understanding of disease and spoke about it in the same language. In this system, the patient was viewed as a patron and had much autonomy as the doctor relied on the patient's fees for his livelihood. In "bed-side medicine", diagnosis was based upon the doctor getting an empathetic understanding of the patient's narratives relating to their sickness.

A major transformation occurred during the second half of the eighteenth century, where bed-side medicine was replaced by "hospital-medicine" as, during this period, continental Europe was almost continually at war. This led to a demand for doctors to serve in the army and in institutions to train competent doctors. It resulted in the emergence of more hospitals which spread through the entire West rapidly and subsequently to the areas colonised by the West.

As the name suggests, the typical setting for "bed-side medicine" was domestic, wherein the patient seemed to be more autonomous and had more power, whereas the setting for "hospital-medicine" was in the wards of the hospital where the hospital came to assume a dominant position. "Hospital-medicine" further placed the doctor in the dominant position as the doctor (Foucault, 2008) now no longer had to consider the patient as a "patron" as everyone was treated for free in the hospitals and the doctor depended upon the hospital authorities to look for remuneration (MacLeod and Lewis, 1988).

The disease was no longer a general state of imbalance, but a specific state reduced to an individual's body part or parts. Its impulse was to localise disease to a specific organ or tissues of the patient's body. "Hospital-medicine" was carried out by way of three techniques.

The first involved subjecting the patient to rigorous physical examination with the help of instrumental aids, of which the stethoscope was the most significant. Second, if the sickness proved fatal, the patients' bodies were sent for post-mortems to relate bodily symptoms to morbidity alterations as evident from the deceased's organs. Finally, the results were subjected to statistical analysis to establish patterns and draw conclusions.

This made the hospital an ideal place for such scrutiny and rendered the patient extremely powerless, whereas it placed the doctor into a very dominant position due to their authority over medical knowledge and diagnostics. "Bed-side medicine" laid more emphasis upon the prognosis of the disease, whereas "hospital-medicine" was concerned with diagnosing the disease and classification of morbidities (Arnold, 1993, p. 53; Pickstone, 2009).

This led to a widespread realisation that the hospital setting was the best place for medical students to gain and imbibe varied diagnostic and therapeutic skills. According to Foucault (2004)in the "Birth of the Clinic", hospitals in the latter part of the eighteenth century saw the emergence of the "clinical gaze" – a way of looking at the patient and "seeing" disease which no longer dealt with lifestyle or environmental changes but focused on the organic changes occurring in the spaces of the body. Foucault asserts that knowledge and power are intimately linked, which resulted in medical practitioners developing a new discourse of the disease, which gave them a new authority in their clinical relationship. Thus, the patient became a teaching material that could be probed and examined.

He mentions a tactic, the "contract" that legitimatised the exploitation of patients' bodies to the "medical gaze" in return for free medical attention. Thus, medicine saw a radical shift by introducing a new way of seeing, which turned the patient's body into objects tending to be reductive. This practice made medicine more labour intensive, and to fulfil these requisites; women were imbibed as nurses. Thus, nurses came to be widely referred to as the physicians "operational right arm" (Sandelowski, 2000).

The nursing profession as we see today had evolved from the extension of values and ideas imbibed in this profession which dates to the mid-nineteenth century (when "nursing" started gaining a "professional status"). During that time, Florence Nightingale and her nurse colleagues struggled to raise the professional status of nursing by attempting to establish nursing as a legitimate work profession for women. This was important to combat the arguments and doubts raised about women's abilities to treat the war wounds of the soldiers from the Crimean War and the American Civil War. Nursing was therefore considered as a task suited for women due to their very "feminine" nature. Thus, this profession got embodied into the Victorian ideology of what "befits" a woman. Immediately, this equation was included in the literature on nursing.

Nursing is distinctly woman's work ... Woman are peculiarly fitted for the onerous task of patiently and skilfully caring for the patient in faithful obedience to the physician's orders. Ability to care for the helpless is woman's distinctive nature. Nursing is mothering. Grownup folks when very sick are all babies. (*Hospital*, 8 July 1905, p. 237)

(Garmanikow E. in Kuhn and Wolpe, 1978, p. 110)

This effort proved to be successful in granting the nursing profession as some form of professional status, however, by the end of the twentieth century, the image of "being a nurse" was always associated with "being a female" (Breu, G., 1980). Women's ideological belief and segregation into traditionally female jobs in "nursing" results in lower status being accorded with predominantly female occupations, which are also generally considered as less prestigious than other male-dominated occupations. The prevalence of this attitude in society has served to keep women as a reserve army of labour. The most notorious example of this belongs to the World War II era, when most of the females were employed in factory work because men left for military purposes and then on their return, women were hustled back out of their jobs (Blau F.D. in Freeman, 1995; Rothman,1978). In recent times, this ideology seems to govern wage levels for women in labour markets as jobs traditionally labelled as predominantly "feminine jobs" remain underpaid. The concept prevails that women can do with less income than men because they will be supported by a man (O'Leary in Kaplan A.G. and Bean J.P., 1974; Rosalyn Fraad Baxandall, 1976).

Despite many hindrances, the Nightingale nurse, a product of the Victorian era, continued caring for the sick. During those times, due to the societal structure based upon the principles of non-participation of women in the labour market, most often, the women who participated in nursing were destitute, prostitutes, and drunken women. To free itself from a maligned image, emphasis was placed on "femininity", and the Victorian values demanded "ladylike" behaviour. However, to date, the promiscuous image continues to survive along with the angelic image (Ehrenreich and English, 1973).

As healing started leaning towards being more technical and lucrative, it attracted more men into taking up this as a profession. What had been considered art started getting gradually moulded into a form of science, resulting in separating the boundaries between caring and curing. Curing was brought under the domain of medicine which saw the dominance of men physicians who learnt from medical colleges in which women were not considered. Nursing was left with its nurturance skills and continued caring for the sick. The most potent stereotype which has continued throughout literature and history is that – "Nurses are women; men need not apply!" (Muff, 1982).

Nursing, with its emphasis on caring, has not been an economically rewarding profession. The profession was founded on religious orders, which led to the societal belief that nurses would receive heavenly rather than earthly rewards. Florence Nightingale always demanded that nurses be well compensated. However, this profession built on saintly values always remained chronically underpaid as nurses were deprived of bargaining powers possessed by other professional groups (Hughes, 1980; Muff, 1982, pp. 101–106). This social construction of the female role has been described by Hearn (1982) as the "patriarchal feminine", feminine because it accords with the feminine, "caring" stereotype; patriarchal, it reinforces female subordination.

It has been argued that in parallel to Foucault's "clinical gaze", there is a "therapeutic gaze", which observes and interprets the needs and problems of the sick by considering not just the physical but also the psychosocial aspects of the illness. The clinical and social histories are intermeshed into patients' accounts, which convert these accounts into "therapeutic sensibilities". In it, the patient is not subjected to a mere interrogation but is also made to feel cared in terms of "getting to know" by including a mix of questions that address the body–mind duality with a tender touch of care (Hardey and Mulhall, 1994; Bunton and Petersen, 2002). What is significant about this position in nursing is the extent to which the rhetoric of nursing at least addresses the duality of the "body" and "mind". The present study argues in favour of the significance of this care component by bringing in the views of nurses about caregiving and how it differs from a mere diagnosis.

Cheek (1999) mentions the analysis of Parker and Wiltshire, which states that the nurse's work is more of an emotional and empathetic one which forms the "nursing gaze/nurses gaze".[1] This gaze is not just limited to reducing the patient to an object of enquiry but is concerned with an understanding and reasoning of the diseased condition in which the patient and the nurse are moulded together as one. This form of understanding is quite often considered unprofessional and has been taken for granted as having a more subjective look that is not valued highly. This stands true especially when nursing has been carried out under the subjugation of modern medicine, which leans towards empiricism to prove its scientific worth and maintains its dominance as a discipline.

The literature highlights that there has been a consistent effort to fit "nursing" into being either art or an emerging science over the years. Nursing's quest for achieving a professional status has been extremely challenging because there is a limit to which nursing practice can fit within the dominant views of medicine (Huston, 2014). Such a process illustrates the extent to which empirically oriented disciplines have dominated other disciplines which follow non-reductivist and non-positivist lines of enquiry. The subjective realities like how a sick person feels and understands the illness or how an interpersonal exchange of care makes people feel better or worse remain of less concern in these enquiry forms (Adams and Nelson, 2009).

As argued by Barnard and Gerber (1999), incomplete care provision through health systems, which are not theoretical but tangible, is mostly derived from a short-sighted perception of nursing care which completely undermines the ability of nurses to engage with other human beings as they struggle with suffering. It remains important to note that "caring" in nursing is not a singular entity and cannot be reduced to quantifiable components. This concept of "care" probably remains inadequately researched and understood. It has been seen that, in health care, instrumental, technical, "masculine" behaviours addressed to specific "cures" of diseases are more valued and funded than expressive, social, "feminine" behaviours addressed to care of the whole person.

As Miller (1978) rightly pinpoint her notion that, by projecting into what is called women's work

> some of its most troublesome necessities, male-led society may also have simultaneously and unwittingly, delegated to women, not humanity's lowest needs but its "highest necessities" – that is, the intense emotionally connected cooperation and creativity necessary for human life and growth.
>
> (Miller, 1978, pp. 25–26)

While emphasising the "care" aspect of nursing, we argue that the human aspect must be preserved, recognised, and respected and adequately rewarded. Nurses and women, in general, have been performing the vital work of caregiving; we must demand its recognition and high value and not simply treat it as a gender attribute.

The Social Construction of the Nursing Profession in India: Made to Migrate

The development of an ideology of nursing care based upon dedication to the poor and salvation of the soul resulted in caring work being considered menial work, worthless, requiring no ability, no knowledge, and remained socially and economically unrecognised (Reverby, 1987).

Literature shows that nursing involves dealing with patients' bodily fluids; in Indian society, it was associated with "purity and pollution". Thus, the profession saw the entry of nurses who were less affected by the fears of pollution and caste constraints, i.e., the Christians and Hindus who were in the lower rung in the caste order.

This association with menial work presented a threat to the social identity of the upper caste Hindus, thereby making it an inappropriate choice of employment for them. These beliefs, which are deep rooted in the Indian society, led to the distortion of the public image of the nursing profession in India, which continues to beleaguer it even today (Thomas, 2006; Alonso-Garbayo and Maben, 2009; Nair, 2012; Percot and Rajan, 2007).

The historical predisposition of terming nursing as a lowly profession has contributed to being a major reason for Indian nurses to emigrate to destination countries where nursing is perceived as a desirable and respectable profession (Nair, 2012).

The research findings presented in this chapter draws on interviews with 27 female nurses. The interviews were conducted at different periods between the years 2016 and 2017. Of the 27 participants, 19 were Christians, whereas the remaining 8 were Hindus. Out of the Christian nurses, 18 nurses belonged to Kerala, and the rest were from Maharashtra. The chosen field location was across hospitals in Mumbai. The sample tried to maintain an equal representation of nurses from public hospitals, missionary hospitals, and private–corporate hospitals with at least a BSc. (Bachelor of Science) nursing degree. Nursing Director's, Matron's, and Nursing Tutors were purposely included in the research. It was believed that their seniority and experience would bring in the added dimension required to justify the research findings. Irrespective of the fact that it was decided as part of the methodology to include only those nurses who had completed B.Sc. nursing degrees as part of our sample, this criterion had to be relaxed in the field as almost all the senior nurses from the government hospital, and the mission hospital had completed a General Nursing and Midwifery (GNM) course (12th grade + 3 years) from nursing schools. It was associated with the hospital ever since. However, a few of them had also managed to pursue and complete a PBB.Sc. (Post Basic Bachelor of Science in nursing) degree program. The government sponsors the nurses who complete a minimum of ten years in the nursing job to get a PBB.Sc. degree. They get a full fee waiver to pursue this degree. As only a few senior nurses from the government hospital and mission hospital had a B.Sc. degree, experienced senior nurses with a GNM degree were also included in the study. The rest of the sample was of younger nurses, i.e., those who had started working from 2000 onwards.

Findings from Engaging with Research Participants

"We Also Suffer the Disease with the Patients …" – What It Means to "Care" in Nursing

The senior nurses from the public hospital and mission hospital viewed "caring in nursing" as a service to God and fitted their descriptions of personal attributes with the role of being a nurse. These nurses said that they chose nursing as they wanted to care for other people and gave them a feeling of fulfilment and being close to God. They emphasised being available for their patients not just physically but also emotionally and empathetically.

> Well, I don't know, may be just that making patient's feel that they are cared … that someone cares that they should get well soon … attending to all the basic needs … not just assisting them physically but also

emotionally ... being compassionate. We lean it as a service to patients and in turn a service to God!

(Senior nurse, public hospital)

And;

On similar lines, a senior nurse from the mission hospital expressed:

Nursing care is a duty rather than a profession ... it's a service to God ... putting others needs before your needs. We have to go beyond the professional boundaries and get into the personal boundaries and making this happen requires a lot of skill in the form of gradual building of trust so that very intimate details are shared with us and only being patient and listening can also relieve the patient a lot ... so being caring, understanding the needs of the patients emotionally engaging with them ... I believe that an individual is blessed to be a nurse and follow her passion to care for others ... it has been in my nature ... yes ... I cared for my grandparents ... both alright ... for like a long time ... I was always with them and then physically they became weak and more than that they needed someone by their side all the time and then I understood that it's not just physical help but mental as well ... emotional help I mean [sic]that which matters.'

(Senior nurse Tutor, mission hospital)

One of the most striking aspects of the narrative accounts of the senior nurses was the general agreement regarding the ethos of nursing as being centric to "being of service to the patients and in turn also serving God." They also mentioned that the trust they shared with the patients created emotional bondage between them and kept them motivated to perform their caring duties. Their accounts of caring tended to focus on things that they did for making their patients feel better by alleviating their suffering and the affirmation that they received in the form of appreciation from their patients. Emotional caring in nursing also stands out strongly when the nurses mentioned negotiating their feelings after the demise of their critically ill patients and praying to God before their patients' surgeries.

A senior nurse shared:

I think a good nurse is the one who suffers the disease along with the patient ... as the patient starts getting better, the nurse also starts feeling better ... so do you understand now? I meant that other professions like that of being a doctor, for example, doctor can be a little strict or can talk less as caring is not something that is taught to them [doctors] they are only for giving medicines. But the first thing we are taught is to be for the patient holistically ... means emotionally, spiritually, and physically. Some critically ill patients are in bad condition, some can be very old also with families neglecting them. But we are like family to them as they share some stories with us as there is no one to talk to and we laugh and smile with them. They instantly feel better, we know they are going to die and sometimes we feel relieved after their death as they are relieved from the pain … it's it's … like seeing the patients suffering itself is very painful … don't get me wrong … I hope you understand.

(Senior nurse, public hospital)

And;

It's about service to got … nursing care is about creating that bond and trust between you and the patient. Some of my patients never listened even to their family members but did listen to me when I asked them to take medicines. Now do you understand why it happens? Sometimes I feel tired but that smile on my patients face and that is all I require to keep going! … Its not just work but it's creating that communication and bond with the patient. Listening to them, attending to them in the middle of the night, staying awake for them, praying for them before their surgeries … so we are not external but are like family to them.

(Senior nurse, mission hospital)

The communication did not always require verbal one for the nurses to understand their patients' medical requirements. Even a single glance at the patient who has a foot injury was enough for one of the nurses to arrange for a bed with a lesser height for her patient so that it is not difficult for the patient to climb onto the bed. Thus, showcasing non-verbal empathetic skills and corroborating the importance of the "nursing gaze" meet the patients' requirements. A senior nurse expressed:

Looking at the patient and understanding what the patient is going through. Now if a patient with cellulitis on the foot comes in, I do not need to ask him what is happening. I will automatically give him a low (lesser in height) bed so that it is not difficult for him to climb it. Touching the patient and checking for fever … earlier we used to give sponge baths and bedpans to the patients. Now the aaiya bai (nurse's aide) does it. Else there was so much more touching and attending to each need even the minute one … just smiling and asking if the patient is doing well. Most importantly feeling miserable when a patient does not get well and suffers.

(Senior nurse, public hospital)

Amongst the younger generation nurses, some agreed to the idea of nursing as "a service to God" and a "calling", but others mentioned it as a profession that enables them to care for the sick. There was no talk of virtue script surrounding this profession, and the responses were brief. Nevertheless, even if they were more inclined towards considering it as a profession as against considering it "a duty", many pointed out that nursing requires good intentions and that caring for someone is a labour intensive and tough task.

A young nurse from mission hospital said:

> It's caring as a service. And its physically challenging for a nurse also. We have to continue double shifts and have to stay awake all night ... stand for really long hours.
>
> (Young nurse, mission hospital)

And;

> Care of sick and empathy.
>
> (Young nurse, corporate hospital)

And;

> Being of service to the patients and in turn to God himself ... trying to connect emotionally with people and only a person with good values can do it well.
>
> (Young nurse, Mission hospital)

Most of these new-generation nurses expressed similar thoughts of "being of service" to patients. The similarity in responses amongst the younger nurses can be attributed to the common "Nightingale values" taught during a compulsory course in their initial years of B.Sc. nursing. During the interviews, a younger corporate hospital nurse mentioned:

> It's about caring for the patients and helping them with their needs. It's taught to us during the first semester itself.
>
> (Young nurse, corporate hospital)

Again, a young nurse from the public hospital shared:

> We are all taught about nursing being equal to caring. That's the first thing we learn as we enter nursing.
>
> (Young nurse, public hospital)

"This Is a Noble Profession, and It Rewards You Both Personally and Professionally" – Senior Nurses Choice of Nursing as a Career

Most of the senior nurses from the public hospital and mission hospital recognised themselves as coming from marginalised families with meagre means of survival for themselves and their siblings. From the narratives, it seems clear that the main thought that drove their decision to choose nursing as a career was to make themselves financially independent at a young age, which would enable them to provide for their families.

My mother was a nurse, and I had seen that she took responsibility of the entire family. I mean the financial responsibility. Father died[sic] when I was very young, and I had three siblings. Nursing gave my mother a career else [sic]we would have not even got to eat.

(Senior nurse, mission hospital)

And;

I had no idea of nursing. But my family condition was extremely poor … I was searching for a job! My best friend had a nursing job and took responsibility of her family. So I decided to take up nursing on her advice.

(Senior nurse, public hospital)

Not just a provision of financial stability but a deep sense of satisfaction was also associated with this profession. A senior public hospital nurse shared her thoughts as:

I wanted to help my mother with the finances and I earning quickly [sic] would also help my younger siblings. At the same time, the peace of mind that you get after you see an almost dying patient get cured … well … it can't be described … it can just be felt!

(Senior Nurse, public hospital)

A point that remains noteworthy is that most senior nurses from the public hospital and the mission hospital had completed a GNM nursing course. They attributed this to the fact that this course was completely free; they did not have to bear any expenses and added it provided them with a job towards the end of the course.

I could be a nurse because during the GNM course we don't have to pay anything in government nursing schools, and mostly government schools give GNM degree.

(Senior nurse, public hospital)

And;
Similar thoughts were shared by a senior nurse from the mission hospital:

The GNM nursing course was free means[sic] we did not have to pay anything even a single rupee towards fees, food, accommodation which can lead to major expenses during studies. We just had to pay very negligible amount of fees towards the mark-sheets … like really basic some fifteen rupees or something. Everything was taken care of by the nursing school. Even today, GNM nursing course remains free. During our times, there was only one college which offered B.Sc.

degree, and even there some fees had to be paid. It must not have been much during that time but still the idea of getting a free admission and later on which also gives you jobs[sic] felt good to the parents ... you know we were five siblings, and I was the eldest so if parents[sic] pay for my education who will pay for theirs (siblings)? And no, ... it would not have been possible for them to pay for me. We barely survived ... so after I finished, two of my younger sisters also followed me and joined this GNM course.

(Deputy Director nursing, mission hospital)

Although these narratives demonstrate the idea that the families inspired these nurses' career to move past financial struggles and provision for the so-called "financial stability during poverty", almost all the senior nurses from the public hospital and the mission hospital mentioned very staunchly that they never consciously planned this career for inordinate monetary returns or financial benefits. The narratives reiterated the desire to make a difference in peoples' lives and help others at the forefront of the participant nurses' stories.

I joined nursing for[sic] I wanted to help my family, but the thought of only earning money never came to me. It gives me pleasure to see the patients' get back to their feet. Our times were different ... we were never money-minded! ... The satisfaction that this job gives is of the higher [sic]order ... actually, it is considered as a job now, but during our times the emphasis was on being in service of the patients' as a service to God himself!

(Senior nurse, mission hospital)

And;
On similar lines, a senior nurse from the public hospital expressed:

This is a noble profession, and it rewards you both personally and professionally ... like you see a smile on the patients' face when he leaves the hospital feeling better, and you know that the smile is because maybe the patient feels relieved from pain ... so it's a great opportunity as a career as you are the reason of somebody's smile. We get those blessings and of course some amount of money to feed our families.

(Senior nurse, public hospital)

Almost all the senior nurse participants' narratives closely revolved around the traditional and stereotypical understanding of nursing and reflected a desire to be caring and help their patients. They had a strong conviction that it was a divine influence that chose them for a job that was altruistic in spirit, making them feel even more joyous and passionate about their profession. A senior public hospital nurse shared:

Nursing is different even from medicine such that with all my experience of all these years I have seen that a patient can talk freely only with a nurse and never with a doctor. So, it is the compassion that we have for them that generates the trust. The care that we offer to them daily creates a bond of compassion and love which is also a very important factor in [sic]recovery of a patient. Nursing has been considered as a service to god, and I think it's true because you help people recover. It is not work but worship.

(Senior nurse, Matron, public hospital)

And;

Being a nurse means being responsible and one should feel happy about it as it simply means that you are the one chosen by God to help the sick and the poor and to be of service to them. Now days we get paid well, but there were times when nurses were not paid, and yet they served the sick selflessly. It makes me extremely happy that I am in divine service and that perhaps keeps me going! I never thought of making money from my service irrespective of having four children to feed. I knew that God would take care of them and I just took pleasure in treating my patients and so did he (God) take care of my children.

(Senior nurse, mission hospital)

During the conversation, most senior nurses from the public hospital recalled the incidences of being strongly opposed by their parents and extended family members while contemplating their nursing careers. They further shared that the opposition from the families was well attributed to the fact that these senior nurses from the public hospitals were all Hindus, and nursing was stigmatised and considered synonymous with menial work within their religious order. Nursing work also required working in shift duties at odd hours and thus was associated with women of immoral character. As a result of the nature of this work lacking social status, their parents would be held in contempt and treated as inferior in their social circle.

My parents were just not ready to see me be a nurse and especially my father who felt that his daughter will have to touch the bodies of naked male patients and will have to deal with the sputum and faeces and urine and what not! ... Like so much of dirty-work is involved is what they felt! ... but my friend had taken up nursing and was in the final year and even her mother was a nurse so they had to intervene and explain it to my parents that it's not just about faeces and urine, but it's a noble profession which not everyone can take up ... This friend had lost her dad, and they were three siblings and only because of her mother was a nurse were they able to survive, and her aunt was a nurse too. My mother hesitantly agreed. However, my father didn't! ... he[sic] asked me to leave the house if I wished to do nursing … and then … I left! Yes, I left the house and stayed at my friend's house for about six months and then gradually my father maybe came to terms with my career … and it must have been because of the determination I showed.

(Senior nurse, public hospital)

And;

Clearly it is too much of hard-work that goes in, but we have to work in shift that has always been there, and it will always be … now during those times, first of all, a woman working was something not like its seen today and on top of that working at nights means obviously staying away from home all night nobody[sic] to see as what she does … neighbours would ask as why she doesn't opt for a fixed time? Some aunt's would also ask this question … Does it look good that a young unmarried girl is out of house during nights? Will it not be difficult for you to find a good husband for her? You understand? One of my Uncles even declared that my father was not man enough to have not managed [sic]from stopping his daughter from taking up such work which questions her character. So, the conversation was basically on these lines like maybe she has a loose moral character, and that is why your daughter is in nursing … so my parents avoided these people, and I felt that strongly! I was not immoral, and hence it didn't budge me, but obviously, I felt bad about such discussions.

(Senior nurse, public hospital)

Also, the people who persuaded them to take up this career were mostly friends who had completed their nursing course or had family members like mothers and aunts who were practising this profession for a long time. These women were holding nursing jobs and were the ones who were able to drive their families out of poverty to some extent.

However, in contrast to these narratives stood the narrative responses of the senior-generation (MH) nurses while they recalled the incidences of being supported by their parents and extended families when they were contemplating nursing as a career choice. These senior nurses from the mission hospital mentioned that it was mostly their mothers, teachers, and aunts who persuaded them to choose nursing as a career. It is important to note here that all the nurse participants in the mission hospital were Christians and the caste hierarchy and the notions of pollution and menial work are not so prominent in this religion. These nurses recalled choices being limited to either being a "teacher" or "a nurse" during their times. In some cases, the mothers and aunts were nurses, whereas they were not in a few others. They also shared that these professions were considered both gender-appropriate and affordable during their times, hence being popular among women.

My mother gave me clearly two options as, either be a nurse or be a teacher. My aunty was a nurse. See,[sic] and my mother didn't have an option herself. These were two professions where education was literally free and we obviously could not afford. Also most importantly, this feeling of being of service to other and then in turn to God himself was always at the back of her mind.

(Senior nurse, mission hospital)

And;

Be a nurse or be a teacher! You will hear this story from almost 80 percent of nurses of our times OK. It was the cheapest option available. We didn't pay anything for GNM course, no hostel fees, nothing. Also, during those times, girls didn't used to study also. Plus these professions were considered to be appropriate for a girl child. We used to church[sic], so that feeling of service comes to us very early. So that also influences our decisions.

(Senior nurse, mission hospital)

However, during the interviews, quite a few senior nurses expressed concern about inadequate career advancement opportunities and very low salaries in this profession. These concerns echoed through the narratives of almost all the senior nurse participants from the public hospital.

Earlier till very recently, the hospital used to sponsor GNM nurses with more than 10 years of service to go and do PBB.Sc.. (Post Basic Bachelor of Science in nursing) but now they do not even do that. So who is going to like to get stagnated especially in the age of so much advancement happening? … I have also completed my PBB.Sc. through this scheme only else who would have paid such high fees? I was sponsored completely. We don't have many government colleges providing PBB. Sc ….here … I think there is only (names a public hospital with a B.Sc. nursing college attached to it) with hardly any seats and then we had to approach private colleges. Along with me, some other sisters have finished PBB.Sc. which was sponsored. Rest of them (other nurses) could not do it as the fees in private colleges are very high such that no nurse can self-sponsor. Now with even this opportunity gone …, No funding no career development.

(Senior nurse, public hospital)

And;

Our times were different … in the sense that everything was not so expensive, but now you see it's all so costly! This issue of nurses not being paid enough was always there, and I feel it remains today as well.

Today after working for 32 years and I tell you ... 32 years is a really big time to be in nursing which is a physically also challenging job, I am being paid sixty thousand rupees that too because it is a government hospital because of the pay commissions revisions and all. ... Otherwise, the salaries were very less[sic] they still are in private and other places.

(Senior nurse, public hospital)

And;

They call it a noble profession but don't increase the salary of these noble people (nurses)! I also have to pay my bills and educate my children ... the salary increments take a long time, and now that is the reason why nurses are coming on[sic] the streets for asking good pay. By that, I don't mean that we want lakhs of rupees like some of the other professionals get also ... but be considerate of us ... that's all.

(Senior nurse, public hospital)

Irrespective of mentioning some of these specific negative features of nursing work and enduring hardships about these features, the senior nurse's narratives still emphasised self-sacrifice for the good of others.

All the senior nurses from the corporate hospital had specific managerial designations. The Nursing Director directed a senior nurse to arrange for the nurses to be interviewed based on their duty hours. She very clearly insisted that I do not ask the questions about choosing nursing as a career and the ethos of this profession to these senior nurses as she felt that they were too time consuming and could be better fitted for the younger nurses. She mentioned that these senior nurses shouldered some form of managerial positions, which kept them very busy, hence sitting out through the interview would be difficult for them. Also, she mentioned her rationale behind directing me not to ask the questions related to the "care in nursing" and "choice of nursing as a career" to the senior nurses because all of them were holding managerial positions in this hospital, and she felt that the younger nurses would be appropriate participants as they were directly dealing with patients. This might have also been because I was only permitted to conduct the interviews against the fact that I submit a copy of my interview schedule to the Nursing Director. I felt that she assumed that because she was permitting me to conduct interviews within her hospital, it was all right for her to trim my interview guide to suit the comfort and ease of the participant nurses from her hospital. I very strongly sensed that this scenario was choreographed, and it was predetermined on the part of the Nursing Director and her team (of senior nurses) as to which questions to engage with during the interview. We had to comply with their rules else, we would have been denied permission to conduct the interviews with the nurses from their hospital. This would result in losing out on rich information from the narratives of the younger nurses, which gave an important dimension to this research.

"A Profession That Is Never Affect by Recession and a Pathway to Overseas Job Opportunities" – Young Nurses Choice of Nursing as a Career

The most striking aspect of the narratives of the young nurses across all the hospitals was that they were straight to the point and expressed that they chose this B.Sc. nursing education with a common foregrounded idea that closely revolved around the employment opportunities that this career would offer. Knowledge about ample job opportunities, especially abroad, was the deciding factor for nursing career choice. The following expressions highlight their future intentions to shift abroad for job opportunities.

> While growing up in Kerala, I have seen that nursing is one profession that is never affected by recession and is a pathway to overseas job opportunities ... lots of jobs are available in countries abroad. My intention was to go abroad after nursing, and that's what made me choose this.
>
> (Young nurse, mission hospital)

And;

> There are a lot of opportunities in foreign countries for nurses. My aunty is a nurse in the UK since a long time, and two of my cousins are in Ireland, so I had decided that I will also leave. Actually, I am in the process of getting the final documents ready, and I will be leaving this job next week.
>
> (Young nurse, corporate hospital)

And;

> I had planned to move abroad after finishing nursing and taking experience, so I had joined nursing. I was not sure as till when I would live there but yes ... I was going to leave when suddenly the marriage happened, and now I am here.
>
> (Young nurse, public hospital)

Most of the new-generation nurse interviewees were very specific about their intentions to migrate abroad and mentioned it as the driving factor in taking up nursing as a career. However, a unanimous response that echoed throughout all the participant's responses was that they had intentionally chosen this career by weighing the employment opportunities provided.

> If you are a graduate from other stream, now a days it's like compulsory that you should have a Master's degree in order to get some kind of a job. But nursing is a field where it's alright if you don't do a M.Sc. as

only the ones who want to teach take opt for it. Today no graduation gives you a job as easily as B.Sc. nursing [sic] does.

(Young nurse, mission hospital)

A young nurse from the corporate hospital shared how she was forced into this career by her father, influenced by the idea of getting a "stable job" that this career provides. She expressed:

> I had not decided as what career to take and maybe I wished to pursue arts ... but you see I come from a poor family So, there were two other girls in the neighbourhood where we stayed, who took up nursing and then one left for Saudi and was sending money back home and suddenly everyone could see a change in their standard of living and the other girl also managed to make her family condition better. So my parents also felt as what is a career in arts going to pay me! So, I was literally forced by them into nursing college. In the first month itself, I said, I will not be able to pursue this career like it was very strict reporting on time in the college and when you're disinterested, it's in a way painful. ... but somehow my father was persistent, and he always told me that this is going to give me a stable job and additionally we had paid so much towards the fees. I had no choice but to stay.

(Young nurse, corporate hospital)

The most striking aspect of these narratives was that nursing as a career choice was the parents' decision that was imposed upon them and influenced primarily by the motive to bring economic stability to the families. However, economic constraints within the households emerged as being particularly important when determining the choice of profession. Most of them associated this career with employment opportunities, which opened employment opportunities abroad while providing secure financial prospects. They expressed resentment about their salaries, further associating it with the stigma attached to choosing nursing as a career. They further mentioned migrating overseas as a beneficial option and stated that better salaries and better professional status were the main draws to migrating overseas.

> At least in government, it is fine but what about the private clinics and hospitals? There exploitation is so deep rooted! They hardly pay the nurses anything. And how many government jobs are there, so nurses have to take up private jobs and then gone[sic] ... I mean what should I say? Every now and then there are strikes for an increase in the payment, and now all of us support each other because if we don't, no one else will care. Trust me ... This is too much of hard work that we put in ... plus the most disheartening thing is that even the patients don't

respect us many times. They will start shouting if we are late to attend them ... if a nurse speaks from a distance, they feel she is not empathetic but if we touch them for their good, they feel that our occupation is bad as being a woman she is touching males also.

(Young nurse, corporate hospital)

And;

A young nurse from the mission hospital expressed her concern as:

See nursing is still treated very disrespectfully as a profession in our society. It pains me when people look down upon us and say that are oh yeh to nurse hai (she is just a nurse) like in a way to embarrass me. Do people realise that, if they get admitted the doctor is not the one who is going to be by their side all the time? And I don't think this mentality is going to change anytime soon, so it's better to leave this country and go where this profession is respected. My friend tells me not to be upset and just leave this place as there is respect there [abroad] and enough of money. What are the nurses paid in India? You go to the private hospitals and ask those nurses ... they will tell you such heart breaking stories as how they are exploited so much and made to overwork and yet[sic] paid nothing!

(Young nurse, mission hospital)

And;

You see the tone of the patient's when they talk to the doctor and talk to a nurse ... we can immediately feel the change ... they will be so humble and nice in front of him (doctor), and they treat us like some people doing lowly jobs. Nursing is not seen as a good career, and plus there is no satisfactory payment here. I was against this profession because the society only outcasts you and decides the good and bad professions ... but as my parents felt that this will give us money and give me a job, I am here.

(Young nurse, public hospital)

The narratives also paint a disheartening picture of the crass-societal attitudes towards "caring in nursing" wherein the nurses find it extremely heart-wrenching when they are labelled as women involved in lowly jobs. That nursing is predominantly gendered work, and caring includes touching the patients, staying on duty for long hours, and on night duties; these activities have been culturally associated with promiscuity in India, resulting in the nurses being treated as women with low morality.

The paradox being that these are the same patients whose pain and discomfort these nurses alleviate. This societal attitude that has lowered the status of nursing and its attractiveness as a career to people of high status does remain a factor of utmost importance when a nurse decides to emigrate from India.

Most of the young nurse interviewees had attended private fee-paying nursing colleges. The amount that they quoted towards paying their B.Sc. nursing fees for the entire course varied between Rs 4.5 and 7 lakhs. Most of these nurses who were educated in private colleges mentioned that the finances to support their B.Sc. education were obtained through bank loans. Their responses also reflect the collective decision-making process that occurs at the household level where an investment in nursing education is considered to bring in high financial returns for them and their families as it is considered to get them a job relatively quickly, which would also help them pay off their loans.

> See, after you finish your B.Sc. you don't get more than 4 to 6 (Rs.4, 000-6, 000) anywhere in the South (South of India). And this is the same everywhere. So we take these loans from banks or relatives, and the overall cost of the B.Sc. differs from institution to institution, but it definitely goes in[sic] a few lakh rupees in private colleges. We are all middle class people, and some are lower down (in the class order) so when will we repay the loans, and we have our expenses also to take care of from the salary that we get ... many nurses send money back home as families are dependent on them. There are no government jobs as well. I mean here (In India) there is no value of nurses. We also have to pay our bills, isn't it?
>
> (Young nurse, corporate hospital)

And;

> I have taken a loan from my aunt who is a nurse. Yes, I have taken it for my education. So, it was decided that I go to her in Muscat and work there and repay the loan. Then I am free to return. I will come and work here only. Here there is a lot of honesty. We care a lot for patients, and we are taught good values here. Here everyone is God-fearing, so everyone behaves well. Patients from all religion come to us and before every surgery that is conducted, we pray with the patient. So, the patient also feels very good. They [the authorities from the mission hospital] also care a lot for us also. Sisters live like one big family. They provide us food in minimal rates, so obviously, it shows that they care for our health. In other hospitals, nobody cares for nurse's health. Accommodation is also free here. They understand we have difficulties back at home and hence we migrate for earning more money to pay off loans [sic]. Also, all nurses are from Kerala, so I feel nice that there are people around me from my place.
>
> (Young nurse, mission hospital)

And;

> Once I settle my home in village, I will come back and continue working here only ... they care for us a lot ... and some sisters also help with

money like no one feels like they are away from home. I have to get my sisters married and responsibility of paying at home ... some monetary responsibilities and them I am free.

(Young nurse, mission hospital)

The new-generation nurses, especially from the corporate hospital, explained the decision to migrate abroad to acquire returns on the investment that they had made in the form of taking loans for undergoing nursing training in private nursing colleges, an investment that they feel has very fewer financial returns if they were to stay in India. A few other nurses considered earning money for repaying their educational loans, building houses for their families, and supporting sibling's education as the main reasons to migrate overseas. These new-generation nurses from the mission hospital seemed to be migrating to shoulder their family responsibilities and expressed a desire to return to India once their monetary needs get fulfilled.

Discussion

What Do Nurses Do? And How Can We Avoid the Crippling of "Nursing Care"

From our study, it remains evident that the senior nurses have chosen nursing as a career based on the intertwining of the threads about the traditional and stereotypical understanding of nursing being a virtuous profession. They provide a strong justification towards the realisation of financial security, which this profession provides, especially towards overcoming the economic constraints faced by their families. In our sample, most of the senior nurse interviewees had completed their GNM training, wherein they had to refrain from paying any registration and course fees or charges towards food and accommodation during their entire tenure of studying in the nursing school. This availability of an economically less invasive educational opportunity that would secure them guaranteed employment so that they start earning for their families at a very young age can be visualised as a very determining factor that drove most senior-generation nurses to take up their chosen profession. The idea behind choosing free education in nursing enabled them in making savings in the family budget. This is suggestive of a need, driven not just by personal economic motives but also on the families' factual socio-economic condition, which required them to take up the chosen career to make a living for their impoverished families to sustain marginally. This shows how such a profession encourages the economic mobility of women from more vulnerable sections of society.

As the interviews with the senior nurse interviewees evolved towards recognising the underlying ethos of this profession, choosing nursing seems to be narratively grounded in their perceived virtues and personal characteristics. The interviewees described their personalities of being motherly, caring, loving, and empathetic as closely adherent to the ethos of nursing. They expressed that the patient's and their family members' report that the services provided in the form of emotions are critical towards patient care. The nurses mentioned doing much physical work and looking at the gait of their patients and accordingly deciding upon the arrangement of low-lying beds, touching the patients gently while taking the temperature and engaging in encouraging talks as some of the components aimed at improving patient care. From the responses of the senior nurses, it remains evident that on the path to healing, nurses are responsible for patient care 24 hours a day which involves a lot of physical work and emotional engagement with the patients for their speedy recovery. The narratives of the senior nurses constantly kept moving back and forth between making sense of their careers around the virtue script and earning a living for their respective families.

However, the senior nurse interviewees also specifically quoted some of the negative features of nursing work, such as the humiliation and stigma attached to this profession, the workload demands, the lack of career advancement opportunities, and a very slow increment in salaries. However, they positioned the image of nursing as a "calling" that they seem to embrace as an acceptable sacrifice given the associated reward of personal satisfaction for being of help to others. Although it is appreciable that these nurses demonstrate a certain kind of training that adheres to the virtue script which seems well-intentioned to make the healthcare delivery system more humane, this specific aspect of "caring" is often interpreted in a sentimental manner (Deegan, 1980; Adams and Nelson, 2009).

Unfortunately, these services of caring are little appreciated and have been associated with negative factors. The ideal image of the nurse being "motherly" has resulted in nurses being put on the pedestal till the sickness fades. There are ample instances when the same nurse is subjected and made to feel like an immoral woman for coming in physical contact with the patients while she performs her caring duties. Abiding by this approach contains a danger of "care", going unrecognised and hence being "undervalued". This is reflected through the research findings as the nurse interviewees express vulnerability on account of inadequate salaries irrespective of them being engaged in caring labour.

Although the notion of "being a good nurse" who is recognised for being motherly and having caring attributes seems ideal, these ideals prescribe a sex role to these females who only fit into jobs labelled as "women's work". These jobs are considered an extension of women's work at home due to the nurturance skills these nurses portray as if they are biologically destined for that place in the economy (Muff, 1982, pp. 101–106). This ideology of women's work helps create and perpetuate a notion of it being less skilled than it comes naturally to the female gender. The belief that a nurse is synonymous with being a female still prevails.

The narratives related to negative attitudes towards nursing came out most strikingly from almost all the senior-generation nurses who univocally express strong resentment towards the association of nursing labour with stigma and humiliation. For this generation, nurses had to struggle against prevalent attitudes towards the profession that gave it a "bad name". They recall when they chose to take up nursing as a career much against family members and acquaintances because they believed that this profession was menial. This feeling echoes through almost all the interviews conducted with the nurses across the institutions except the mission hospital nurses. This also highlights the general invisibility of the aspect of care which is not given its due importance. The narratives reflect that gender and the unspoken prejudice continue in the background of caring working in nursing. These findings stand in similar lines with the work published by George (2005); Lawler (2006); Shuriquie, While and Fitzpatrick (2008); Reddy(2015), wherein the author's account of nursing is considered as a low-status job in India because of it being associated with touching the most "untouchable" parts of the patient's bodies. In communities where strict social norms govern the interaction between the sexes, women's proximity to men through nursing work has resulted in accusations of "immorality" and "prostitution" (George, 2005; Nair, 2012).

Similarly, it bears a close resemblance to the findings of a study published by Ray (2016), wherein the author argues that work that has been intimately connected to bodily services has always been stigmatised; hence, as nursing work perfectly fits into this category, it remains stigmatised, undervalued, and hence ill-paid. As these caring activities are intangible products, they fall under the umbrella of "care" as against "work" (which produces tangible products with a definite exchange value). Thus, as these activities do not produce any obvious immediate, measurable results, they get taken for granted, exploited, and rendered invisible.

Here, we need to divert our attention to why certain forms of work are considered valuable activities, whereas others like care get devalued. To answer this, we must understand that "value" as a social construct describes what is desirable in a society based on society's political philosophy wherein various forms of work take on value only in each system of hierarchies and categories (Graeber, 2001). Hence, activities with a "value" are considered worthy, leading to a socially desirable end of being wealthy, honourable, and prestigious. As Marx's value theory of labour suggests, in the capitalist "market" system of value, where the labour is "commodified", the only value that is legitimately recognised is the economic value, where "work" produces tangible, lasting products that can be exchanged, calculated, and measured. So, in this system, "only certain forms of labour (obviously labour that contributes to producing marketable commodities) produce value in the first place" (as quoted in Graeber,(2013, p. 224). Therefore, work that has no immediate and measurable economic benefit remains undervalued and monetarily less compensated.

While choosing nursing as a career, the role of the family in the decision-making remains significant in the case of the younger nurses. The narratives evolved from choosing nursing primarily for economic reasons to interpreting the meaning of career choice in relation to enhancing one's position in the social world by procuring overseas employment. The young nurse interviewee's narratives revolved around choosing the nursing profession primarily for job security and migrating overseas. Many revealed that their families forced them to choose this career because of the abundance of employment opportunities leading to secure financial prospects. This can also be associated with their self-intents and the aspirations of their family members to secure overseas lucrative job opportunities, which the nurses did not shy away from stating clearly while making their motives obvious while deciding upon the nursing career. They undoubtedly reiterated negotiating the subverted public image of nursing as a stigmatised job, with the perception of it not just being "a job" but "a job with overseas migratory prospects". This may also explain why there is a forced pursuance for choosing this career from the younger generation nurse's families. They see nursing education and training as an investment that would provide them with a high salary and a gateway that opens overseas migratory opportunities.

The new-generation nurse participant's responses about the resolute stigma attached to this profession reflect the fact that a mixture of shame and humiliation still prevails in the society, which they must deal with daily. They also expressed strong resentment about their salaries and the stigma attached to this profession, further considering them as the driving factors for overseas migration. Some of the younger generation nurses also complained of the discriminatory treatment meted out to them by the patients under their care. The nurses describe instances when they are held in contempt by the patients who look down upon their profession, indicating that nursing in India remains an overwhelmingly ill-regarded profession. The research findings align closely with the findings by Reddy (2008); Johnson, Green and Maben,(2014), wherein many new-generation nurses spoke about migration overseas as an option to escape the infamy that surrounds this profession. Although caste discrimination is no longer legal in India, cultural stigmas are complex and are not easily erased (Sweas, 2013). Many researchers have primarily reported this stigmatisation as a "push factor" for nurse migration from India (Margaret Walton-Roberts in Rajan, 2010; Margaret Walton-Roberts, 2015).

The astute narratives of many young nurses to migrate abroad for better financial prospects and better social acceptance reflect a desire to shed the baggage of being an outcast in a society that denies recognition of caring activities. These findings also challenge claims laid by Garner, Conroy, and Bader,(2015), wherein the authors conclude that perhaps the nursing profession is being re-shaped in India as a respected career because of the internal job opportunities garners. These findings further fall in line with the research findings of Johnson, Green, and Maben (2014), who state that the renegotiation of stigmatised identity is at the heart of career advancement strategies being adopted by contemporary nurses. An upward movement in an "economic space" is a key factor in achieving "status renewal" in society. Globalisation seems to have given this opportunity to these nurses to display their competencies, which give them an edge to do away with traditional social hierarchies.

According to Reynolds et al. (2013), the entry of private sector nursing institutions is responsible for producing 90% of nurses. This has been correlated with a growth in student debt wherein most young nurses admitted to having taken loans to pay towards the high fees during their student tenure as a nursing graduate (Dinesh Unnikrishnan, 2012). Migration abroad seems like the only reasonable option as it boasts lucrative salaries for nurses who can pay off their loans.

Private capital recognises the opportunity to promote and attend to such demands by promising the younger nurses to pay high fees and provide them training that helps them emigrate abroad (Levitt and Rajaram, 2013; Margaret Walton-Roberts, 2015). Consequently, this sets a vicious loop that replicates market tendencies with very little room left for accommodating the altruistic spirit. Thus, in a society that still disregards care and considers it as menial work, the nurses endeavour to rid themselves of an imposed inferiority by the invisible nature according to their "care-giving" services by identifying with the dominant views of medicine. This will certainly result in the "nursing gaze" and "caring service" get further submerged within the curing practices.

Conclusion

Whereas policy-level discourses around nurse migration in India have focused on individual "push" and "pull" factors that decide nurse emigration, this research calls for expanding this discourse by bringing in discussions about career advancement opportunities, professional status, and improved incentives and economic rewards. This is certainly not going to change the entire ongoing scenario of nurse migration but can be a positive step in the direction of "managed migration" wherein the nurses will get a fair chance to decide if they wish to be working in their own countries and will not be pushed to envisage a permanent move abroad. The research also found that many younger nurses also planned to return to India after working a few years abroad. This can be seen as an opportunity to inoculate this health workforce back into the health system, which provides a "morally habitable" West, Griffith, and Iphofen (2007) work environment for the Indian nurses as against being raised on patrifocal roots (Nair and Percot, 2010). Thus, using intersectionality, this research reiterates that the skills necessary for nursing practice do not simply arise out of a natural feminine sense of sympathy and willingness to be a nurturer nor are they merely degraded skill sets. They are distinct nursing skills acquired by nurses through clinical practice, education, and training, which typically the other health workers do not possess. The stereotypes of nurses grew out of femininity and their conformity towards caring, ultimately becoming tools for their oppression. The argument here is not that nurses should completely reject caring work, but we defend the humane values and practice of traditional nursing to assimilate their economic and social mobility better.

This calls for a new and transformative progressive vision that draws a common line to articulate and demand adequate economic support for the actual caring work of the nurses because when nurses do a good job, the healthcare delivery system does become better (Adams and Nelson, 2009).

Note

1 Examples of nursing gaze can include recognising signs of complications during recovery from surgery, incipient bedsores and pain, difficulty in swallowing food or medication, or problems arising during self- or homecare. While it is essential for nurses to have information about medical needs, the medical model should not be the sole guide for the planning of nursing care (Reed J. and Watson D. cited in Griffiths (1998).

References

Adams, V. and Nelson, J. A. (2009) 'The economics of nursing: Articulating care', *Feminist Economics*, 15(4), pp. 3–29. https://doi.org/10.1080/13545700903153971.

Alonso-Garbayo, Á. and Maben, J. (2009) 'Internationally recruited nurses from India and the Philippines in the United Kingdom: The decision to emigrate', *Human Resources for Health*, 7(1), p. 37. https://doi.org/10.1186/1478-4491-7-37.

Arnold, D. (1993) *Colonising the body: State medicine and epidemic disease in nineteenth-century India*. Berkeley, CA: University of California Press.

Barnard, A. and Gerber, R. (1999) 'Understanding technology in contemporary surgical nursing: A phenomenographic examination', *Nursing Inquiry*, 6(3), pp. 157–166. https://doi.org/10.1046/j.1440-1800.1999.00031.x.

Baxandall, R. F. (1976) *America's working women: A documentary history 1600 to the present*, ed. R. F. Baxandall. Random House, New York: Random House Publishing.

Breu, G. (1980) 'The one in suit and tie is a nurse, too', *People Weekly*, 30 June, p. 46.

Bunton, R. and Petersen, A. (2002) *Foucault, health and medicine*. Taylor and Francis. https://doi.org/10.4324/9780203005347.

Cheek, J. (1999) *Postmodern and poststructural approaches to nursing research, postmodern and poststructural approaches to nursing research*. SAGE Publications (EBSCO Academic Collection). https://doi.org/10.4135/9781452204895.

Crenshaw, K. (1989) 'Demarginalizing the intersection of race and sex: A Black feminist critique of antidiscrimination doctrine, feminist theory and antiracist politics', *University of Chicago Legal Forum*, 1989. Available at: https://heinonline.org/HOL/Page?handle=hein.journals/uchclf1989&id=143&div=&collection= (Accessed: 4 August 2019).

Deegan, M. J. (1980) 'Feminism, technology and nursing', *Humboldt Journal of Social Relations*, 7(2), pp. 87–97. Available at: https://www.jstor.org/stable/pdf/23261725.pdf.

Dinesh, U. (2012) *Banks feel the heat of bad study loans, mint*. Available at: https://www.livemint.com/Money/1Zenj5AbyxeZs6E1fHixkN/Banks-feel-the-heat-of-bad-study-loans.html (Accessed: 4 May 2020).

Ehrenreich, B. and English, D. (1973) *Witches, midwives, and nurses: A history of woman healer*. New York: The Feminist Press.

Foucault, M. (2004) *The birth of biopolitics: Lectures at the college de France 1978–79, economy and society*. https://doi.org/10.1057/97802305941 80preview.

Freeman, J. (1975) *Women: A feminist perspective* (5th ed.). Mountain View, CA: Mayfield Pub. Co.

Garner, S. L., Conroy, S. F. and Bader, S. G. (2015) 'Nurse migration from India: A literature review', *International Journal of Nursing Studies*, pp. 1879–1890. Elsevier Ltd. https://doi.org/10.1016/j.ijnurstu.2015.07.003.

George, S. M. (2005) *When women come first: Gender and class in transnational migration, when women come first: Gender and class in transnational migration*. University of California Press. https://doi.org/10.1177/009430610603500311.

Gill, R. (2016) 'Scarcity of nurses in India: A myth or reality?', *Journal of Health Management*, 18(4), pp. 509–522.

Graeber, D. (2001) *Toward an anthropological theory of value the false coin of our own dreams* (1st ed.). New York : Palgrave Macmillan US: Imprint: Palgrave Macmillan.

Graeber, D. (2013) 'It is value that brings universes into being', *HAU: Journal of Ethnographic Theory*, pp. 219–243. School of Social and Political Sciences. https://doi.org/10.14318/hau3.2.012.

Griffiths, P. (1998) 'An investigation into the description of patients' problems by nurses using two different needs-based nursing models', *Journal of Advanced Nursing*, 28(5), pp. 969–977. https://doi.org/10.1046/j.1365-2648.1998.00739.x.

Hardey, M. and Mulhall, A. (1994) *Nursing research: Theory and practice*. Boston, MA: Springer. https://doi.org/10.1007/978-1-4899-3087-3.

Hearn, J. (1982) 'Notes on patriarcy, professionalization and the semi-professions', *Sociology*, 16(2), pp. 184–202. https://doi.org/10.1177/0038038582016002002.

Hughes, L. (1980) 'The public image of the nurse', *Advances in Nursing Science*, 2(3). Available at: https://journals.lww.com/advancesinnursingscience/Fulltext/1980/02030/The_Public_Image_of_the_Nurse.6.aspx.

Huston, C. J. (2014) *Professional issues in nursing: Challenges and opportunities, Wolter Kluwer*. Philadelphia, PA: Lippincott Williams& Wilkins.

Jewson, N. D. (1976) 'The disappearance of the sick-man from medical cosmology, 1770–1870', *Sociology*, 10(2), pp. 225–244. https://doi.org/10.1177/003803857601000202.

Johnson, S. E., Green, J. and Maben, J. (2014) 'A suitable job?: A qualitative study of becoming a nurse in the context of a globalising profession in India', *International Journal of Nursing Studies*, 51(5), pp. 734–743. https://doi.org/10.1016/j.ijnurstu.2013.09.009.

Kaplan, A. G. and Bean, J. P. (Eds.). (1974) *Beyond sex-role stereotyping: Readings towards a psychology of androgyny*. Boston, MA: Brown, and Co.

Kuhn, A. and Wolpe, A. M. (1978) *Feminism and materialism: Women and modes of production, feminism and materialism: Women and modes of production*. London: Taylor and Francis. https://doi.org/10.4324/9780203094082.

Lawler, J. (2006) *Behind the screens: Nursing, somology, and the problem of the body.* Sydney: Sydney University Press.

Levitt, P. and Rajaram, N. (2013) 'Moving toward reform? Mobility, health, and development in the context of neoliberalism', *Migration Studies*, 1(3), pp. 338–362. https://doi.org/10.1093/migration/mnt026.

MacLeod, R. M. and Lewis, M. J. (1988) *Disease, medicine, and empire : Perspectives on Western medicine and the experience of European expansion.* Routledge, London: Taylor & Francis Group.

Margaret, W. R. (2015) 'International migration of health professionals and the marketisation and privatisation of health education in India: From push-pull to global political economy', *Social Science and Medicine*, 124, pp. 374–382. https://doi.org/10.1016/j.socscimed.2014.10.004.

Miller, J. B. (1978) *Toward a new psychology of women.* London: Penguin Books.

Muff, J. (1982) *Socialisation, sexism, and stereotyping: Women's issues in nursing.* Toronto, ON and London: The CV Mosby Company.

Nair, S. (2012) *Moving with the times: Gender, status and migration of nurses in India.* Routledge, India: Taylor & Francis.

Nair, S. and Percot, M. (2010) 'Transcending boundaries: Indian nurses in internal and international migration', *esocialsciences.com*, Working Papers. Available at: https://www.researchgate.net/publication/46476400_Transcending_Boundaries_Indian_Nurses_in_Internal_and_International_Migration (Accessed: 18 March 2021).

Noddings, N. (1984) *Caring: A feminine approach to ethics & moral education* (1st ed.). Berkeley, CA: University of California Press.

Percot, M. and Rajan, S. I. (2007) 'Female emigration from India: Case study of nurses', *Economic and Political Weekly*, 42(4), pp. 318–325.

Pickstone, J. V. (2009) 'Commentary: From history of medicine to a general history of "working knowledges"', *International Journal of Epidemiology*, 38(3), pp. 646–649. https://doi.org/10.1093/ije/dyp185.

Rajan, S. I. (2010) *India migration report 2010: Governance and labour migration.* New Delhi: Routledge.

Rao, K. D., Shahrawat, R. and Bhatnagar, A. (2016) *Composition and distribution of the health workforce in India: Estimates based on data from the national sample survey,* WHO South-East Asia journal of public health. Available at: http://www.who-seajph.org (Accessed: 16 April 2021).

Ray, P. (2016) "Is this even work?': Nursing care and stigmatised labour', *Economic and Political Weekly*, 51(47), pp. 60–69.

Reddy, S. (2008) *Women on the move: A history of Indian nurse migration to the United States.* New York: New York University.

Reddy, S. K. (2015) *Nursing and empire: Gendered labor and migration from India to the United States.* Chapel Hill, NC: University of North Carolina Press.

Reverby, S. (1987) 'A caring dilemma: Womanhood and nursing in historical perspective', *Nursing Research*, pp. 5–11. https://doi.org/10.1097/00006199-198701000-00003.

Reynolds, J. et al. (2013) 'A literature review: The role of the private sector in the production of nurses in India, Kenya, South Africa and Thailand', *Human Resources for Health*, p. 14. BioMed Central. https://doi.org/10.1186/1478-4491-11-14.

Rothman, S. M. (1978) *Woman's proper place: A history of changing ideals and practices, 1870 to the present.* New York: Basic Books.

Sandelowski, M. (2000) *Devices & desires: Gender, technology, and American nursing, the university of North Carolina Press.* Chapel Hill, NC: University of North Carolina Press.

Sen, G. and Iyer, A. (2012) 'Who gains, who loses and how: Leveraging gender and class intersections to secure health entitlements', *Social Science & Medicine*, 74(11), pp. 1802–1811. https://doi.org/10.1016/j.socscimed.2011.05.035.

Shuriquie, M., While, A. and Fitzpatrick, J. (2008) 'Nursing work in Jordan: An example of nursing work in the Middle East', *Journal of Clinical Nursing*, 17(8), pp. 999–1010. https://doi.org/10.1111/j.1365-2702.2007.01973.x.

Springer, K. W., Hankivsky, O. and Bates, L. M. (2012) 'Gender and health: Relational, intersectional, and biosocial approaches', *Social Science and Medicine*, pp. 1661–1666. https://doi.org/10.1016/j.socscimed.2012.03.001.

Sweas, M. (2013) 'Caste off: Catholic Dalits (untouchables) in India are divided over how to improve their lot', *US Catholic*, 78(3), pp. 23–27.

Thomas, P. (2006) 'The international migration of Indian nurses', *International Nursing Review*, 53(4), pp. 277–283. https://doi.org/10.1111/j.1466-7657.2006.00494.x.

Walton-Roberts, M. and Rajan, S. I. (2013) 'Nurse emigration from Kerala: 'Brain circulation' or 'trap'', in S. I. Rajan (Ed.), *India migration report 2013: Global financial crisis, migration and remittances* (pp. 206–223). New Delhi: Routledge.

Walton-Roberts, M. and Rajan, S. I. (2020) 'Global demand for medical professionals drives Indian abroad despite acute domestic health-care worker shortages', *Migration Information Source.* January 23, 2020. https://www.migrationpolicy.org/article/global-demand-medical-professionals-drives-indians-abroad.

Walton-Roberts, M., Runnels, V., Rajan, S. I., Sood, A., Nair, S., Thomas, P., Packer, C., Mackenzie, A., Murphy, G. T., Labonté, R. and Bourgeault, I. L. (2017) 'Causes, consequences, and policy responses to the migration of health workers: Key findings from India', *Human Resources for Health*, 15(1), 28.

West, E. A., Griffith, W. P. and Iphofen, R. (2007) 'A historical perspective on the nursing shortage', *Medsurg Nursing*, 16(2), pp. 124–130. Available at: https://www.researchgate.net/profile/Edith-West/publication/6289848_A_historical_perspective_on_the_nursing_shortage/links/53f7af2c0cf24ddba7da9993/A-historical-perspective-on-the-nursing-shortage.pdf (Accessed: 4 May 2021).

WHO and SEARO. (2019) 'The decade for health workforce strengthening in the SEA region 2015–2024: Mid-term review of progress, 2020', New Delhi PP – New Delhi: World Health Organization. Regional Office for South-East Asia. Available at: https://apps.who.int/iris/handle/10665/333611.

Young, R. et al. (2020) 'Health systems of oppression: Applying intersectionality in health systems to expose hidden inequities', *Health Policy and Planning*, 35(9), pp. 1228–1230. https://doi.org/10.1093/heapol/czaa111.

6 Indian–EU Healthcare Workforce Migration in Data 2000–2019

Gunjan Sondhi

Introduction

This chapter provides country-level data on internationally mobile health workforce between India and the European Union (EU) for the period 2000–2019 to support evidence-informed policy-making to ensure safe migration and decent work for the migrant health workforce. The predominantly descriptive analysis draws on the unique Organisation for Economic Co-operation and Development (OECD) Health Workforce Database (HWD) that harmonises data from OECD countries on migrant and non-migrant health workforce. Through the analysis of international migration of the health workforce, the discussion aims to (a) encourage further research on India–EU migration corridor and (b) highlight the strengths and limitations of the HWD to support evidence-informed policy-making.

The global demand for health professionals was expected to increase even before the COVID-19 pandemic. The pandemic has made visible a potential crisis in the health force labour force and the dependency on internationally trained doctors and nurses. Migrant doctors and nurses constitute increasing proportions of health professionals in OECD countries. In 2010/2011, foreign-born doctors and nurses accounted for 22% and 14% of all doctors and nurses currently working within OECD countries (OECD 2019). Foreign-trained doctors and nurses make up 17% and 6%, respectively, of total doctors and nurses in OECD countries in 2012–2014.[1] Nursing in particular is a profession highly entangled within infrastructures of international mobility (Walton-Roberts 2021). According to the state of the world's nursing report 2020, one nurse out of every eight practises in a country other than their country of training or birth (World Health Organization 2020).

The United States and the United Kingdom are the top two receiving countries while India and the Philippines are the largest sending countries for doctors and nurses within OECD countries. In many of the receiving countries, foreign-trained doctors usually face greater challenges as they need to apply for work permits or undertake exercises for equivalence qualifications due to lack of portability of skills. The limited portability of skills of migrant doctors and nurses leads to loss of skills, further exacerbating the challenges posed

DOI: 10.4324/9781003315124-6

by shortages in the health workforce. While a majority of the movement has been of trained medical professionals for work, an emerging mobility also streams for initial and further training as international students from India to places such as Canada, Ireland, Poland, and Romania (OECD 2019). This is because a "western" experience and training is ascribed greater value than non-western and non-anglophone. Moreover, there is a sending country premium that impacts the ascribed value of the received training. Students from Norway, Sweden, and France who obtain their medical degrees from countries such as Poland and Romania do not face a devaluation of their training and certificates unlike other international graduates (OECD 2019), thus further complicating the issues around portability of skills, as it isn't only the country of the training, but also nationality and race.

Additionally, this crisis has specific gendered implications as women make up the majority of the health workforce and hence are disproportionately on the frontlines (Pozzan and Cattaneo 2020). As research on nursing migration has long shown, women are also disproportionately responsible for unpaid care work (Percot and Rajan 2007; Yeates 2004; Kofman and Raghuram 2015). Overall, health worker migration, particularly of nurses, is highly feminised – with women making up 72% of the skilled health workers (Pozzan and Cattaneo 2020; Ciccarone 2015). However, there is limited global gendered data to inform policies and programs that are aimed at the migrant health workforce.

Taken together – portability of skills and gendered implications – this geography of skills (Raghuram 2021) produces national, gender, class, and racial hierarchies within the global health workforce. This is of course made more complex through other intersecting social locations such as religion, colonial linkages, and other regional/cultural affiliations. This hierarchy of the migrant health workforce is well documented especially within nursing (Nair 2020; Percot and Nair 2011; Oda, Tsujita, and Rajan 2018; Smith and Mackintosh 2007; Kofman and Raghuram 2015). Based on the geographies of skills (Raghuram 2021) – such as the place of training, qualification, and years of experience, many of the nurses potentially end up undertaking non-nursing work, but work which is still considered work in the healthcare sector as care aides, live-in caregivers, or other named categories which vary depending on the country of destination. Within this geography of skills is also the regional specification of both receiving and sending countries. Such a movement of nurses from India are likely to originate from Kerala, a state in the south of India, or from Punjab, a state in the north of India. Little is known about the regional specifications of international mobile doctors from India.

All of this combined the impact of the flows of migrants from both the sending and receiving country perspectives. And simultaneously, these flows shape the policies and programs of the countries within bilateral corridors. With the increasing recognition of the global shortage of health professionals and the need for cooperation and long-term investments training a health workforce (World Bank 2020a; 2020b; IOM 2020; Ratha 2021), there is an increasing need for reliable and global data that can be used to develop evidence-informed policies and programs ensuring that migration is safe and secure and migrants are afforded the opportunities for decent work – key components of the sustainable development goals. This global demand is shaping the flows from India despite the shortages in the national health workforce sector (Walton-Roberts and Rajan 2020).

Migration of healthcare professionals from India – as trained doctors and nurses – is entangled in the colonial history of bilateral movements between India and Britain for training, and work, which in the mid-twentieth century extended to include other anglophone countries such as the US. South Asian-trained doctors have been credited for their significant impact on shaping Geriatric medicine as a discipline within the UK NHS (Bornat, Henry, and Raghuram 2011). The migration of doctors from India has long been a discussion within academic and policy spheres (Khadria 1999, 2004; Khadria and Perveen Kumar 2012) including several pieces that have been published in this series such as by Bhattacharjee (2018) examining the India–EU corridor. Migration of nurses from India and its impact on both sending and receiving societies has been well documented especially across India–Canada (Walton-Roberts 2012; Walton-Roberts et al. 2017) and India–Gulf Cooperation Council (GCC) corridors (Percot 2006; Percot and Rajan 2007; Ray 2019). The Kerala migration survey has been a key instrument in capturing and understanding the dynamics of this migration of migrant workforce from sending country's perspectives (Rajan 2021), and it remains one of the few resources to undertake longitudinal quantitative analysis of the migration workforce flows which is crucial for evidence-informed policy to ensure safe and secure migration and decent work.

Among these health migration flows, European countries make up a smaller group of receiving countries of Indian-trained doctors and nurses and thus far have received limited attention (Percot 2012; Gallo 2005; Kodoth and Jacob 2013; Stievano et al. 2017). The healthcare labour market sector in the EU has always experienced labour shortages. Reports published by the EU commission have pointed to the labour markets experiencing shortages. In light of the increasing global demand, the EU countries are certainly not an exception. The EU has sought out India as a strategic partner (Jain and Sachdeva 2019; Stefan 2017), which includes looking to the Indian workforce to fill the EU's labour market shortages. In light of the evolving demands for trained health workforce and shifting relations between India and the EU, it is important that policies and programs developed within this relationship are evidence-informed to ensure safe and secure migration and decent work. For this purpose, reliable national and sub-national level data is imperative, especially on the health workforce. This data is also crucial to start developing a macro-level understanding of the migration flows along the India–EU corridor from the receiving country's perspective.

To fully understand the complex and entangled landscape of international health workforce mobility along the India–EU corridor, this chapter maps the current trends and patterns. The next section discusses the data sources and definitions used and the strengths and limitations of the data sources. The third section provides a gendered overview of the India–EU migration flows over the last decade. The fourth section describes the stocks and flows of Indian-trained doctors and nurses across the EU by focusing on country case studies of Germany, Italy, and Ireland. The fifth section closes this chapter by offering avenues for future research on India–EU migration, the strengths of the data presented for evidence-informed policy-making, and lastly it recognises the chapter's analytical limitations to descriptive data.

Data Sources and Definitions

OECD

There is limited data available on migrant healthcare workers. In response to this gap, the OECD started a database that consolidates and harmonises the data of the health workforce – Health Workforce Database (HWD), of which migration is the component. The key data presented in this discussion has been extracted from the OECD health workforce migration database. This captures both migrant and non-migrant labour force. The EU member states comprise a large part of the OECD countries and consolidate its own data definitions

From a receiving country perspective, immigrant doctors and nurses are an increasing share of health professionals working in OECD countries. There are two groups of immigrant health professionals: foreign-born and foreign-trained. Foreign-born health professionals are those who are born in a country different from the one they are practising in. This does not reflect their country of training. This means that someone who moved into a country during their younger years would still be counted as foreign-born. Foreign-trained refers to those health professionals who are working in a country different from the one in which they received their training.

A key difference is that foreign-born health professionals may not need to apply for work permits, or undertake exercises for equivalence qualifications. Foreign-born health professionals' qualifications may have been acquired in the country in which they are practising. In 2010/2011, Foreign-born doctors accounted for 22% of all doctors, and foreign-born nurses made up 14% of all nurses actively working within the OECD countries (OECD 2019).

Data and Definitions on Doctors (OECD Health Statistics 2020, Definitions, Sources, and Methods)[2]

The stock data described below include the number of doctors who have obtained their first medical qualification (degree) in another country and are entitled to practise in the receiving country. The annual flow data on foreign-trained doctors include the number of doctors who have obtained their first medical qualification (degree) in another country and are receiving a new authorisation in a given year to practise in the receiving country.

	Stocks	*Flows*
Include	• Foreign-trained doctors who have obtained any type of registration to practice in the receiving country • Medical interns and residents who have obtained a medical degree in another country but have not yet obtained a (full) registration to practice in the receiving country.	• Foreign-trained doctors coming in the country under all types of registration status (full, temporary, limited, provisional, or conditional registration). *Source*: professional registers • Foreign-trained doctors coming in the country under a permanent or temporary working permit. *Source*: working permits delivered to immigrants • Medical interns and residents who have obtained a medical degree in another country but have not yet obtained a (full) registration to practice in the receiving country.
Exclude	• Foreign-trained doctors who are registered to practice in the receiving country but are practising in another country (temporarily or permanently)	

Data and Definitions on Nurses

The stock data described below includes the number of nurses who have obtained a recognised qualification in nursing in another country and are working as a nurse in the receiving country. The annual flow data on nurses counts the number of nurses who have obtained a recognised qualification in nursing in another country and are receiving a new authorisation in a given year to practice in the receiving country.

	Stocks	*Flows*
Include	• Foreign-trained nurses who have obtained any type of registration to practice in the receiving country. • Nurses who have obtained a recognised qualification in nursing in another country but have not yet obtained a (full) registration to practice in the receiving country.	• Foreign-trained nurses in the country under all types of registration status (full, temporary, limited, provisional, or conditional registration). Source: Professional registers. • Foreign-trained nurses coming in the country under a permanent or temporary working permit. Source: Working permits delivered to immigrants.
Exclude	• Foreign-trained nurses who are registered to practice in the receiving country but are practising in another country (temporarily or permanently).	

As this data collection is recent, there are known issues of data comparability among countries, especially across EU member states.[3] Thus far, data for only a select EU member states is available to help identify Indian-trained doctors and nurses. Hence, the data presented in this chapter does not represent the key receiving countries. Rather, these are the only countries for which substantial data was available – Belgium, Germany, Ireland, Italy, and Norway.

While helpful, the dataset can offer more details to support a deeper analysis. It is also not possible to undertake OECD wide gender analysis on this dataset. While individual countries may offer gendered data, this has not been made available through the OECD web portal. As this data collection and consequently the database matures, a deeper analysis of this migrant workforce ought to be possible.

EUROSTAT

In addition to the key OECD database, discussion in the section "India–EU Migration – a Gendered Overview" on India–EU migration is based on data compiled and presented in Eurostat.

The Eurostat database is the most complete, including statistics on the number of female migrants from India to each of the EU-27 countries. It identifies four categories of migration reasons for first permits: work, education, family reunification, and "other reasons", and this report is organised around these categories. When Indian migrant health workers – coming from a third country (outside of the EU member states) – enter the EU they are usually required to obtain a visa/permit to enter an EU member state. These first permits – granted for a minimum of three months – show the annual flow of migrants entering the EU countries for work, education, family, and other reasons. Other reasons include international protection, residence without the right to work (e.g., pensioners), or people in the intermediate stages of a regularisation process. While this is an important category and is included in the figures below, the chapter does not include a discussion of this category.

There is limited gendered data analysis. Comparable data on Indian female migration to the EU-27 is not easy to obtain. Each country has its own data collection, analysis, and reporting system that are then merged into international databases. There is also a great deal of variety between individual country statistics with respect to quality, completeness, gender disaggregation, and base year for which data is reported (Raghuram and Sondhi, 2019). The gendered data analysis of stocks and flows of Indians into the EU is derived from two key tables. The *migr_pop3ctb* provides gendered stock data; the m*igr_Resfas* tables provides gendered data on flows – first permits. Lastly, a third table *migr_resfirst* is used. The tables are identified alongside the figures.

The discussion in the following sections starts by presenting a gendered breakdown of the population of India-born in EU countries using the Eurostat datasets. The next set of discussion on the migrant health workforce is drawn exclusively from the OECD HWD.

India–EU Migration – a Gendered Overview

Migration flows and stock are both crucial for the measurement of migration but cannot be directly compared. Flow data shows migrant entrants, i.e., residence permits granted in each year, while stocks show the number of migrants in a country.

Over the past decade, the total Indian population (stock) in EU-27 has increased from 275,000 in 2011 to 478,349 in 2020, accounting for approximately 1% of total foreign-born population in the EU (Figure 6.1).

Women made up approximately 43% of the total Indian-born population. The percentage varies across EU member states. In 2020, the member states with near gender parity in their Indian-born population were Iceland (52%), Denmark (49%), Switzerland (49%), Belgium (48%), and France (48%). The top five countries with the largest population of Indian-born are Italy, France, Netherlands, Spain, and Sweden. These member states also have a high female proportion (see Figure 6.2).

Over the past decade, the population of Indian-born in the EU member states has increased and the streams through which migrants enter the EU countries have also evolved during this time across all categories except employment. The proportion of Indian migrants entering the EU for *employment* held steady at 38% of the total flows between 2015 and 2019. By contrast, the proportion of Indians entering as *family* migrants fell from 38% of total Indian migrants in 2015 to 32% in 2019, and migration for

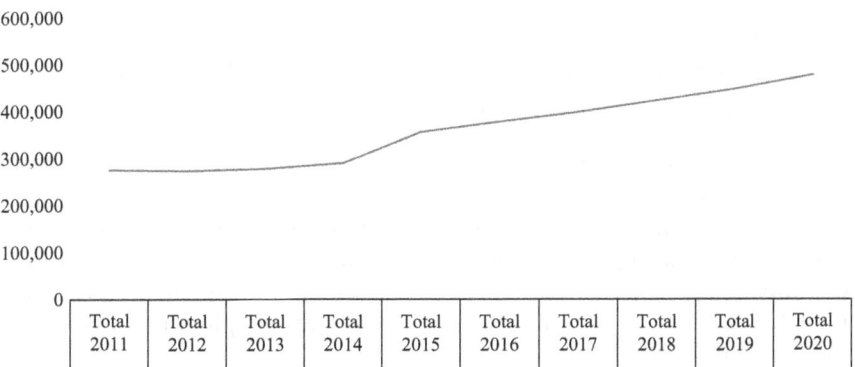

Figure 6.1 Total Indian-born population in EU-27, 2010–2020.

Source: Eurostat (online data code: migr_pop3ctb).

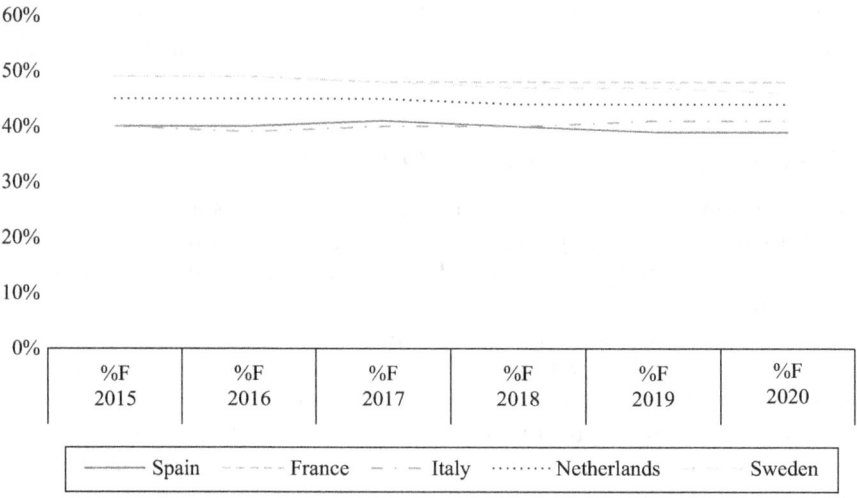

Figure 6.2 Percentage females as total Indian-born population in EU-27 by sex, 2020.

Source: Eurostat (online data code: migr_pop3ctb).

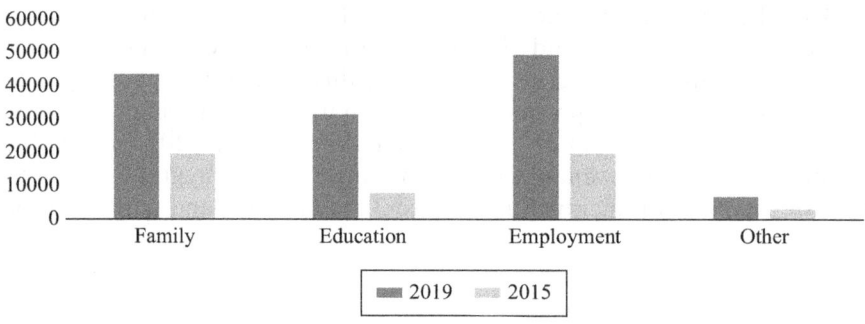

Figure 6.3 Residence permits issued to Indians by reason, 2015 and 2019.

Source: Eurostat (online data code: migr_resfirst).

education increased from 15% of total annual flows in 2015 to 25% in 2019 (Figure 6.3).

Women overall account for approximately 40% of the total annual flows.[4] They make up the largest proportion of migrants entering under the family category (75%), as shown in Figure 6.4 on first permits issues in 2019. By contrast, flows for education (70%) and employment (82%) are skewed towards men (Figure 6.5).

The highest proportion of men are in the new countries of migration such as Latvia (85%) and Lithuania (85%). Countries such as Italy, which already have significant numbers of employed female migrants due to a longer history of migration (ref), have comparatively more gender balanced

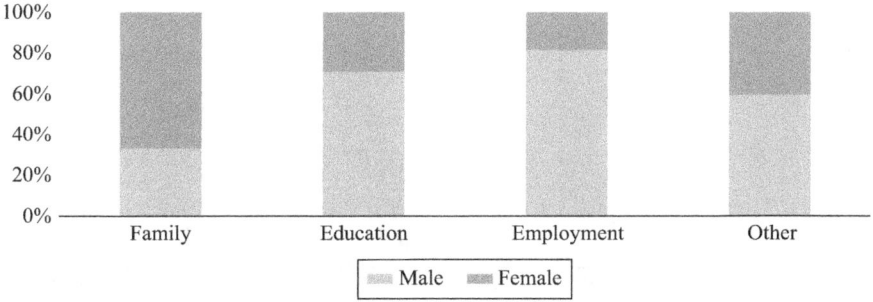

Figure 6.4 First permits issued to Indians, by reason and sex, 2019.

Source: Eurostat (online data code: Migr_Resfas).

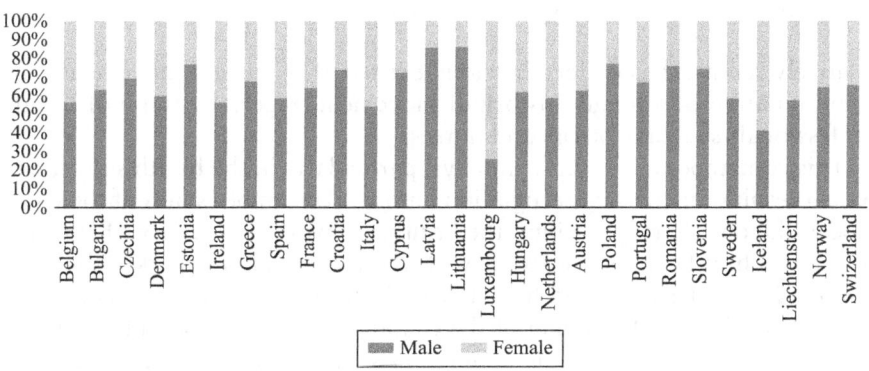

Figure 6.5 First permits issued to Indians, by sex, 2017.

Source: Eurostat (online data code: Migr_resfas).

profiles with regard to Indian migrant flows (see Figure 6.6). This is especially the case where there are also significant flows of women moving as family migrants (Figure 6.6).

The above description is to give an idea of what the stocks and flows of the Indian-born population in the EU looks like. Unlike the US and the UK, the EU is not a common or popular destination for Indians.

Indian Healthcare Professional Migrants in EU-27

The mobility from India to the EU has been varied – spread across the categories of work, study, family, and other. The following discussion focuses on a subsection of the mobility for work of doctors and nurses. It may appear that the increasing movement along the EU-India corridor is a "relatively" recent phenomenon by comparison to the longer linkages to move to the US, the UK, and GCC for nurses for instance. However, further examination shows that while the increase in the number of people moving is

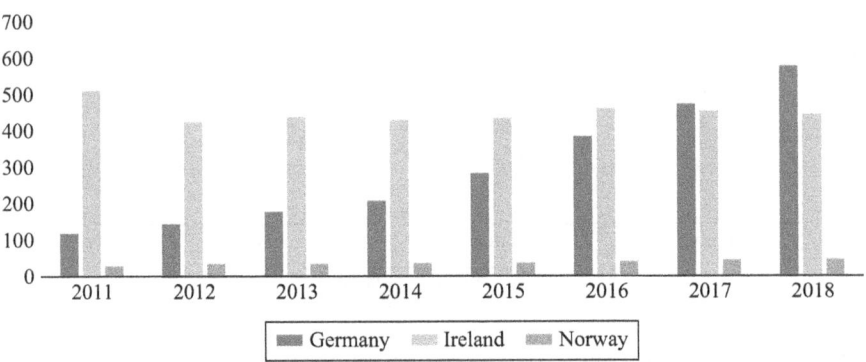

Figure 6.6 Stock of Indian-trained doctors 2011–2018.

Source: OECD health workforce migration database.

relatively recent, the corridor has long existed. The current movements are a continuation of a longer history of movement, especially those of health professionals such as doctors and nurses.

This contemporary increase in flows, particularly in the health sector, has been a result of increasing recognition among EU member states of their significant labour shortages within the healthcare workforce. Across EU member states, healthcare is the sector with the largest labour market shortage (Gupta 2013). This demand has increased during the pandemic. However, as mentioned at the beginning of the chapter, there is a geography of skills (Raghuram 2021) – meaning a migrant's nationality, ethnicity, gender, place of training/qualification all combine to shape whether their skills and knowledge are recognised, and then if they are able to deploy them fully. For instance, in Norway, all health personnel are required to seek an authorisation or licence from the sectoral professional body – Norwegian Registration Authority for Health Personnel (Bhattacharjee 2013; Brenne and Jensen 2013). However, before the migrant can enter the country, they also need to meet the criteria as setup within the national migration policies/programs. It is the entanglements of these professional, sectoral, and national structures of the receiving countries that shape who enters, under which category, and for how long. Depending on where the migrant sits within the hierarchy of healthcare work – doctors, nurses, carers, care aides, and general healthcare workers reflects the differentiated national labour market demands, the migration requirements and the requirements of the regulatory body. The hierarchy also determines whether the migrant is classed as highly skilled or low skilled migrant. These are determined by demands and structures of the local labour markets of the receiving country rather than migrant qualifications. These inequalities are important considerations as we explore in detail below the stock and flows of Indian-trained doctors and nurses over time, and delve into the three country case studies: Germany, Italy, and Ireland.

Stock of Indian-Trained Doctors and Nurses in EU-27

Over the past decade, within the EU-27 group of countries Germany, Ireland, and Norway are noted receiving countries for Indian-trained doctors. Figure 6.6 shows the number of Indian-trained doctors between 2011 and 2018 (Figure 6.7).

Germany is notable here as there has been a continual increase of Indian-trained doctors in Germany over the past 20 years (Figure 6.8), while Norway, with its much smaller stock of Indian-trained doctors, is a relatively new receiving country. The three countries among the EU-27 countries have been identified in Figure 6.9. These three countries – Germany, Ireland, and Norway – do not necessarily represent the countries with the largest number of Indian-trained doctors. Rather, they represent the availability of the data in the OECD health workforce database (HWD). Due to

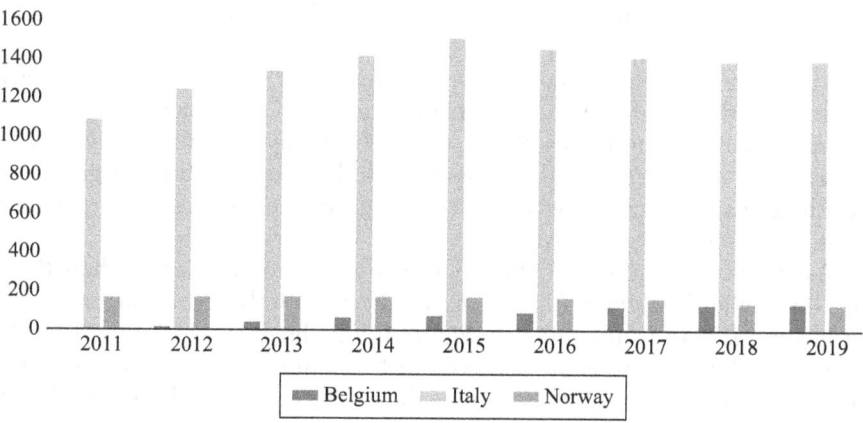

Figure 6.7 Stock of Indian-trained nurses 2011–2019.

Source: OECD health workforce migration database.

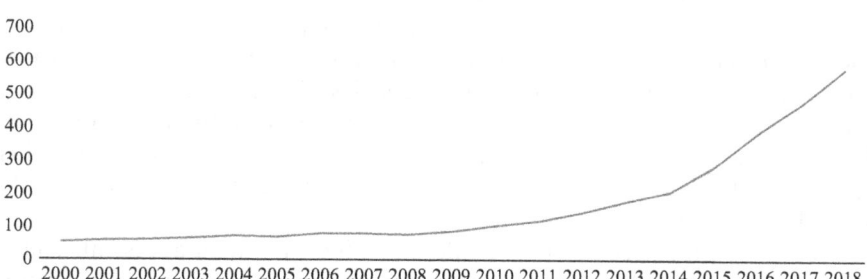

Figure 6.8 Stock of Indian-trained doctors in Germany 2000–2018.

Source: OECD health workforce migration database.

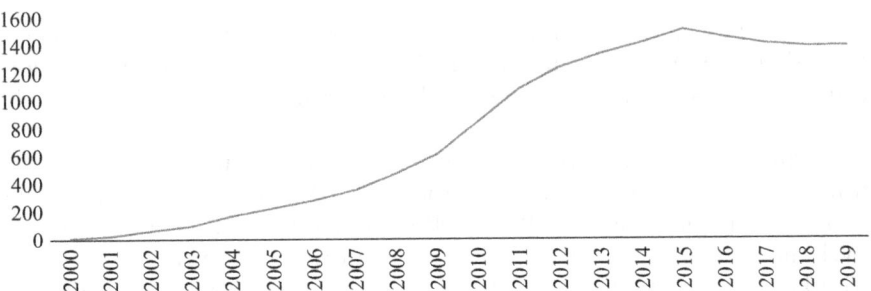

Figure 6.9 Stock of Indian-trained nurses in Italy 2000–2019.

Source: OECD health workforce migration database.

the newness of the database, it currently has significant gaps in the available data. Hence, this chapter explores three countries for which sufficient data is available.

This also limits cross-country comparisons as well as those between nurses and doctors for the same sets of countries. Consequently, there isn't comparable data for stocks of nurses for Germany, Ireland, and Norway. Instead, by looking at available data for Italy, Norway, and Belgium, we see that, unsurprisingly, the stocks of foreign-trained nurses are larger than those of foreign-trained doctors.

As shown in Figure 6.7, the stock in Italy is notably larger than those in Norway and Belgium. This is in part because Italy has a longer history of hosting Indian-trained nurses (Figure 6.9). This is discussed more in the sections below. There is no discussion of the annual flows of doctors and nurses across EU-27 countries. This is due to the limited and poor quality of the flow data currently available in the database.

A third limitation of this database is the absence of sex-disaggregated data. While we do not have the HWD does not have this data, it would not be incorrect to say that the stocks and flows of nurses are likely to be dominated by women since women make up the majority of the nursing workforce. Similarly, men make up the majority of the physicians in the health workforce (Boniol et al., 2019). This gendering of the health workforce also impacts the migrant categories. For instance, while women labour migrants within the global care chain (Yeates 2004) are likely to be embedded within the lower end such as domestic workers, or care aids (the hierarchy of nursing), men are likely to be embedded within the highly skilled as doctors.

Nursing is not necessarily considered as highly skilled across all countries. For instance, in Germany, nursing and midwifery are not considered as skilled professions due to their local apprenticeship structures. This leads to the devaluing of skills of migrant women who are tertiary level educated trained and experienced nurses (Raghuram and Sondhi 2019;

Raghuram 2021). By contrast, in Norway, the definition of a skilled worker or specialist includes vocational training at the upper secondary level including health workers with appropriate training, completed education/degree from university such as nursing. Hence, someone who may be considered as a skilled worker in Norway might not be considered as one in Germany due to different labour market and qualification structures.

However, other factors also impact the entry of doctors and nurses into specific countries. The case study of Italy below also offers us an example on how religious affinity may also play a role in shaping the movement of nurses from India to the EU.

Germany

There is a long history of migration of health workforce migration from India to Germany. During the 1960s–1970s, nurse migration from Kerala to Germany was a key flow of the corridor (Faist, Aksakal, and Schmidt 2017). However, this route was closed in the 1970s as West Germany decided to close its border to immigration. This meant that many Indian nurses were unable to extend their visas during that time, and neither could they benefit from family reunification programs at that time. In 2000, Germany started to reopen its labour market to highly skilled migrants – particularly IT professionals from India. Alongside the IT stream, there has been a slow increase in the number of Indian-trained doctors working within the Germany health workforce (Figure 6.8) as evidenced by the increasing stock of Indian-trained doctors. It is important to note that these are not annual flows. A limitation of the OECD database does not allow for further examination of these stocks, and neither is data for nurse migration into Germany available.

Despite the increasing numbers of the India-trained doctors visible in Figure 6.8, research has highlighted that there is limited migration of Indian healthcare professionals into Germany, particularly nurses. This is due to the mandate from the World Health Organization which has listed India as being on the list of human resources crises within the health sector. Hence, Germany has not proposed or signed any agreements with India for recruitment of health workforce (Gereke 2013). In principle, Germany differs from the other two countries' cases in this chapter – Italy and Ireland – two countries which have a greater dependence on the migrant health workforce comprised of non-EU third-country nationals.

Italy

Like Germany, the migration of Indian nurses into Italy is part of the long history of movement along the India–Italy corridor. Indian migrant nurses

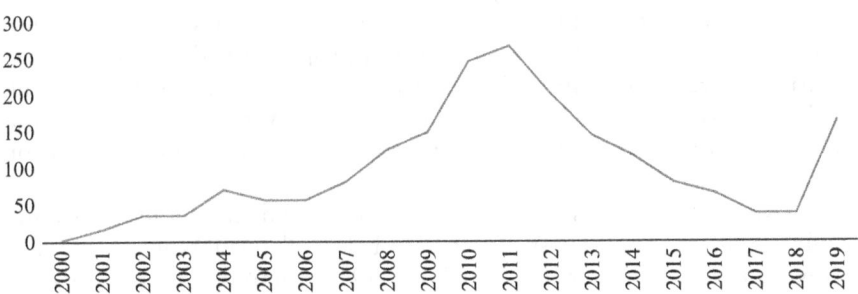

Figure 6.10 Annual flow of Indian-trained nurses in Italy 2000–2019.

Source: OECD health workforce migration database.

in Italy primarily come from Kerala, a state in South India (Gallo 2005), or from Punjab, a state in north India in, which has a long history of out-migration of nurses, including to the Gulf countries, the US, and the UK. It is salient that a number of the nurses are Catholic, making it easier for Italians to accept nurses (and carers) from this region of India.

However, this trend is changing. Between 2000 and 2010, there was an upward trend in the annual flows of Indian nurses into Italy as evidenced in the increasing stocks and annual flows (Figure 6.10). However, since 2011, there has been a steep decline in the annual flows.

This sudden decline in the flows has started to influence the stocks as well since 2016 as seen in Figure 6.11.

There appeared to be a change in the trend in 2018; however, the impact of COVID is likely to shape the future trend of this flow, and consequently the stocks of Indian nurses in Italy.

Ireland

Thus far, we have seen stock data for doctors in Germany, and stock and flow data for nurses in Italy. In this section, we compare the limited annual flow data on Indian doctors and nurses in Ireland.

Over the years, Ireland has undertaken several special initiatives to attract qualified workers in the health sector to cover the projected short-ages of doctors and nurses (Talbot 2013). As part of one of the initiatives in 2011, it recruited over 200 doctors non-EU foreign-trained doctors, of which nearly 25% were Indian-trained (see Figure 6.12). Ireland's foreign-trained doctors are largely third-country nationals from India, Pakistan, South Africa, and Sudan. Between 2000 and 2010, foreign-trained doctors as a percentage of the health workforce increased from 13% to 33%, mak-ing the second most dependent OECD country on foreign-trained health workforce (Brugha, McAleese, and Humphries 2015). In 2014, nearly 35%

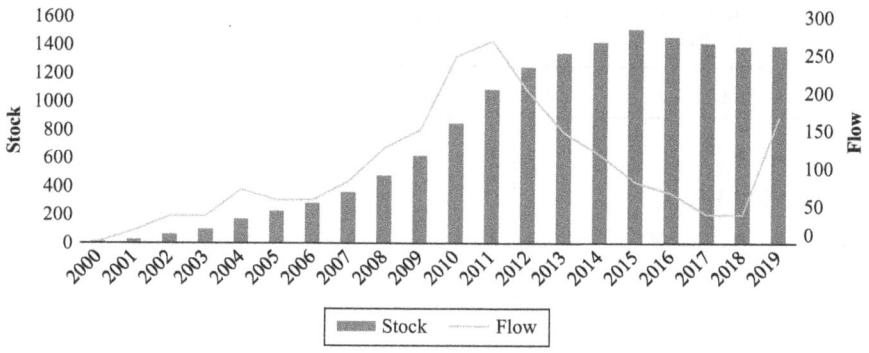

Figure 6.11 Comparison of stocks and flow of Indian-trained nurses in Italy 2000–2019.

Source: OECD health workforce migration database.

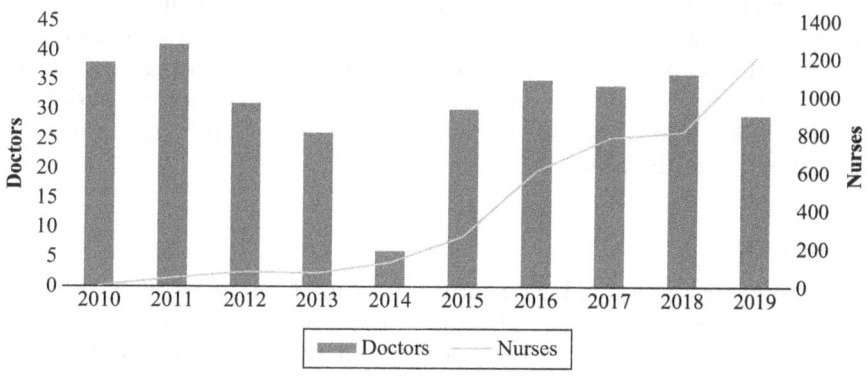

Figure 6.12 Annual flow of Indian-trained doctors and nurses in Ireland 2010–2019.

Source: OECD health workforce migration database.

of the health workforce of Ireland was composed of international medical graduates (Brugha, McAleese, and Humphries 2015).

Figure 6.12 and Table 6.1 show that the numbers of doctors entering Ireland annually have remained more or less the same over a period of 10 years (other than a sharp drop in 2014), but nurse migration has increased steadily through the period 2010–2019. During 2000–2009, Ireland undertook large-scale recruitment of nurses recruiting nearly 12,000 nurses from India and the Philippines (Brugha, McAleese, and Humphries 2015). Figure 6.12 shows that over the past decade, the flows of nurses from India have been on a steady increase. The data prior to 2010 is unavailable in the OECD database; hence, there is discrepancy between data from other studies and the OECD database, and thus another limitation of the HWD.

Table 6.1 Annual Flow of Indian-Trained Doctors and Nurses in Ireland 2010–2019

	Doctors	Nurses
2010	38	5
2011	41	45
2012	31	77
2013	26	71
2014	6	126
2015	30	266
2016	35	612
2017	34	786
2018	36	816
2019	29	1206

Source: OECD health workforce migration database.

While recruitment of doctors and nurses has been more or less steady, research has shown that Ireland has faced retention challenges due to limitations on the scope of practice, as well as barriers to securing long-term residency in Ireland. Hence, Ireland is likely to be a stop on a multinational migration (Paul and Yeoh 2021) career pathway of health professionals rather than the destination.

Conclusion

This chapter has presented descriptive statistics from the OECD health workforce migration database. The aim of the discussion has been to point to the need to (a) open up further research on India–EU corridor and (b) examine the strengths and limitations of the OECD health workforce database to support evidence-informed policy development for safe and secure migration and decent work. This chapter starts to map out the trends of this India–EU mobility to open up avenues for future research.

The contemporary crisis has forced international, regional, and national stakeholders to think more of the migrant health workforce beyond the development-deficit models of brain or care drain to consider more carefully and responsibly the safety and security of migrants and migration processes, as well as issues around decent work along the mobility corridors and in the receiving countries.

Through the case of health workforce migration, the chapter has shown that the movement between the India–EU corridor is not new. Its trends and patterns (even with limited data) reflect both existing corridors such as Italy and Germany, but also emerging such as Ireland and Norway.

While the data in this database is limited, it does provide a window into existing and emerging trends and patterns of migration between India and the EU. The chapter has shown three types of comparisons that can be undertaken with the current data set. For the case of Germany, the stocks of doctors over a 20-year period were examined. The case of Italy focused on nurses rather than doctors compared both stocks and flows of nurses over a 20-year period. Lastly, the Irish case provided a unique opportunity to compare the trend of annual flows of doctors and nurses. Hence, the database offers various possibilities of undertaking occupational, spatial and temporal comparative work to identify national-level patterns of migrant health workforce, particularly along the India–EU corridor.

However, due to the relative newness of this database, there are several limitations for migration analysis, particularly one that focuses on movement from India to EU member states. The three limitations identified in this chapter are: missing data, inconsistent data (between individual country sources and data available in the HWD), and lastly the absence of sex-disaggregated data. The latter missing data therefore limits deeper gendered analysis of health workforce migration both in this specific content of India–EU mobility and also globally. This absence sex-disaggregated data is of particular relevance due to the dominance of women within the health workforce globally both migrant and non-migrant.

Despite its limitations, the database opens up several avenues for future research employing diverse methodologies. Firstly, an improved database will lead to improved quantitative analysis of the migration of the health workforce, especially gendered analysis. The existing body of research on Indian nurse migration – which has remained mostly microlevel, can now extend the analysis by looking at receiving country data. The data on migration of doctors can also benefit from gendered analysis to complement the gendered analysis of mobility within the nursing profession. Lastly, the database could offer an opportunity to examine multinational migration trajectories that nurses and doctors may undertake.

Second, for every country case presented in this chapter, several questions have been raised regarding the specificities and commonalities across EU member states. While some context of each receiving member state is provided, the in-depth analysis of the structures within which the migrations occur has not been examined. Thus, the undertaking analysis for instance of the national labour markets and professional bodies that impact entrance and retention of migrant health workforce would highlight the barriers and enablers at the level of both member states and the EU.

As a final point, it is important to say that not all health workforce is captured under the movement of doctors and nurses. For instance, migrant women are employed as care workers in a range of EU countries. Many of them are trained as nurses but are deskilled after migration as they navigate the intersecting hierarchy of health work and care work, and are then employed as live-in care workers, or care aides. Hence, it is important to recognise the limitations of quantitative-only analysis and reliance on one type of database. The OECD HWD is a useful starting point, especially as it enables cross-country comparison. However, this quantitative analysis needs to be complemented with qualitative methodologies to ensure that a deeper and productive analysis of this stream is usefully undertaken to improve our understanding and improve policies and programs that support the migrant workforce.

Acknowledgements

This chapter forms one of the background pieces for a report produced for the ILO-India led by Professor Parvati Raghuram. The report identifies the existing and emerging mobility streams of women within the India–EU corridor. The author would also like to thank Dr Caterina Mazzelli and Dr Johanna Waters for their support during this project.

Notes

1 https://www.who.int/hrh/com-heeg/International_migration_online.pdf.
2 http://www.oecd.org/health/health-data.htm.
3 For details on comparability issues, please see data definitions document https://ec.europa.eu/eurostat/cache/metadata/Annexes/hlth_res_esms_an13.pdf.
4 Author's calculations based on data available in Eurostat table: Migr_Resfas, available here: https://ec.europa.eu/eurostat/databrowser/view/migr_resfas/default/table?lang=en.

References

Bhattacharjee, Ayona. 2013. 'Migration of Indian Health Professionals to Selected European Nations : The Case of Denmark, Netherlands, Norway, Sweden'. https://cadmus.eui.eu/handle/1814/29469.

———. 2018. 'Migration of Indian Health Professionals to the European Union: An Analysis of Policies and Patterns'. In *India Migration Report 2018: Migrants in Europe*, edited by S. Irudaya Rajan. London: Taylor & Francis.

Boniol, Mathieu, Michelle McIsaac, Lihui Xu, Tana Wuliji, Khassoum Diallo, and Jim Campbell. 2019. *Gender Equity in the Health Workforce: Analysis of 104 Countries*. Working Paper 1. Geneva: World Health Organisation. https://apps.who.int/iris/bitstream/handle/10665/311314/WHO-HIS-HWF-Gender-WP1-2019.1-eng.pdf.

Bornat, Joanna, Leroi Henry, and Parvati Raghuram. 2011. 'The Making of Careers, the Making of a Discipline: Luck and Chance in Migrant Careers in Geriatric Medicine'. *Journal of Vocational Behavior* 78 (3): 342–50. https://doi.org/10.1016/j.jvb.2011.03.015.

Brenne, Geir Tore, and Helge Hiram Jensen. 2013. 'An Overview of Highly-Skilled Labour Migration to Norway : With a Focus on India as Country of Origin'. https://cadmus.eui.eu/handle/1814/29933.

Brugha, Ruairí, Sara McAleese, and Niamh Humphries. 2015. *Ireland: A Destination and Source Country for Health Professional Migration*. European Union. https://www.who.int/workforcealliance/031616-108IrelandStudy.pdf?ua=1.

Ciccarone, Giuseppe. 2015. 'Personal and Household Services - Italy'. *Brussels: European Commission*. https://www.epsu.org/sites/default/files/article/files/EEPO-TR-PHS-Country-Report-Italy-06-15-EN.pdf.

Faist, Thomas, Mustafa Aksakal, and Kerstin Schmidt. 2017. *Indian High-Skilled Migrants and International Students in Germany: Migration Behaviours, Intentions, and Development Effects*. Bielefeld: Universität Bielefeld, Fak. fürSoziologie, Centre on Migration, Citizenship and Development (COMCAD). https://www.ssoar.info/ssoar/bitstream/handle/document/51856/ssoar-2017-faist _et_al-Indian_high-skilled_migrants_and_international.pdf?sequence=1.

Gallo, Ester. 2005. 'Unorthodox Sisters: Gender Relations and Generational Change among Malayali Migrants in Italy'. *Indian Journal of Gender Studies* 12 (2–3): 217–51. https://doi.org/10.1177/097152150501200204.

Gereke, Johanna. 2013. 'Highly-Skilled Indian Migrants in Germany'. *CARIM-India*, EUI. https://citeseerx.ist.psu.edu/viewdoc/download?doi=10.1.1.899.3966 &rep=rep1&type=pdf.

Gupta, Pralok. 2013. 'Facilitating Migration between India and the EU : A Policy Perspective'. https://cadmus.eui.eu//handle/1814/29468.

Irudaya Rajan, S., ed. 2021. *India Migration Report 2020: Kerala Model of Migration Surveys*. Abingdon, Oxon; New York, NY: Routledge.

IOM. 2020. 'COVID-19 and Women Migrant Workers: Impacts and Implications'. Geneva. https://publications.iom.int/system/files/pdf/the-gender-dimensions-of-the -labour-migration.pdf.

Jain, Rajendra K., and Gulshan Sachdeva. 2019. 'India-EU Strategic Partnership: A New Roadmap'. *Asia Europe Journal* 17 (3): 309–25. https://doi.org/10.1007/ s10308-019-00556-0.

Khadria, Binod. 1999. *The Migration of Knowledge Workers: Second-Generation Effects of India's Brain Drain*. London: SAGE.

———. 2004. 'Migration of Highly Skilled Indians: Case Studies of IT and the Health Professionals'. April. https://doi.org/10.1787/381236020703.

Khadria, Binod, and Perveen Kumar, eds. 2012. *India Migration Report 2010–2011: The Americas*. New York: Cambridge University Press.

Kodoth, Praveena, and Tina Kuriakose Jacob. 2013. 'International Mobility of Nurses from Kerala (India) to the EU: Prospects and Challenges with Special Reference to the Netherlands and Denmark'. 2013/19. CARIM-India Research Report. European University Institute. https://mea.gov.in/images/pdf/Internation alMobilityofNursesfromIndia.pdf.

Kofman, E., and P. Raghuram. 2015. *Gendered Migrations and Global Social Reproduction*. Basingstoke: Springer.

Nair, Sreelekha. 2020. *Moving with the Times: Gender, Status and Migration of Nurses in India*. Routledge, New Delhi: Taylor & Francis.

Oda, Hisaya, Yuko Tsujita, and Sebastian Irudaya Rajan. 2018. 'An Analysis of Factors Influencing the International Migration of Indian Nurses'. *Journal of International Migration and Integration* 19 (3): 607–24.

OECD. 2019. *Recent Trends in International Migration of Doctors, Nurses and Medical Students*. Paris: OECD. https://doi.org/10.1787/5571ef48-en.

Paul, Anju Mary, and Brenda S. A. Yeoh. 2021. 'Studying Multinational Migrations, Speaking Back to Migration Theory'. *Global Networks* 21 (1): 3–17. https://doi .org/10.1111/glob.12282.

Percot, Marie. 2006. 'Indian Nurses in the Gulf: Two Generations of Female Migration'. *South Asia Research* 26 (1): 41–62.

———. 2012. 'Transnational Masculinity: Indian Nurses' Husbands in Ireland'. *E-Migrinter* 8 (April): 74–86. https://doi.org/10.4000/e-migrinter.630.

Percot, Marie, and S. Irudaya Rajan. 2007. 'Female Emigration from India: Case Study of Nurses'. *Economic and Political Weekly* 42 (4): 318–25.

Percot, Marie, and Sreelekha Nair. 2011. 'Transcending Boundaries: Indian Nurses in Internal and International Migration'. In S. Irudaya Rajan and Marie Percot (Eds.), *Dynamics of Indian Migration: Historical and Current Perspectives* (pp. 195–228). Delhi: Routledge.

Pozzan, Emanuela, and Umberto Cattaneo. 2020. 'Women Health Workers: Working Relentlessly in Hospitals and at Home'. *International Labour Organisation*. 7 April 2020. http://www.ilo.org/global/about-the-ilo/newsroom/news/WCMS_741060/lang--en/index.htm.

Raghuram, Parvati. 2021. 'Interjecting the Geographies of Skills into International Skilled Migration Research: Political Economy and Ethics for a Renewed Research Agenda'. *Population, Space and Place* 27 (5): 1–14.

Raghuram, Parvati, and Gunjan Sondhi. 2019. 'Skilled Female Migrants in the EU'. *Policy Brief. Germany: Federal Education for Civic Education: Policy Briefs.* http://www.bpb.de/gesellschaft/migration/kurzdossiers/292980/skilled-female-migrants-in-the-eu.

Ratha, Dilip. 2021. 'Staying the Course on Global Governance of Migration through the COVID-19 and Economic Crises'. *International Migration* 59 (1): 285–88. https://doi.org/10.1111/imig.12822.

Ray, Nilanjana. 2019. 'Indian Women as Nurses and Domestic Workers in the Middle East: A Feminist Perspective'. In S. Irudaya Rajan and P. Saxena (Eds.), *India's Low-Skilled Migration to the Middle East*, 339–54. Singapore: Springer.

Smith, Pam, and Maureen Mackintosh. 2007. 'Profession, Market and Class: Nurse Migration and the Remaking of Division and Disadvantage'. *Journal of Clinical Nursing* 16 (12): 2213–20.

Stefan, Marco. 2017. 'Migration versus Mobility in EU External Action towards Asia: A Closer Look at EU Relations with China , India, the Philippines and Thailand'. 2017/01. CEPS Research Reports. Brussels: Centre for European Policy Studies. https://www.ceps.eu/download/publication/?id=9813&pdf=RR%202017-01%20Migration%20vs%20Mobility.pdf.

Stievano, Alessandro, Douglas Olsen, Ymelda Tolentino Diaz, Laura Sabatino, and Gennaro Rocco. 2017. 'Indian Nurses in Italy: A Qualitative Study of Their Professional and Social Integration'. *Journal of Clinical Nursing* 26 (23–24): 4234–45. https://doi.org/10.1111/jocn.13746.

Talbot, Conor C. 2013. 'Highly Skilled Indian Migrants in Ireland'. SSRN Scholarly Paper ID 2335957. Rochester, NY: Social Science Research Network. https://papers.ssrn.com/abstract=2335957.

Walton-Roberts, Margaret. 2012. 'Contextualizing the Global Nursing Care Chain: International Migration and the Status of Nursing in Kerala, India'. *Global Networks* 12 (2): 175–94.

Walton-Roberts, Margaret. 2021. 'Bus Stops, Triple Wins and Two Steps: Nurse Migration in and out of Asia'. *Global Networks* 21 (1): 84–107. https://doi.org/10.1111/glob.12296.

Walton-Roberts, Margaret, and S. Irudaya Rajan. 2020. 'Global Demand for Medical Professionals Drives Indians Abroad Despite Acute Domestic Health-Care Worker Shortages'. *Migration Policy Institute- Migration Information Source* (blog). 21 January 2020. https://www.migrationpolicy.org/article/global-demand-medical-professionals-drives-indians-abroad.

Walton-Roberts, Margaret, Vivien Runnels, S. Irudaya Rajan, Atul Sood, Sreelekha Nair, Philomina Thomas, Corinne Packer, et al. 2017. 'Causes, Consequences, and Policy Responses to the Migration of Health Workers: Key Findings from India'. *Human Resources for Health* 15 (1): 28. https://doi.org/10.1186/s12960-017-0199-y.

World Bank. 2020a. 'COVID-19: Through a Migration Lens'. 32. Migration and Development Brief. World Bank Group. https://www.knomad.org/sites/default/files/2020-06/R8_Migration%26Remittances_brief32.pdf.

———. 2020b. 'Phase 2: COVID-19 Crisis through a Migration Lens'. 30. Migration and Development Brief. World Bank Group. https://www.knomad.org/sites/default/files/2020-11/Migration%20%26%20Development_Brief%2033.pdf.

World Health Organisation. 2020. *State of the World's Nursing Report – 2020*. Geneva: World Health Organisation. https://www.who.int/publications-detail-redirect/9789240003279.

Yeates, Nicola. 2004. 'Global Care Chains'. *International Feminist Journal of Politics* 6 (3): 369–91. https://doi.org/10.1080/1461674042000235573.

7 An Analysis of Nurses' Intention Not to Migrate

Evidence from Nurses in Tamil Nadu

Hisaya Oda, Yuko Tsujita and S. Irudaya Rajan

Introduction

In response to the global demand for nurses and care workers due to ageing in developed countries, as well as the shortage of medical personnel in the Gulf countries, nurses from developing countries, including Indians, have migrated to other countries to fill these demands. Higher salaries, favourable working environments, higher living standards, and geographical proximity in some cases have attracted nurses to these countries (Kline 2003; Kingma 2006; Nair and Webster 2012). The number of Indian nurses abroad was "guesstimated" to be 640,078 in 2011 (Irudaya Rajan and Nair 2013)[1]—a number that is likely considerably larger now. Most of the students we interviewed during our visits to many nursing educational institutions in Kerala and Tamil Nadu said that they would like to migrate temporarily or permanently sometime in the future for work. In particular, almost 100% of the students in private schools revealed their willingness to migrate overseas. India is now one of the major nurse-exporting countries on a global scale and the second-largest exporter of nurses to OECD countries after the Philippines (OECD 2021).

A large number of studies have investigated nurses' overseas migration from various dimensions. Garner et al. (2015) categorized Indian nurse migration literature into four themes: (1) issues related to exponential growth in nurses' migration, (2) factors influencing decisions to migrate, (3) challenges facing migrating nurses before and after migration, and (4) status transformation as both an individual and a nurse after migration. While the existing literature covers a wide range of topics, one important issue has not received much attention: the analysis of non-migrating nurses. To our knowledge, no studies have discussed this issue in detail. There is a common view that Indian nurses tend to migrate abroad. However, contrary to the common perception, the reality is that not all nurses migrate; rather, the majority remain in India.

Non-migrating nurses are not homogenous. In terms of the intention to migrate, there are two types: nurses who have the intention to migrate and nurses who have no intention to migrate. The former includes nurses who

DOI: 10.4324/9781003315124-7

plan to migrate sometime in the near future or are preparing to migrate, and the latter includes nurses who have no intention to migrate at all or who had wished to migrate but have given up for some reason. These types of non-migrating nurses have stimulated the development of our research questions about how they differ from nurses who have migration experience, what factors influence their decisions, and why they choose to stay or leave. In order to understand nurses' international migration more thoroughly, it is crucial to examine who is and who is not migrating. As these are two sides of the same coin, studying one side provides more information about the other.

First, we investigated the relationship between the nurses' intention to/ not to migrate and their characteristics based on our survey data. The study identified what types of nurses intend to go abroad and what types of nurses remain in India. Second, we discuss the reasons for non-migration.

The survey was conducted in Chennai, Tamil Nadu, India, and data were collected from alumni of two nursing schools. Tamil Nadu is one of the south-most states in India, where the country's first nursing school was established and where nursing education has been quite active. The number of seats offered at nursing education institutions in 2019 in Tamil Nadu was 17,835; there were 7,175 seats in general nursing and midwifery (GNM), and 10,660 seats in BSc Nursing[2]. This number is the fourth-largest in India after Karnataka, Madhya Pradesh, and Uttar Pradesh, accounting for around 7.8% of all nursing institutions that offer GNM and BSc Nursing in the country.

This chapter is organized in the following way. The first section explains the data and provides brief profiles of the sample nurses. The second section presents an empirical analysis of the factors that influence nurses' intention to migrate. The third section discusses the reasons for the sample nurses' non-migration. The last section provides concluding remarks.

Data and Profiles of Sampled Nurses

Data Collection

Our study was based on a nurse migration survey from Tamil Nadu, jointly conducted by the Institute of Developing Economies (IDE-JETRO) in Japan and the Loyola Institute of Social Science Training and Research (LISSTAR) at Loyola College in Tamil Nadu, India. The survey began in June 2016 and was completed in December 2017. Alumni of two nursing schools' diploma courses were interviewed, one being a nursing school run by Tamil Nadu's state government (hereafter "government school") and the other being a private school established by a Christian group (hereafter "private school"). Both schools are well renowned and located in Chennai, the capital of Tamil Nadu. In total, 292 female nurses were surveyed: 174 government school alumni and 118 private school alumni. Their graduation years ranged from

1990 to 2015. Among them, 71 nurses had international migration experience or were migrants at the time of the survey. The remaining 221 nurses had no previous migration experience, and 128 of them had no intention to go abroad to work.

We employed a questionnaire to collect information about each respondent's profile, nursing education, career, migration experience, and family profile. Since complete alumni lists were not available for both schools, the study employed a snowball sampling method to collect the sample nurses. Two enumerators were recruited for this survey. The questionnaire survey was administered primarily in person by the enumerators and occasionally by telephone, email, and/or social networking service applications.

A Brief Profile of the Sample Nurses

Table 7.1 shows a summary of the characteristics and international migration experiences of the sample nurses. The nurses were categorized by the type of hospital in which they were working, their religion, and their social class, and were asked about their migration experience. Among them, 147 nurses worked in government hospitals and 145 in private hospitals. Regarding religion, 132 nurses were Hindu, 148 were Christian, and 12 were Muslim. The relatively high number of Christian nurses in the sample reflects the fact that the private school is run by a Christian organization and that it is also the tradition that nurses are mainly from Christian communities. This stems from the fact that Christian missions played an important role in nurses' training in the early days in India (Nair and Rajan, 2017). The nursing profession was not well-received by Hindus because of their caste prejudices and ideology of purity, nor by Muslims mainly because of the practice of *purdah* (Nair and Healy 2006; Simon 2009). Though this tradition is fading away as the economic and social status of nurses rise thanks to international migration opportunities, and therefore the nursing profession attracts many people regardless of their religion. Still, there is a tendency for the proportion of Christians who want to be nurses to be higher than for other religions (Simon 2009; Johnson et al. 2014; Prescot and Nichter 2014; Garner et al. 2015)[3].

Regarding social class (e.g., caste), 21 nurses belonged to the Hindu general castes, 212 to the Other Backward Class (OBC), and 59 to the Scheduled Castes (SC). Hindu general status is considered highest, while SC status is considered lowest. OBC, which is the most voluminous, is placed in the middle of the social ladder. The small number of nurses from the Hindu general castes is an indication of the fact that the nursing profession is still not preferred among the socially high class because of the reason mentioned above. It is still considered an impure job.

Regarding international migration experience, 71 nurses had such experience at least once or were working outside India at the time of the survey, and 221 nurses had no international migration experience. Significantly, a

Table 7.1 Summary of the International Migration Experience of the Sample Nurses

	Type of Hospital		Religion			Social Class			Total
	Public Hospitals	Private Hospitals	Hindu	Christian	Muslim	Hindu General	OBC	SC	
Number of nurses who had migration experience	11	60	25	41	5	8	49	14	71
Number of nurses who had no migration experience	136	85	107	107	7	13	163	45	221
Number of nurses who did not intend to migrate abroad	116	12	68	58	2	7	98	23	128
Number of nurses who had an intention to migrate abroad	5	20	13	11	1	2	14	9	25
Number of nurses who did not disclose their intention	15	53	26	38	4	4	51	13	68
Total	147	145	132	148	12	21	212	59	292
Proportion of nurses who had migration experience	7.5%	41.4%	18.9%	27.7%	41.7%	38.1%	23.1%	23.7%	24.3%
Proportion of nurses who had an intention to migrate among those who had no migration experience	3.7%	23.5%	12.1%	10.3%	14.3%	15.4%	8.6%	20.0%	11.3%

smaller proportion of nurses who were working in government hospitals had migration experience (7.5%, 11 out of 147 nurses) compared to those who were working in the private sector (41.4%, 60 out of 145 nurses).

This study focused on nurses who had never migrated, particularly those who had no intention of going abroad to work. Therefore, non-migrated nurses were further classified into three categories: nurses who had an intention to migrate, nurses who didn't have an intention to migrate, and nurses who did not disclose their intention at the time of the survey. The numbers of nurses in each category (out of the 221 non-migrated nurses) were as follows: 25 (12.9%) intended to go abroad; 128 nurses did not have an intention to migrate; and 68 nurses did not answer this question, 53 of which were nurses in private hospitals. A more detailed analysis could have been performed if this last group had responded to the question. This is a limitation of our study.

A notable characteristic shown in Table 7.1 is that only 5 of the 136 nurses working in public hospitals intended to migrate (3.7%), while 20 of 85 nurses working in private hospitals (23.5%) intended to migrate. Because of this trend, naturally, the ratio of nurses with no intention to migrate working in government hospitals is much higher than that of those working in private hospitals. If the 68 nurses who did not disclose their intention for international migration had answered the question, the difference could be even wider.

Estimation and Results

Dependent and Explanatory Variables

We employed a logit analysis to estimate the factors that influence a nurse's decision not to migrate overseas. The dependent variable was a binary variable that indicated a nurse's intention to/not to migrate; it was assigned a value of 1 if the nurse did not intend to migrate and a value of 0 otherwise. The explanatory variables used for estimation comprised two dimensions: individual characteristics and the type of hospital in which the nurse was working. Variables related to individual characteristics included a nurse's age, marital status, religion, and her social class. Religion was categorized as Hindu, Christian, or Muslim, and the social class was divided—in order from high to low—into Hindu general, OBC, and SC. The hospitals were categorized as either private or public (government hospitals). These variables were selected based on relevant literature (Percot 2006; Percot and Rajan 2007; Thomas 2006; Nair and Percot 2007; Walton-Roberts 2010; Walton-Roberts and Rajan 2013; Garner et al. 2015; Timmons et al. 2016; Walton-Robert et al. 2017; Oda et al. 2018).

Age was a continuous variable, while the others were all dummy variables. Reference categories for marital status, religion, social class, and hospital type were single, Christian, OBC, and private hospital, respectively.

Table 7.2 provides the descriptive statistics and definitions of the explanatory variables.

Estimated Results

The estimated results are reported in Table 7.3. *Odds ratios and corresponding* standard errors (in italics) are shown. Due to possible correlations between religion and social class, each was investigated separately. Thus, the results shown in Column 1 were derived using the religion dummy variables, while those in Column 2 used the social class dummy variables. The significant factors are marital status and hospital type. The coefficient of the marital status variable was found to be greater than 1, meaning that the mobility of married nurses was more restricted than that of single nurses. It is understandable that married nurses, as well as other married women, are generally less mobile because their actions and decisions are constrained to some extent by family matters. This point is discussed in detail in a later section.

The coefficient for hospital type was significantly larger than 1. The odds ratio was significant, and hospital type was the most dominant factor among

Table 7.2 Descriptive Statistics and Definitions of Explanatory Variables

Variable	Obs	Mean	Variable Description
Age	153	38.288 (7.683)	Min: 26 years old, Max: 58 years old
Marital status	153	0.889	The value takes the value of 1 if the nurse is married; =0 otherwise
Religion (Hindu)	153	0.529	The value takes the value of 1 if the nurse is a Hindu; =0 otherwise
Religion (Christian)	153	0.451	The value takes the value of 1 if the nurse is a Christian; =0 otherwise
Religion (Muslim)	153	0.020	The value takes the value of 1 if the nurse is a Muslim; =0 otherwise
Social class (Hindu general)	153	0.059	The value takes the value of 1 if the nurse belongs to Hindu general caste; =0 otherwise
Social class (OBC)	153	0.732	The value takes the value of 1 if the nurse belongs to OBC; =0 otherwise
Social class (SC)	153	0.209	The value takes the value of 1 if the nurse belongs to SC; =0 otherwise
Hospital type	153	0.791	The value takes the value of 1 if the nurse works in a government hospital; =0 if she work in a private hospital

Notes: Standard deviation in parenthesis for the continuous variable.

Table 7.3 Results of Logit Estimation (Odds Ratios)

Explanatory Variables	Odds Ratios 1	Odds Ratios 2
Age	0.952	0.953
	0.046	0.046
Marital status	6.783 **	5.886 **
(Reference category: Single)	5.353	4.639
Religion (Hindu)	0.474	
(Reference category: Christian)	0.319	
Religion (Muslim)	0.155	
(Reference category: Christian)	0.290	
Social class (Hindu general)		0.282
(Reference category: OBC)		0.264
Social class (SC caste)		1.080
(Reference category: OBC)		0.743
Hospital type (Private)	37.795 ***	40.915 ***
(Reference category: public hospital)	27.770	32.194
Number of Observation	153	153
Pseudo R2	0.437	0.435
Log-Likelihood	–38.370	–38.520

Notes: (1) Standard errors in *italic*.

(2) ***, **, and * denote statistical significance at the 0.01, 0.05, and 0.10 level respectively using two-tailed tests.

the explanatory variables. Nurses working in government hospitals did not intend to migrate overseas more often than those working in private hospitals. This finding is in line with those of Thomas (2006), Timmons et al. (2016), Walton-Roberts et al. (2017), and Oda et al. (2018). Each of these studies reported a high incidence of international migration among nurses in private hospitals compared to nurses in government hospitals. In the next section, we discuss why the type of hospital matters in migration decisions.

Other variables were not significantly related to the propensity of nurses to go abroad. Religion and social class are important determinants of an individual's or household's choices in India, including migration decisions (Keshri and Bhagat 2012; Tsujita and Oda 2014). However, statistically significant impacts of religious and social class categories were not observed in our case.

Discussion of Reasons for Non-Migration

We asked nurses who did not intend to migrate why they did not plan to do so. Responses were received from 120 non-migrating nurses: 115 nurses working in government hospitals and 5 nurses working in private hospitals.

The reasons for non-migration are listed in Table 7.4. The most frequently cited reason was that they were simply not interested in migration. Fifty-three nurses working in government hospitals and two nurses working in private hospitals expressed a lack of interest in overseas migration. A substantial number of nurses working for government hospitals prefer

Table 7.4 Reasons for Non-Migration

Reasons	Government Hospital	Private Hospital	Total Response
Not interested in overseas migration	53	2	55
Family matters	30	3	33
Fear of going abroad	26	0	26
Language problems	12	0	12
Didn't have chances	3	0	3
Others	4	0	4

*Multiple answers

Responses received from 120 nurses (115 working in government hospitals, and 5 in private hospitals)

not to work overseas. As discussed in the literature, this preference is due to more favourable working conditions and salaries in the public sector. Oda et al. (2018) pointed out that international migration is not attractive to nurses working in the public sector because they are well paid, their government jobs are secured, and they receive several fringe benefits, including pensions, among other factors. *The Times of India* reported in 2017 that, in state government hospitals in Tamil Nadu, nurses were paid on average 33,045 Indian rupees (INR) per month,[4] while private hospitals paid around 8,000 to 9,000 INR per month.[5] It is not surprising to find that nurses in private hospitals are paid 3,000 INR per month or even less. Some nurses in private hospitals even work without pay to gain the experience needed for international migration; several countries impose a requirement of at least two to three years of nursing experience on migrating nurses (Garner et al. 2015; Timmons et al. 2016). Despite a Supreme Court-appointed committee recommending in 2016 that the minimum salary of nurses in the private sector be comparable to the level of nurses in the government sector, nurses' salaries in private hospitals remain low. This is why many nurses in the public sector have not migrated previously or do not have an intention to go abroad, and it is why nurses in the private sector have migrated or intended to do so. Our survey results clearly align with this tendency.

The second-most common reason for non-migration was family matters; 33 nurses listed this factor as a reason why they did not plan to migrate. Family matters cover a wide range of issues, such as taking care of parents, children, and grandparents, as well as completing household duties. These responsibilities normally increase when one marries and indicate a significantly negative impact of marriage on mobility. This explains why the coefficient of the marital status of nurses was greater than 1. In addition, an imbalance in the intra-household bargaining power between a nurse and her parents might discourage a nurse's overseas migration. There are some parents who would like to keep their daughters at home and do not permit them to migrate. Such a case might be rare in South India, where international migration is active, but it happens in North India. During our survey in Uttar Pradesh, we came across several nurses who would like to go abroad but had been prohibited from doing so by their parents[6].

The third and fourth reasons stated were fears of going abroad and language problems, which are somewhat related. Difficulty communicating in a foreign language may be attributed to the fear of going abroad. In South India, the teaching mode in nursing schools is usually English, but nonetheless, some nurses educated in the South feel reluctant to migrate.[7] Overcoming language problems bears some cost. Many nurses take English classes, such as IELTS preparation courses, to qualify for migration to English-speaking countries. IELTS consists of four components: reading, writing, listening, and speaking. For example, nurses and midwives who wish to work in the UK are required to achieve a minimum IELTS score of 7.0 in each component. It seems that many Indian nurses tend to have difficulty obtaining a 7.0 in the writing component. Migration to other English-speaking countries also requires similar IELTS scores or other types of English proficiency tests.

One may hypothesize that the level of happiness among nurses who intend to migrate is lower than that among those who do not possess such an intention, and thus low happiness levels encourage nurses to migrate abroad; however, the reality is more complex. Table 7.5 shows the happiness levels among the two types of nurses at the time of their interviews. There were no negative responses, except from one respondent who claimed that she was *very unhappy*. The majority of nurses stated that they were either *happy* or *very happy*. Each happiness level was assigned a number from 1 (*very happy*) to 5 (*very unhappy*). The simple sample mean scores were 1.91 for nurses who planned to migrate and 1.85 for nurses who did not. Nurses with no intention to migrate were generally happier, but the difference was not statistically significant, meaning the two types of nurses were equally happy.[8] It can be understood that nurses plan to migrate not because they are unhappy with their current occupation, but because they seek more favourable working conditions and higher salaries. However, caution is necessary when interpreting the result. As noted previously, nurses who work in private hospitals tend to migrate overseas. This may indicate that those

Table 7.5 Levels of Happiness of Nurses Who Did/Did Not Intend to Migrate

	Very Happy	Happy	Neutral	Unhappy	Very Unhappy	Total
Nurses who didn't intend to migrate	50	60	17	0	1	128
Nurses who had an intention to migrate	6	16	3	0	0	25

who were not happy with being nurses in India had already migrated, leaving those who were not unhappy behind. It might be why the two types of surveyed nurses were equally happy.

Conclusion

This study focused on non-migrating nurses and examined what factors influenced their decision to/not to migrate based on our survey data from Tamil Nadu, India. The salary gap between government and private hospitals provides nurses working in private hospitals with a greater incentive to go abroad in search of higher wages, while the majority of nurses working in government hospitals had no such intention. The most frequently cited reason for non-migration was that nurses were simply not interested in going abroad. Nurses who work for government hospitals are relatively well paid, and their jobs are secured. The high opportunity cost of overseas migration discourages these nurses from migrating.

Sample nurses were found to be generally satisfied with their current occupation. The hypothesis that nurses who intend to migrate feel unhappier than nurses who do not intend to migrate has been rejected. Nurses plan to migrate not because they are unhappy with their current occupation, but because they wish to achieve more favourable working conditions and higher wages.

It has often been reported that there is a nurse shortage in India (WHO 2010, Gill 2011, 2016; Walton-Roberts and Irudaya Rajan 2020). According to the World Health Organization, in 2019, India had 3,263,633 nurses, which was equivalent to 2.39 nurses per 1,000 people (WHO 2010). The reported shortage varies from 834,700 to 2,300,800, depending on which ratio of required nurses per 1,000 people is used.[9] In any case, India has faced a shortage of nurses. It is ironic that Indian nurses are filling the shortage in other countries, but India itself faces a serious nurse shortage. Because of the COVID-19 pandemic, every country needs more health workers. The demand for Indian nurses will increase and may create additional shortages. Our study implies that increasing the salary of nurses in private hospitals eventually leads to mitigating the nurse shortage. This is a necessary prescription for India to maintain the standard of public health throughout the country. The Supreme Court has already suggested that private hospitals should increase their wage level, but the implementation is another story, and it needs time to implement.

Notes

1 Irudaya Rajan prefers to use the term "guesstimate" because the number is a product of estimation and a (scientific) guess. It is a difficult task to estimate the number of nurses abroad and there are no such official figures.

2 Data on the number of seats was obtained from the Indian Nursing Council's homepage (http://www.indiannursingcouncil.org/Statistics.asp, accessed on August 18, 2020)

3 Simon (2009) noted that 30% of nursing graduates were from Christian families while Christian represented only 3% of the total population of India.

4 "Private hospital nurses ask for better pay, work conditions." *Times of India*, August 11, 2017 electronic version (accessed on November 11, 2020).

5 This information was obtained during interviews with nurses in Chennai in 2016. Our recent survey in Tamil Nadu and Uttar Pradesh in 2018 showed that nurses were earning 5,000–8,000 INR in private hospitals.

6 A nurse we met in Lucknow, Uttar Pradesh, North India during our visit to a private hospital in December 2018 stated, "Personally, I would like to migrate abroad. I have been dreaming of going to the US or a European country, even to the Gulf. I want to see the different world and have more experience as a nurse. In addition, I can get a higher salary than here. But my parents never allow me to leave. I simply obey them."

7 It seems that many nurses in North India tend to feel language problems more strongly. While interviewing nurses in Uttar Pradesh in December 2018, many claimed they had no plans to migrate. When asked why, several responded that communicating in English is a problem. They asserted that, at school they read English textbooks but are taught in Hindi, thus making them experience difficulty talking with doctors and patients in English abroad.

8 The *t*-statistics for the group sample mean difference was 0.729 with 151 degrees of freedom. The difference was not statistically significant.

9 Based on the author's calculation. If the recommended number of nurses per 1,000 people is 3, the shortage would be 834,700, and if the number is 4, then the shortage would be 2,300,800. Data were taken from the WHO Global Health Observatory website (https://who.int/data/gho: accessed on February 27, 2021).

References

Garner ZL, Conroy SF and Bader SG (2015) Nurse migration from India: A literature review. *International Journal of Nursing Studies* 52 (12): 1879–1890.

Gill R (2011) Nursing shortage in India with special reference to international migration of nurses. *Social Medicine* 6 (1): 52–59.

Gill R (2016) Scarcity of nurses in India: A myth or reality? *Journal of Health Management* 18: 509–522.

Irudaya Rajan S and Nair S (2013) *Assessment of existing services for skilled migrant workers: India project site, ILO promoting decent work across boards: A pilot project for migrant health professionals and skilled workers*. Draft Report submitted to International Labour Organization.

Johnson SE, Green J and Maben J (2014) A suitable job? A qualitative study of becoming a nurse in the context of a globalizing professions in India. *International Journal of Nursing Studies* 51 (5): 734–743.

Keshri K and Bhagat RB (2012) Temporary and seasonal migration: Regional pattern, characteristics and associated factors. *Economic and Political Weekly* 47 (4): 81–88.

Kingma M (2006) *Nurses on the move: Migration and the global health care economy*. Ithaca, NY: Cornell University Press.

Kline D (2003) Push and pull factors in international nurse migration. *Journal of Nursing Scholarship* 35 (2): 107–111.

Nair S and Healy M (2006) A profession on the margins: Status issues in Indian nursing, CMDS Occasional papers series. New Delhi: Centre for Women's Development Studies.

Nair S and Irudaya Rajan S (2017) Nursing education in India: Changing facets and emerging trends. *Economic and Political Weekly* 52 (24): 38–42.

Nair S and Percot M (2007) Transcending boundaries: Indian nurses in internal and international migration, CWDS Occasional papers no. 47, New Delhi: Centre for Women's Development Studies.

Nair M and Webster P (2012) Health professionals' migration in emerging market economies: Patterns, causes and possible solutions. *Journal of Public Health* 35(1): 157–163.

Oda H, Tsujita Y and Irudaya Rajan S (2018) An analysis of factors influencing the international migration of Indian nurses. *Journal of International Migration and Integration* 19 (3): 607–624.

OECD. 2021. *Health Work Force Migration*. OECD Health Statistics. https://doi.org/10.1787/71bb9c24-en (accessed on 30 April 2022).

Percot M (2006) Indian nurses in the Gulf: Two generations of female migration. *South Asia Research* 26 (1): 41–62.

Percot M and Irudaya Rajan S (2007) Female emigration from India: Case study of nurses. *Economic and Political Weekly* 42 (4): 318–325.

Prescott M and Nichter M (2014) Transnational nurse migration: Future directions for medical anthropological research. *Social Science & Medicine* 107: 113–123.

Simon E (2009) Christianity and nursing in India: A remarkable impact. *Journal of Christian Nursing* 26 (2): 88–84.

Thomas P (2006) The international migration of Indian nurses. *International Nursing Review* 53 (4): 271–283.

Timmons S, Evans C and Nair S (2016) The development of the nursing profession in a globalized context: A qualitative case study in Kerala, India. *Social Science & Medicine* 166: 41–48.

Tsujita Y and Oda H (2014) Caste, land, and migration: Analysis of a village survey in an underdeveloped state in India. In Y Tsujita (Ed.), *Inclusive growth and development in India: Challenges for underdeveloped regions and the underclass* (pp. 96–116). Cham, Switzerland: Palgrave Macmillan.

Walton-Roberts M (2010) Student nurses and their post graduation migration plans: A Kerala case study. In S Irudaya Rajan (Ed.), *India migration report 2010* (pp. 196–216). London: Routledge.

Walton-Roberts M and Irudaya Rajan S (2013) Nurse emigration from Kerala: 'Brain circulation' or 'trap'. in S Irudaya Rajan (Ed.), *India migration report 2013: Global financial crisis, migration and remittances* (pp. 206–223). New Delhi: Routledge.

Walton-Roberts M and Irudaya Rajan S (2020) Global demand for medical professionals drives Indians abroad despite acute domestic health-care worker shortages. *Migration Information Source*. Migration Policy Institute. https://www.migrationpolicy.org/article/global-demand-medical-professionals-drives-indians-abroad (accessed on Aug. 25, 2020).

Walton-Roberts M, Runnels V, Irudaya Rajan S, Sood A, Nair S, Thomas P, Packer C, Mackenzie A, Murphy GT, Labonte R and Bourgeault IL (2017) Causes, consequences, and policy responses to the migration of health workers: Key findings from India. *Human Resources for Health* 15(28): 1–18.

World Health Organization (2010) Wanted: 2.4 million nurses, and that's just in India. *Bulletin of the World Health Organization.* http://www.who.int/bulletin/volumes/88/5/10-020510/en/ (accessed on Mar. 5, 2017).

8 Health Worker Mobility from India

Trends and Opportunities for International Cooperation

Rupa Chanda and Sudeshna Ghosh

Introduction

Human resources for health shape not only the lives of real people, those delivering and those receiving health care, but also the sustainability of national health systems, which is so critical for development. As "Development is about more than money, or machines, or good policies – it's about real people and the lives they lead",[1] the health workforce is critical for a country's development. However, the world faces an acute shortage of health workers and this shortfall will only grow. According to a Global Burden of Disease Study (2017), only half of all countries have the requisite health workforce to deliver quality healthcare services to realize Universal Health Coverage (UHC). The World Health Organization (WHO) estimates a projected shortage of 18 million health workers by 2030, mainly in less developed and developing countries, though countries at all levels of development are faced with this challenge to varying degrees. Currently, there is a shortage of 9 million nurses and midwives, a gap that is expected to narrow only slightly to 7.6 million by 2030.[2] Aggravating the problem is the uneven and inequitable distribution of the global health workforce. Africa which bears more than 24 per cent of the global burden of disease, has access to only 3 per cent of health workers while the Americas, with 10 per cent of the global burden of disease has 37 per cent of the world's health workforce.[3] According to the World Bank, the Sub-Saharan region has the lowest ratio of doctors per 1,000 population in the world.[4]

A variety of factors have contributed to the world's health workforce crisis, including inadequate investment in education and training of health workers in some countries, misalignment of education and employment strategies, and poorly managed health systems.[5] Against this backdrop, international mobility of health workers assumes importance. It is both an outcome of and a contributing factor to the shortage of health workers. The significance of cross-border mobility of health workers is evident from the fact that in 2015, as per the WHO, 25 per cent of the medical workforce across 70 countries and 17 per cent in case of 28 OECD countries was trained abroad, comprising of a mix of developed and developing source

DOI: 10.4324/9781003315124-8

countries.[6] In future, as healthcare systems become further burdened by the rising incidence of non-communicable diseases and a growing geriatric population, the demand–supply gap is expected to increase, generating demand for an additional 40 million health workers globally by 2030.[7] In other words, this will require a doubling of the current global health workforce. Clearly, such a gap cannot be bridged by augmenting national health capacity alone. Such trends will only reinforce the reliance on foreign health professionals, making cross-border health worker mobility and how it is managed and strategized even more important in future. The latter in turn will require a good understanding of the patterns of international migration and of the key source and destination countries.

International health worker migration is a complex phenomenon. While flows have traditionally been from low- and middle-income countries to developed countries, driven by traditional push and pull factors,[8] the dynamics today also include movement within regions, including among developing and low-income countries. Recent evidence shows that a large proportion of healthcare workers in not only developed countries but also in developing countries and LDCs is foreign-born and foreign-trained. Reflecting these trends and recognizing the importance of managing these flows in both national and international interest, various bilateral, regional, sub-regional, and international frameworks and agreements have emerged to regulate health worker mobility. These arrangements establish principles for recruitment, market access, employment, welfare, and harmonization of standards. Potentially, such arrangements, if well crafted, could facilitate the cross-border movement of health workers in a mutually beneficial manner for both sending and receiving countries and thus help address the human resources for health crises.

India's role in the international mobility of health workers is critical as it is a key source country for health workers for the world. It is the world's largest source country for physicians and is also among the leading suppliers of nurses to the world. It features among the five leading countries of origin for foreign-born nurses and doctors in the OECD countries and is also a significant supplier of nurses to the Gulf region. According to estimates, between 20 and 50 per cent of Indian health workers aim for overseas employment and about 3 per cent of its registered nurses in India currently work abroad.[9] Hence, India's national policies to develop human resources in healthcare as well as its approach to managing the migration of its health workers through bilateral, regional and multilateral platforms has a bearing on the availability of human resources for health in the rest of the world as well as on the capacity of its own healthcare system.

This chapter provides an overview of the salient features of India's health worker migration to the world and the management of this migration through bilateral and other arrangements. The section "International Landscape of Health Worker Migration and Management" following this introduction, discusses the international landscape of health worker migration and cooperation frameworks that currently exist to address such movement. The section "Global Context of Health Worker Mobility" places India in this global context of health worker migration, focusing on its role as a source country for health workers and outlines important characteristics and trends. The section "Governance Mechanisms and Frameworks" discusses various arrangements India has entered into with destination countries through Memoranda of Understanding (MoUs), bilateral sectoral agreements, and health specific provisions and health sector commitments within broader economic cooperation agreements, and also compares with evidence on the same from other source countries. This section also presents some primary evidence on India's skilling, recruitment, and other initiatives with host countries in the health sector and its overall approach to the migration of health workers. The last section, Concluding Thoughts and Future Consideration, highlights certain issues which India could consider in future to better leverage cooperation arrangements to address health worker mobility related interests and concerns.

International Landscape of Health Worker Migration and Management

In order to understand the global landscape for health worker migration, one needs to recognize the nature of the global labour market for healthcare workers. This market is huge and consists of diverse occupational categories. In 2013, over 43 million people had formal, certified health care skills around the world. Together with all those working in supporting occupations, the number of health workers is estimated to account for around 5 per cent of the paid global workforce, with nurses and midwives constituting the largest occupational group, or almost half of all global health workers, followed by doctors.[10] Associated health professionals – opticians, podiatrists, physiotherapist, pharmacists, emergency service workers, such as ambulance workers, and administrative support staff, account for the remaining health workers.

Global Context of Health Worker Mobility

The healthcare workforce is highly international. In most countries, it comprises locally born and trained staff as well as migrants who are born and/or trained abroad. Five categories of health professionals, namely, dentists, midwives, nurses, pharmacists, and physicians represent the largest share of all regulated health professionals. These are the categories of health workers, especially nurses and doctors, who are the most associated with international migration.[11]

The OECD countries rely heavily on foreign-trained health workers, as highlighted earlier. Among foreign-born doctors working in OECD countries, the five major countries of origin were India, China, Germany, UK, and Pakistan. Among foreign-born nurses, the five major countries of origin were the Philippines, India, the UK, Germany, and Jamaica.[12] With ageing populations, growing affluence, improved health coverage, and increased incidence of non-communicable diseases, the demand for healthcare will continue to grow, resulting in a projected global shortage of 18 million healthcare workers by 2030, up from a shortage of 7.2 million healthcare workers in 2013.[13] As a result, countries have over the years increased their reliance on foreign health professionals to bridge their demand and supply gaps and notwithstanding constraints to such movement that arise from language barriers, national regulatory systems concerning the recognition of qualifications which affect the portability of skills, immigration restrictions, and high regulatory and other compliance costs for migrating individuals and employers. As per the WHO, there has been a 60 per cent rise in the number of migrant doctors and nurses working in OECD countries over the last decade.[14]

The following figures and tables illustrate this growing dependence on foreign-born health professionals in OECD countries.[15] Similar figures are not readily available for other recipient countries, but as the OECD markets constitute a major destination for foreign health workers, the trends for this selected set of countries are representative of the growing importance of international migration of health workers (Table 8.1).

As shown in Figures 8.1 and 8.2, in 2015/16, the dependence on foreign-born doctors was as high as 30 per cent or more, and as much as 50 per cent in certain OECD countries. It was around 20 per cent or more in some countries in case of foreign-born nurses. Further, this dependence

Table 8.1 Share of Foreign-trained Doctors and Nurses in Selected OECD Countries, 2018 (Unless Otherwise Indicated)

Country	% of Foreign-trained Doctors	% of Foreign-trained Nurses
Australia	32.46	18.06
Austria	5.97	
Canada	24.54	8.32
Switzerland	35.35	24.99
Denmark	9.35	1.85
Finland[a]	19.91	1.78
France	11.48	2.87
The United Kingdom	29.23	14.90
Ireland	41.64	
The Netherlands[b]	2.74	1.30
New Zealand	42.46	26.20
Sweden	27.93	3.05
The United States[a]	24.99	6.00

Source: OECD Health Workforce Migration Statistics (accessed April 27, 2021)

[a]Figures are for 2012; [b]Figures are for 2017

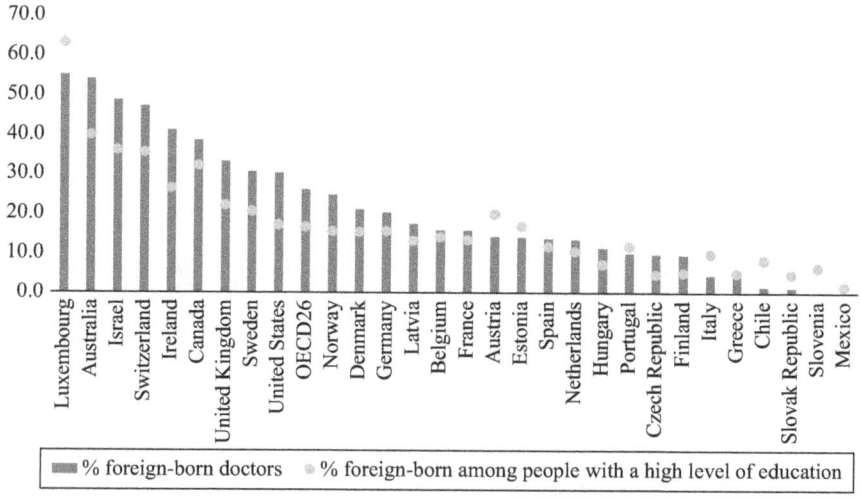

Figure 8.1 Share of foreign-born doctors in 27 OECD countries, 2015/16.
Source: OECD Health Workforce Migration Statistics (accessed April 27, 2021).

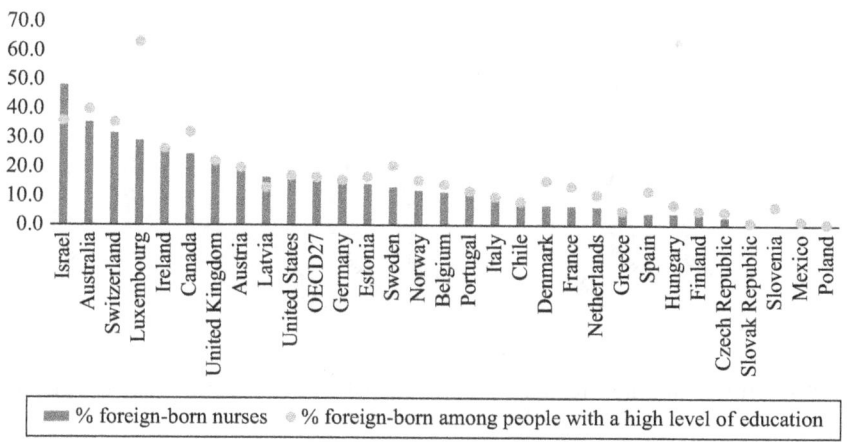

Figure 8.2 Share of foreign-born nurses 2016.
Source: OECD Health Workforce Migration Statistics (accessed April 27, 2021).

increased significantly over the 2010/11 and 2015/16 period with as much as 30 per cent or more of the growth in the number of practising doctors and nurses being attributable to foreign-born professionals. In some OECD countries, as much as 50 per cent of the increase was due to foreign health professionals, reflecting the contribution of migrating healthcare workers (Figures 8.3 and 8.4).

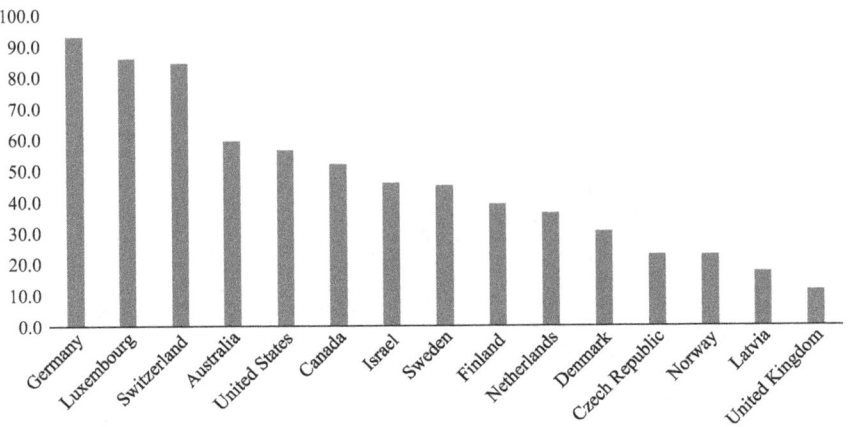

Figure 8.3 Growth in practising doctors between 2010/11 and 2015/16 attributed to foreign-born doctors in 15 OECD countries.

Source: OECD Health Workforce Migration Statistics (accessed April 27, 2021).

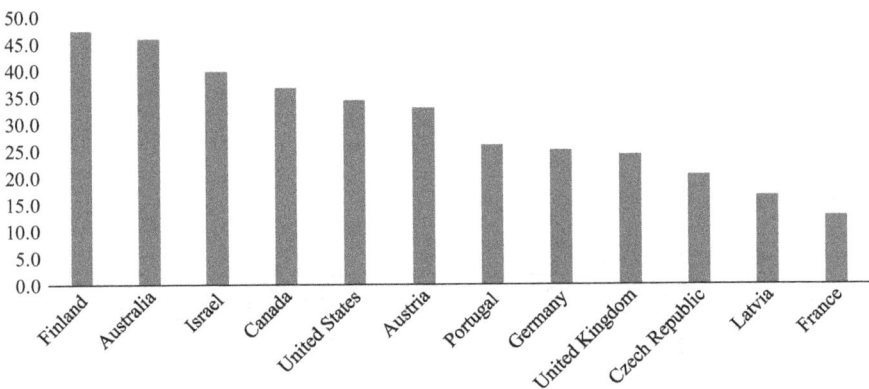

Figure 8.4 Growth in practising nurses between 2010/11 and 2015/16 attributed to foreign-born nurses in 12 OECD countries.

Source: OECD Health Workforce Migration Statistics (accessed April 27, 2021).

Governance Mechanisms and Frameworks

The growing dependence on foreign health professionals indicates that health workers are a global public good, a shared resource that must be appropriately managed in the interests of both sending and receiving countries. Reflecting this recognition, a variety of multilateral, regional, and sub-regional arrangements have emerged to govern the mobility of health professionals. This is because in addition to national policies and regulatory frameworks adopted by countries to mitigate the challenges associated with the migration of health workers, several issues such as recruitment practices, wages and working conditions, repatriation, recognition, and certification, among others, require the cooperation of both receiving and sending countries.

Multilateral Arrangements

Several global frameworks illustrate the governing principles and underlying philosophy of such arrangements.[16] Some important ones include the WHO Global Code of Practice which was adopted in 2010 as a key global governance instrument to better understand and manage health worker migration, the Commonwealth Code of Practice for the International Recruitment of Health Workers, the National Health Service (NHS) Guidelines, the Melbourne Manifesto, the Alliance Code, and the Global Compact on Safe, Orderly and Regular Migration by the OECD, and the International Organization for Migration (IOM). The WHO Global Code adopted by its member states stresses that countries should implement effective health workforce planning, education, training, and retention strategies in order to sustain a health workforce that is appropriate for the specific conditions of each country and to reduce the need to recruit migrant health personnel. It also calls for bilateral agreements and consistency across government agencies. While the WHO Code speaks to all parties involved in foreign recruitment, including private agencies, it is a voluntary process driven by member nations. Countries are supposed to provide updates through the reporting mechanism every three years, but there is wide variance in compliance and compliance approaches. The Alliance Code is a multistakeholder voluntary code which concerns the migration of nurses to the US. It is aligned with the principles of the WHO Code for Ethical Recruitment of Health workers but also includes country-specific aspects pertaining to the domestic health care market, immigration and labour law, so that it is applicable to any country. There are also other platforms which address health worker migration and recruitment, including the 2016 UN High-Level Commission on Health Employment and Growth and the ILO, OECD, WHO International Platform on Health Worker Mobility.

The ethos of these codes is to discourage the international recruitment of health personnel from countries that face acute shortage and instead to encourage improved education and training, better retention strategies, and better distribution of health workers to ensure a sustainable healthcare system. Ethical recruitment which safeguards the interests of sending countries and the rights of recruited health workers is a key concern. These governance instruments also encourage destination countries to collaborate with source countries on training, technology and skill transfer, recognition of qualifications, return and circular migration, and sharing of information and best practices, so that the international migration of health personnel is mutually beneficial. Member states, international organizations, international donor agencies, and others are encouraged to support developing countries that experience critical health workforce shortages by providing financial and technical assistance. Some codes such as the NHS and the Melbourne Manifesto discourage active international recruitment of healthcare personnel from developing countries unless there is an explicit government-to-government agreement or a MoU with the source countries. Some include guidelines advising recruiting countries to develop more training posts at home so as to reduce reliance on international recruitment from developing countries, to establish active links with training institutes and schools in source countries to augment capacity in the latter, and to encourage health professionals to return to their home countries.

One multilateral instrument which is binding and has a potential bearing on the mobility of health workers (mode 4) is the General Agreement on Trade in Services (GATS).[17] Under the GATS countries can make binding market access and national treatment commitments on the mobility of foreign health workers. The GATS also has provisions for the mutual recognition of qualifications and for harmonizing domestic regulations through discussions in the Working Party on Professional Services. Till date, however, the agreement has had no impact on mobility of health workers as very few countries have scheduled health services in their list of sectors tabled for negotiations and even where scheduled, countries have made no liberalization commitments in mode 4. Progress on Mutual Recognition and Domestic Regulations has also been slow.

Regional Arrangements

There are several initiatives at the regional and sub-regional levels to manage health worker mobility and capacity in mutual interest. These initiatives address different aspects, such as recruitment, standards and qualifications, visas, mutual recognition, training, capacity building, regulatory cooperation, data sharing, return, and reintegration. Some examples include initiatives in the CARICOM, ASEAN, EAC, and Mercosur regions.

For instance, the CARICOM region has taken significant steps to collaborate on mobility of health workers and their training and credentialing processes to facilitate such exchange and movement. There is a clear overall goal of managing human resources of health more effectively keeping in view both intraregional flows and migration to countries outside the region. There has been progress in developing regional associations and bodies which play an active role in the harmonization efforts as well as in establishing minimum standards for licensing of nurses and for recognition of doctors trained outside the Caribbean Association of Medical Councils system and in developing a model curriculum through a participatory approach at the country level. Skills, networks, and partnerships developed through returning migrant health workers (nurses) have been used to strengthen standards and capacity in the region, indicating that migration has been seen in a holistic manner, both in terms of outflows and inflows and that return migration related benefits have been leveraged. The Managed Migration Program includes arrangements between countries for subsidized training and for information sharing. The coordination efforts have also extended to other health professionals such as pharmacists and regulatory authorities (for medical products) with efforts to establish harmonized norms for inspection, distribution, registration and quality control for medicines, and related information sharing and technical support.

Similarly, in the Mercosur region, there have been regulatory cooperation efforts to address issues of mutual recognition, accreditation of qualifications, information sharing, and harmonization of related legislations and systems, that have a bearing on the mobility of health workers and medical students. These efforts have been institutionalized through the creation of regional bodies, platforms for dialogue, and coordination mechanisms which govern migration, education, and healthcare. The focus has primarily been on educational qualifications and the validation and acceptance of credentials among member countries, with efforts mostly targeted at upgrading the qualifications of nurses in the region in order to meet domestic needs and address the consequences of migration. These efforts have also been assisted by Pan American Health Organization (PAHO), a regional body of the WHO which has supported nurses' associations and governments in the region in their efforts to upgrade educational facilities and standards for nurses.[18]

Another regional example is the East African Community (EAC) which has focused on health sector regulation and harmonization given the serious shortage of qualified medical specialists in the region and pressures arising from out-migration from the region. Several regional boards and councils have been established, including for nursing and midwifery, radiographers and radiologists, physiotherapists and occupational health practitioners, environmental health practitioners, and for allied health professionals. The focus has been on standardization of training and qualifications in order to ensure quality, enhance capacity, and facilitate intraregional mobility. These efforts have helped improve access to quality healthcare and education services. Economies of scale have been attained through regional investments like the EAC Regional Centres of Excellence. Intraregional movement of health professionals and students has been made easier, with universities finding it easier to request teaching staff from each other following harmonization. More doctors are now registered in other EAC member countries.

The ASEAN region has likewise taken steps to facilitate the mobility of health workers and the cross-border trade in health services. In particular, 3 MRAs facilitate the mobility of health professionals in the regional health labour market by enabling designated health professionals to practise in another ASEAN country without needing to pass other market access assessments before being registered to practice.[19] These MRAs allow mutual recognition of medical, dental, and nursing practitioners and promote circular mobility and temporary migration. Further, excepting limitations imposed by immigration regimes, there are no limits on the number of health workers who can migrate to other ASEAN countries.

In addition to formal regional integration agreements, there are also regional networks and arrangements which address the intraregional mobility of health workers. Some such examples include the Regional Network For Equity In Health In East And Southern Africa (EQUINET),[20] the Pacific Code of Practice for Recruitment of Health Workers in the Pacific Region to provide a framework for better managing the loss of skilled health workers through migration, the African Health Professions Regulatory Collaborative (ARC) launched in 2011 to support countries in East, Central, and Southern Africa, and the New Partnership for Africa's Development (NEPAD) Health Strategy which prioritizes human resource development and retention and migration strategies in health services.

Bilateral Arrangements

Countries have entered into Bilateral Labour Agreements (BLA) to manage their health workforce and migration. Over 120 separate bilateral agreements, both intraregional and cross-regional, have been notified to the WHO Secretariat as part of the national reporting on the WHO Global Code of Practice for the International Recruitment of Health Personnel.[21] These include formal agreements, MoUs, and concerted management agreements (Dhillon et al., 2010).

Table 8.2 highlights the key features of selected bilateral agreements concerning health worker migration. As is evident, these agreements aim to facilitate the movement of health professionals in a transparent and orderly manner and also touch upon aspects such as circular migration, recognition of qualifications, and regulatory cooperation to streamline administrative processes, exchange information and ensure the safety and welfare of migrant health workers.

As is evident from the above MoUs and partnership arrangements, the focus is on facilitating mobility and serving mutual interests in terms of capacity building and training, without undermining ethical and welfare considerations. How effective these agreements have been, is very difficult to gauge as systematic evidence is not available reviewing their performance and implementation.

Health Worker Mobility from India

India is a major source country for health professionals for the world and also for particular countries and regions given its large pool of health workers and their competence in English. It has been the world's largest source country for immigrant physicians since its independence in 1947. We discuss

Table 8.2 Selected Bilateral Agreements on Health Worker Migration and Their Key Features

Agreements	Features and Status
Germany–Vietnam (2012)	• For a period of 4 years.[22] • Commissioned by the *German Federal Ministry of Economics and Technology*, implemented by GIZ in collaboration with the *Vietnamese Ministry of Labour, Invalids and Social Affairs*. • Selected 100 Vietnamese nursing graduates for six months training in German language and culture, followed by a 13-month programme in cooperation with Goethe institute in Hanoi before going to Germany for 2 years. • In Germany, nurses are provided with one-on-one support for a year • During the 2016–2019 period, more than 300 Vietnamese nurses were successfully placed.[23] 195 completed the required training and started working as nurses and geriatric nurses, while 125 were still in training in 2019.
Germany–China (2013)	• Similar to Germany–Vietnam agreement. • Pilot project recruited 150 nursing graduates from China (Dumont, 2016).
Germany–various countries	• "Triple Win" project by the German Society for International Cooperation (GIZ) bilaterally with Philippines, Georgia, Vietnam, and Tunisia • Project enables mobility skills partnerships but with controls to address equity concerns • Germany and the Philippines (2013) agreement describes the framework, rights and obligations for German hospitals and Filipino nurses, in line with the WHO Global Code of Practice, relevant ILO Conventions, international human rights, and anti-discrimination provisions.
Economic Partnership Agreements (EPA) between Japan and Indonesia (2008), Philippines (2009), Vietnam (2008)	• Japan agreed to accept 1,000 Indonesian nurses. • Agreed to admit a specified number of Filipina and Vietnamese nurses • Health professionals from these countries required to learn Japanese, clear the nursing medical examination conducted in Japanese language in a maximum of three attempts (Carzaniga et al., 2019). • By 2018, approximately 1,118 nurses and 2,740 care-workers entered Japan between 2008 and 2016 under the three EPAs[24]
New Zealand–Malaysia (2009)	• Malaysian doctors allowed to work in New Zealand, subject to conditions on work location, approval of transfers, maximum duration of stay (10 years), passing qualifying examination in English language (Carzaniga et al. 2019).
Ghana–Netherlands (2002–12)	• Short term practical internships to enable knowledge transfer for Ghanaian medical residents in the Netherlands (Connell, 2010). • The Netherlands agreed to develop a centre for medical equipment in Ghana.
UK–South Africa (2003)	• MoU to restrict active recruitment of South African health professionals by NHS • Number of registrations by South African trained doctors declined as a result from 3206 in 2003 to 4 in 2004 (Blacklock et. al, 2012)

Source: Compiled based on various sources

the trends in health worker migration from India to the world and to specific regions and groups of countries to highlight the salient characteristics.

Trends by destination markets and regions

It is estimated that between 20 and 50 per cent of Indian health workers aim for employment overseas and around 3 per cent of the registered nurses in India, work abroad currently. Outflows to the Gulf and OECD countries are significant and several facts and figures reveal this importance. For instance, India features among the top five countries of origin for foreign-born doctors in OECD countries, along with China, Germany, UK, and Pakistan. It also features among the top five source countries for foreign-born nurses in the OECD along with the Philippines, India, the UK, Germany, and Jamaica. In the US, 6 per cent of all immigrants registered as nurses were from India, after the Philippines (28 per cent) in 2018, while 22 per cent of all registered immigrant physicians were from India, followed by China (6 per cent).[25] Indian-trained nurses accounted for 2–3 per cent of the nursing workforce in the case of Australia, Germany, Ireland, Italy, Maldives, and Singapore. In the UK, Indians represented the top non-British nationality for the NHS) in 2019.[26]

Tables 8.3 and 8.4 show the relative importance of India as a source country for foreign-trained doctors in selected OECD countries. As shown, India accounts for the largest number of doctors in all the countries, particularly in the case of the US and the UK. Its contribution is several times that of the next source country. In the case of nurses, India is an important source country for Australia, UK, and Ireland, though second to the Philippines for Canada and the UK. It is worth noting, however, that although there is a clear upward trend in the stock of nurses from India, there is a significant deceleration in the annual inflows of foreign-trained nurses from India into the US and the UK over the past decade, which may possibly reflect factors such as changes in immigration policies and also in recruitment practices due to the implementation of the aforementioned codes and protocols regarding the recruitment of health workers.

Table 8.5 further highlights the share of Indian nurses in the total stock of foreign-trained nurses and in the total number of practising nurses in selected OECD countries in 2016. It shows that Indian nurses accounted for around 10 to 20 per cent of all foreign-born nurses in several English-speaking OECD countries, although the share was much lower at around 1–5 per cent in the stock of practising nurses. Within the OECD, Ireland is an emerging market for Indian-trained nurses, with 35 per cent of nurse recruitment into that country coming from non-EU sources between 2000 and 2010.

Table 8.6 provides the latest figures for registered doctors and nurses in the UK who have received their primary medical qualifications in another country. India stands out as a significant source country for both categories of health workers.

Table 8.3 Stock of Foreign-trained Doctors in Selected OECD Countries (Numbers), 2014–19

Year		2014	2015	2016	2017	2018	2019
Country	*Country of Origin*						
Australia	Canada	113	106	118	124	125	–
	China	579	618	644	643	673	–
	India	4,481	4,821	5,037	5,182	5,336	–
	Ireland	997	1,044	1,104	1,179	1,236	–
	Malaysia	247	263	296	328	359	–
	Philippines	527	561	592	596	614	–
	South Africa	1,780	1,836	1,844	1,816	1,846	–
	Sri Lanka	1,358	1,467	1,582	1,607	1,659	–
	United Kingdom	4,563	4,837	5,209	5,577	5,892	–
	United States	156	171	170	168	165	–
Canada	Australia	432	461	489	523	590	–
	Brazil	155	165	170	181	194	–
	Canada	0	0	0	0	0	–
	China	400	390	392	406	414	–
	Cuba	52	52	53	57	57	–
	France	469	458	444	448	431	–
	Germany	225	226	227	236	233	–
	India	1,998	2,036	2,088	2,150	2,163	–
	Indonesia	9	9	10	10	11	–
	Ireland	1,513	1,558	1,621	1,731	1,884	–
	Italy	121	115	121	126	126	–
	Malaysia	13	13	14	14	15	–
	Mexico	182	184	184	193	187	–
	Philippines	268	267	259	257	263	–
	Russian Federation	234	240	247	250	254	–
	Singapore	30	26	25	25	26	–
	South Africa	2,612	2,631	2,642	2,688	2,651	–
	Sri Lanka	239	238	233	241	238	–
	The United Arab Emirates	19	21	25	26	34	–
	The United Kingdom	2,143	2,106	2,090	2,167	2,118	–
	The United States	974	1,032	1,088	1,144	1,218	–
Ireland	Australia	114	117	111	118	119	108
	Brazil	6	6	8	9	13	17
	Canada	7	6	6	6	7	9
	China	14	35	39	45	53	55
	Cuba	10	14	19	18	23	25
	France	21	25	24	27	26	27

(*Continued*)

Table 8.3 Continued

Year		2014	2015	2016	2017	2018	2019
Country	Country of Origin						
	Germany	103	96	95	100	95	100
	India	430	434	460	453	443	437
	Indonesia	..	1	1	1	2	2
	Italy	75	89	110	122	113	123
	Malaysia	6	10	10	17	18	23
	Mexico	8	9	10	13	18	15
	Philippines	11	13	14	13	14	15
	Russian Federation	27	32	38	45	49	50
	Singapore	–	–	–	–	–	1
	South Africa	662	643	683	716	734	769
	Sri Lanka	4	3	5	7	7	8
	The United Arab Emirates	4	4	8	10	15	19
	The United Kingdom	661	701	731	758	766	842
	The United States	37	36	42	42	41	45
United Kingdom	Australia	496	496	491	539	522	561
	Brazil	71	81	93	93	109	135
	Canada	33	40	36	41	42	41
	China	106	136	161	194	229	284
	Cuba	35	30	33	36	41	43
	France	127	120	128	127	116	120
	Germany	1,349	1,199	1,214	1,180	1,175	1,196
	India	17,011	15,119	15,517	15,685	15,870	17,737
	Indonesia	1	1	1	4	7	8
	Ireland	1,860	1,738	1,770	1,763	1,755	1,838
	Italy	947	1,040	1,099	1,117	1,152	1,203
	Malaysia	60	59	68	83	99	118
	Mexico	29	26	27	30	37	44
	Philippines	73	73	76	73	90	119
	Russian Federation	442	420	429	443	453	521
	Singapore	29	29	24	28	26	25
	South Africa	1,427	1,314	1,327	1,324	1,298	1,321
	Sri Lanka	1,372	1,225	1,243	1,209	1,200	1,306
	The United Arab Emirates	39	40	52	72	92	141
	The United Kingdom	–	0	0	0	0	0
	The United States	62	51	58	60	64	70

(Continued)

Table 8.3 Continued

Year		2014	2015	2016	2017	2018	2019
Country	Country of Origin						
United States	Australia	1,109	1,140	1,187	–	–	–
	Brazil	1,408	1,417	1,455	–	–	–
	Canada	8,081	7,918	7,765	–	–	–
	China	5,556	5,671	5,772	–	–	–
	Cuba	1,194	1,244	1,294	–	–	–
	France	700	675	645	–	–	–
	Germany	2,452	2,428	2,437	–	–	–
	India	46,447	46,137	45,830	–	–	–
	Indonesia	115	116	112	–	–	–
	Italy	2,446	2,364	2,270	–	–	–
	Malaysia	62	62	70	–	–	–
	Mexico	10,214	10,089	9,923	–	–	–
	Philippines	10,902	10,536	10,217	–	–	–
	Russian Federation	5,927	5,978	6,021	–	–	–
	Singapore	203	210	213	–	–	–
	South Africa	1,406	1,345	1,290	–	–	–
	Sri Lanka	533	501	475	–	–	–
	The United Arab Emirates	64	72	78	–	–	–
	The United Kingdom	4,600	4,589	4,635	–	–	–

Source: OECD Health Workforce Migration Statistics (accessed April 27, 2021)

Further occupational breakdown by source country of foreign-born health workers in OECD countries shows that India provides a wide range of health providers, including technicians, therapists, pharmacists, dentists, and support personnel, in addition to doctors and nurses. Table 8.7 provides a comparative picture of India's contribution to the health workforce in OECD countries relative to other leading developing source countries.

Apart from the English-speaking OECD destinations, Indian health professionals also have significant presence in the Gulf Cooperation Council countries. Although data for these countries is not systematically available, various sources reveal the importance of the India–Gulf corridor, particularly for key source states such as Kerala. According to government records, in 2018, of the 5,562 nurses emigrating from India under the ECR category (which mainly applies to the Gulf and the Middle East), 4,719 were from the state of Kerala followed by Tamil Nadu with 435 nurses, highlighting the importance of Kerala as a source state.

Table 8.4 Stock of Foreign-trained Nurses in Selected OECD Countries (Numbers), 2014–19

Year		2014	2015	2016	2017	2018	2019
Country	Country of origin						
Australia	Canada	514	502	530	539	519	–
	China	1228	1283	1328	1397	1307	–
	India	7713	8468	9169	10052	10663	–
	Ireland	2039	2090	2088	2108	2123	–
	Malaysia	202	177	177	183	180	–
	Philippines	5734	6235	6941	7835	8552	–
	South Africa	1879	1884	1871	1813	1743	–
	Sri Lanka	83	84	85	86	78	–
	The United Kingdom	14916	14562	14452	14370	14125	–
	The United States	543	515	548	547	555	–
Canada	Australia	378	383	404	402	402	–
	Brazil	56	62	77	86	106	–
	Canada	0	0	0	0	0	–
	China	1373	1346	1322	1300	1249	–
	Cuba	20	22	25	29	28	–
	France	1162	1255	1241	1239	1275	–
	Germany	211	216	208	193	186	–
	India	2756	3215	3894	4413	4880	–
	Indonesia	0	0	0	0	0	–
	Ireland	164	151	165	145	140	–
	Italy	28	31	34	45	50	–
	Malaysia	28	27	26	25	23	–
	Mexico	17	15	14	16	15	–
	Philippines	9890	10319	10872	11244	11621	–
	Russian Federation	126	113	115	123	126	–
	Singapore	59	64	62	62	59	–
	South Africa	240	231	230	219	213	–
	Sri Lanka	69	71	72	78	75	–
	United Arab Emirates	20	19	19	22	24	–
	The United Kingdom	3493	3254	2998	2774	2579	–
	The United States	2146	1988	1953	2051	2057	–
The United Kingdom	Australia	1568	1441	1288	1168	1124	1220
	Brazil	17	18	19	21	23	27
	Canada	248	251	256	237	236	245
	China	302	307	302	290	288	289
	Cuba	1	1	1	1	1	7
	France	154	195	207	191	173	160

(*Continued*)

Table 8.4 Continued

Year		2014	2015	2016	2017	2018	2019
Country	Country of origin						
	Germany	479	494	477	428	394	389
	India	16502	16892	17213	17578	18801	21029
	Indonesia	10	10	10	10	10	10
	Ireland	1765	1858	1811	1733	1693	1661
	Italy	1395	3314	4702	4192	3817	3575
	Malaysia	121	116	112	109	110	114
	Mexico	3	3	3	3	3	2
	Philippines	22581	23248	24483	25806	28320	30653
	Russian Federation	21	20	20	20	19	19
	Singapore	157	157	152	150	164	174
	South Africa	3441	3337	3209	3090	3051	3007
	Sri Lanka	192	190	191	191	187	191
	The United Arab Emirates	12	12	15	22	43	77
	The United States	371	353	358	360	382	434

Source: OECD Health Workforce Migration Statistics (accessed April 27, 2021)

Table 8.5 OECD Foreign-Trained Nurses: Share of Indian Nurses Among Total Foreign-Trained Nurses and Total Practising Nurses in Destination Countries, 2016

Destination Country	Number of Foreign-Trained Nurses from India	Total Foreign-Trained Nurses in Destination Country	% of Indian Nurses among Total Foreign-Trained Nurses	Total Practising Nurses in Destination Countries	% of Indian nurses among total practising nurses
UK	16931	105811	16	516,974	3.3
Australia	9173	51438	17.8	281,752	3.3
Canada	3215	30184	10.7	353,738	0.9
New Zealand	2373	12894	18.4	48,256	4.9
Italy	1455	23308	6.2	326,841	0.4

Source: OECD Health Workforce Migration Statistics (accessed April 27, 2021)

Table 8.6 Registered Doctors and Nurses in the UK by Country of Primary Medical Qualification (Numbers), 2021

Country	Doctors	Nurses
Australia	2,456	1,309
India	29,822	24,866
Ireland	4,892	21,971
Philippines	346	33,595
USA	347	467
China	971	292
France	600	209
Japan	56	103
South Africa	5,123	2,983
Canada	198	276
Malaysia	336	123
Brazil	427	29
Germany	3,217	412
Sri Lanka	3,258	190

Source: GMC (2020) for doctors, https://www.nmc .org.uk/about-us/reports-and-accounts/registration -stat for nurses (accessed April 27, 2021)

In 2018, the majority of ECR nurses from India were headed to Saudi Arabia and 57 per cent of nurses migrating from Kerala were residing in Gulf countries in 2016, with Saudi Arabia being the top destination. Information from Indian state-run agencies such as NORKA, ODEPC, OMCAP, OMCL, TOMCOM, and UP Financial Corporation through which international recruitment of nurses takes place suggests that a very high share of nurses from India head to the Gulf countries, though there is a decelerating trend in recent years.[27] The Kerala Migration survey estimates an external emigration rate of 19.4 per cent for medical doctors from Kerala, with Gulf countries being a leading destination.

These trends in health worker mobility from India are driven by poor salary and working conditions and limited career advancement and professional development opportunities in India, inadequate investment in healthcare, and bureaucratic bottlenecks, and growing international residency and training opportunities often through corporate partnerships, among others. They are also driven by growing demand in many destination countries and changes in immigration policies to encourage foreign health workers. Several countries have encouraged health worker migration from countries like India in recent years. The UK, for instance, introduced a fast-track visa for medical professionals in November 2019 to address shortages in its National Health Service. Projections indicate that, notwithstanding policies to increase the number of domestic graduates and indigenize the

Table 8.7 Number of Foreign-Born Health Workers, By Source Country and Occupational Category in OECD Countries, 2016

	Place of Birth					
	South Africa	*China*	*India*	*Japan*	*Malaysia*	*Philippines*
Health occupations	2760	5155	7985	500	950	20095
Physicians, dentists, and veterinarians	1625	985	2285	90	215	530
Optometrists, chiropractors, and other health diagnosing and treating professionals	20	145	90	15	–	25
Pharmacists, dietitians, and nutritionists	140	415	415	25	75	345
Therapy and assessment professionals	240	145	305	30	15	170
Nurse supervisors and registered nurses	275	820	1675	35	255	6350
Medical technologists and technicians (except dental health)	175	830	725	25	140	2350
Technical occupations in dental health care	35	190	85	135	35	210
Other technical occupations in health care (except dental)	85	810	470	65	100	1295
Assisting occupations in support of health services	165	815	1935	80	115	8820

Source: OECD Health Workforce Migration Statistics (accessed April 27, 2021)

health workforce and uncertainties about immigration policies in certain destination markets, the global pull for healthcare workers from India will continue. The conditions driving emigration of health workers from countries like India will also remain. Hence, the strategic management of such mobility and the role of international cooperation through sector-specific agreements, MoUs, broad-based economic partnership arrangements and frameworks, will become all the more important. This is particularly so for a country like India where there have been concerns about brain drain due to the emigration of health workers.

Impact of COVID-19

The recent pandemic has further highlighted the importance of human resources for health. Since the outbreak of COVID-19, the demand for

Indian health workers has increased around the world. The latter is evident from certain recruitment statistics and policies.[28] For example, according to the Kerala Government-run Overseas Development and Employment Promotion Consultants (ODEPC), between August 2020 and February 2021, the organization sent over 420 nurses to the UAE, Saudi Arabia, Oman, and the UK compared to 300 nurses in all of 2019–20. In February alone, ODEPC sent 253 nurses abroad, 6 times more than its usual monthly deployment numbers. Of these, 153 went to the UAE, 50 to the UK, and the remaining to Saudi Arabia and some European countries. Hundreds of other nurses have also been recruited and are expected to be deployed once they receive their visas.[29] According to ODEPC, the salary offers from Dubai have more than doubled. With the increased focus on strengthening health infrastructure due to the pandemic, demand for Indian nurses has risen from many other countries too, including Ireland, Malta, Germany, the Netherlands, and Belgium, some of whom would be recruiting Indian nurses for the first time. There is demand for Indian nurses for geriatric care in old-age homes in some countries and for Intensive Care Units (ICUs). The UK has expressed its intent to employ 50,000 nurses by 2025 mainly from India and the Philippines.

This rising demand is reflected in countries extending additional benefits relating to food, accommodation, transport, allowances, relaxation of requirements for entrance exams, extended visa facilities, and reduced immigration costs following the COVID pandemic. Several Gulf countries have relaxed certification and entrance exam requirements to help nurses move more quickly. The UK government has reduced visa charges and waived the immigration health surcharge for healthcare personnel and their dependents. As India is already faced with a shortage of health workers, particularly nurses,[30] such measures are only likely to aggravate the shortfall in India, making migration management all the more important at this juncture.

India's Approach to Managing Health Worker Mobility

The emigration of health workers, particularly doctors and nurses, has for long created concerns in India about its impact on national health capacity and quality. In 2016, India's human resources for health was 3.3 for qualified allopathic doctors and 3.1 for nurses and midwives per 10,000 population, much below the WHO's benchmarks of 22.8 and its skilled health care personnel per 10,000 residents stood at 28.52 compared to 52.82 globally.[31] On the other hand, there is also a push to export health workers, particularly in certain states, to capitalize on growing overseas demand to provide employment opportunities and also benefit from associated remittances and earnings for source regions. Reflecting this tension, India's approach to the management of health worker mobility involves a mix of both regulating and restricting outflows on the one hand and initiatives to facilitate outflows of health workers on the other.

At the multilateral level, India has been very supportive of the international protocols concerning health worker mobility. It has endorsed the 63rd World Health Assembly resolution on the Global Code of Practice for the Ethical International Recruitment of Health Personnel, to protect the rights of migrant health workers and to mitigate the potential negative impact of international health worker migration. The Government of India has indicated that the code should cover recruitment of all categories of health workers in a fair and transparent manner, while also upholding the migrants' legal obligations towards their home countries. India is also a signatory to the Commonwealth Code of Practice for the International Recruitment of Health Workers which discourages recruitment from countries facing shortage of health workers and establishes guidelines for international recruitment of health workers. Hence, the focus has mainly been to stem unethical practices in the recruitment of its health workers. In its unilateral and bilateral approaches to health worker migration, however, the tension between facilitation and regulation is evident. The following discussion outlines some of the unilateral measures and bilateral approaches to managing health worker migration.

Unilateral Measures

India has taken many unilateral policies over the years to regulate these outflows. For instance, in 2011, citing the shortage of doctors due to emigration, the Ministry of Health and Family Welfare decided to stop issuing No Obligation to Return to India (NORI) certificates which are needed by medical graduates applying for a J-1 visa to the US. To regulate the outflow of nurses, bureaucratic restrictions have been used such as the imposition of bonds requiring service in the country after training which did not prove to be successful. This was followed by the inclusion of nurses in the Emigration Check Required (ECR) category in April 2015 for nurses going to 18 specified countries mainly in the Middle East and Gulf region. It requires nurse recruitment to be channelled through six state-run employment agencies and permits work to be undertaken only on international contracts approved by government authorities. The latter policy was also motivated by the need to curb the exploitation of nurses by recruiting agents and intermediaries and to make the recruitment process more transparent. The government has also proposed a streamlining of the emigration clearance system and regulation of recruitment intermediaries who are currently outside the purview of the 1983 Emigration Act in the case of health worker migration.[32] Proactive measures have also been taken at the state level to curb emigration. For instance, the state of Kerala mandated that those working in private hospitals be paid a minimum wage of Rs.20,000 per month to reduce the incentive to seek overseas employment. Some destination countries have also taken steps. For instance, in

2018, Kuwait's health ministry decided to recruit directly from government agencies. Such as NORKA Roots and ODEPC to curb the exploitation of candidates by private recruitment agencies and to make the process more transparent under the eMigrate system which fully automates the actions of all key stakeholders such as the Indian Missions, the employers, recruiting agencies, emigrants, and the Protector General of Emigrants and links them on an electronic platform.[33]

There is no systematic evidence available, however, to confirm that such regulations and measures taken unilaterally have been successful in reducing migration costs, addressing ethical concerns, and balancing national with partner countries' interests. With pull and push factors continuing to incentivize the out-migration of health workers, such restrictive regulatory approaches are unlikely to effectively stem outflows or address associated concerns. Moreover, they lack an overall policy framework and seem largely ad hoc. Against this backdrop, cooperation frameworks and bilateral arrangements that take into consideration mutual concerns and interests, assume importance.

Bilateral Partnerships and Cooperation Frameworks

At the bilateral level, India has entered into several partnership agreements with key destination countries. For instance, the Indian Ministry of Health and Family Welfare has health cooperation arrangements in the form of MoUs and Joint Declarations of interest with the Government of Australia, Palestine, Spain, Morocco, Italy, Germany, Poland, Norway, and Switzerland, among others. India has also signed MoUs with several West Asian countries to strengthen bilateral engagement in the health and medicine sectors. But for the most part, these arrangements mainly address aspects such as research, medicines, devices, strengthening of health systems, and do not address the mobility of health personnel specifically. The few that do address health worker mobility are the arrangements with Denmark, UK, and Japan, though the former two are no longer valid. In its labour mobility partnership with the Government of Denmark, the aim was to facilitate safe and legal migration of workers from India. In the bilateral agreement between India's Ministry of Health and Family Welfare and the Regional Office of the Department of Health, UK, which was valid till 2003, the aim was to facilitate sustainable recruitment and employment of health professionals from India and provide an opportunity to the latter to enhance their skills and explore best practices in healthcare delivery. This agreement enabled the UK to recruit registered nurses and other health professionals such as biomedical scientists, radiologists, physiotherapists, and other allied health professionals from India, except from four Indian states.[34]

A more recent example is the cooperation memorandum signed between India's Ministry of Skills Development and Entrepreneurship (MSDE) and the Government of Japan in 2017 for a Technical Internship Training

Program (TITP). The aim is to exchange technical intern trainees between the two countries with National Skill Development Council of India (NSDC) as the implementing and monitoring agency, through sending organizations listed in India.[35] The courses include Japanese language and culture training and sector-specific training as per Japan's requirement with certification being provided on successful completion. This programme covers one health sector related occupation which is that of care-workers. The concerned courses are for front line health workers, general duty assistants and home health aides for deployment in hospitals, sanitariums, and old-age facilities.[36] There has been some progress in this partnership programme. NSDC was invited by Japan International Trainee and Skilled Worker Cooperation Organization (JITCO) and the Japanese Embassy to conduct the first TITP awareness workshop in 2017. In the care-worker category, nine interns were trained and sent to Japan by Navis Nihongo in early 2019.

Another more recent cooperation initiative with Japan is the Basic Framework for Partnership for Proper Operation of the System Pertaining to "Specified Skilled Workers". This memorandum of cooperation was signed between India and Japan in January 2021 and would enable Indian workers skilled in nursing to work in Japan, provided they know the Japanese language. The aim is to enhance people-to-people contact and to foster the mobility of skilled workers through an institutional mechanism for partnership and cooperation between the two countries. These Indian workers would be granted a new status of residence of "specified skilled worker" by the Government of Japan.[37]

There are a few other bilateral MoUs which currently do not cover health personnel but offer scope to do so in future. For instance, India's MoU with Australia in the field of health and medicine is broadly on cooperation across a range of issues, including communicable and non-communicable diseases, digital health, and medical devices and pharmaceuticals, but does not list health worker mobility. However, it has a provision to cover "any other area of cooperation decided mutually between the two countries" and is thus potentially extendable to addressing health worker mobility. Likewise, another bilateral arrangement where there is a scope to cover health worker skilling and mobility is the Indo-German Programme for Vocational Education and Training (IGVET). The aim of this programme is to develop cooperative training opportunities by piloting such training in clusters of companies in a specific region or sector, which is represented by a chamber of industry body.[38] The Ministry of Skill Development and Entrepreneurship (MSDE) is the nodal ministry, and the counterpart is the German Federal Ministry for Economic Cooperation and Development (BMZ). At present, this programme covers sectors such as automotive, construction, retail, and life sciences, but does not cover any occupational category under the health sector. According to experts, this programme can be a useful model for skilling and for providing apprenticeship opportunities to selected health sector workers in future.

Overall, India's engagement on health worker mobility and related issues of ethical recruitment, welfare, return, reintegration appears to be limited under its bilateral arrangements. Its MoUs and cooperation frameworks tend to be quite loose and broadly worded. Details of MoUs and agreements between state-level recruitment agencies and West Asian governments, are not available publicly to gauge the coverage of issues. What is evident, however, is that in recent years, there is a shift towards training and capacity building under these cooperation frameworks. Thus, there seems to be a growing emphasis on deployment alongside developing domestic capacity and upgrading of quality, including certification of training in consultation with partners. The MSDE has emerged as an important focal ministry in such endeavours and innovative training and apprenticeship arrangements are being framed. However, the coverage of the health sector is very limited till date and within health, the focus has been on care-workers and not occupations such as nurses or technicians, to avoid regulatory overlap in certification and training with professional councils governing these other health care occupations.

Trade and Comprehensive Agreements

India has also approached health worker mobility in the context of its preferential trade agreements. Under these agreements, commitments have been made in mode 4 for the temporary mobility of service providers, including in the health sector, and provisions have been included to facilitate mobility and mutual recognition of qualifications with partners. Table 8.8 presents the mode 4 commitments India has received from partner countries in mode 4 of health services under several of its Free Trade Agreements (FTAs).

As can be seen, all market access commitments by India's FTA partners are unbound for movement of health workers under all the applicable subsectors, except as scheduled in the horizontal commitments under mode 4.[39] Hence, FTA partners have not been willing to facilitate mobility of health workers from India. Under the India–ASEAN FTA, ASEAN member countries have made commitments in a variety of health services subsectors but for mode 4, they have left their commitments unbound, referring to their horizontal commitments or scheduling limitations relating to licences, place of practice, and nature of work (charitable purposes only, ownership and management of private hospitals). However, some of the ASEAN members have made horizontal market access commitments for intra-corporate transferees and selected categories of providers in the health services sector. There are a few exceptions. For example, in the case of veterinary services, Korea has made an unrestricted commitment for the mobility of veterinary service providers from India. National treatment commitments are relatively less restrictive, with full commitments in case of certain categories of health workers, and in some cases subject to conditions of practice. In the India–Malaysia CECA, Malaysia has provided national treatment for

Table 8.8 Partners' Scheduled Commitments in Health Worker Related Service Sectors/Subsectors in FTAs with India

| Sector/Subsector | Limitations on | |
	Market Access (MA)	National Treatment (NT)
India–Singapore CECA: Singapore Commitments		
Medical and dental services; Services provided by midwives, nurses, physiotherapists, para-medicals	Unbound#	Unbound
Veterinary Services	Unbound#	Unbound
Hospital Services	Unbound#	Unbound
Other Human Health Services: ambulance services, acute care hospitals, nursing homes, and convalescent run on a commercial basis	Unbound#	Unbound
India–Japan CEPA: Japan Commitments		
Medical and dental services; Services provided by midwives, nurses, physiotherapists, para-medicals	Unbound.	Unbound. None for physiotherapists and dieticians.
Veterinary services	None.	None.
Hospital Services	Unbound.	None.

(Continued)

Table 8.8 Continued

Sector/Subsector	Limitations on Market Access (MA)	National Treatment (NT)
India–Malaysia CECA: Malaysia commitments		
Medical and dental services; Services provided by midwives, nurses, physiotherapists, para-medicals		
Specialized Medical Services covering forensic medicine, nuclear medicine, geriatrics, microvascular surgery, neurosurgery, cardiothoracic surgery, plastic surgery, clinical immunology and oncology, traumatology, anaesthesiology, intensive care specialist, child psychiatry, and physical medicine	Unbound#	None except: Practice only in private hospitals of at least 70 beds;- Practice to be only at a specified location and change in location requires approval; setting up of individual or joint group practices is not permitted. *Related Additional Commitment by Malaysia is that the qualifying examination to determine the competence and ability to supply the services for the purposes of registration with professional bodies will be conducted in English.*
Veterinary Services	Unbound#	Unbound#
Hospital Services	Unbound#	Unbound#

Source: Based on Schedules of Commitments in India's FTAs with selected partner countries

Note: # Except as specified in horizontal commitments

contractual service suppliers and independent professionals for specialized medical services, veterinary services, dental specialists (for institutions of higher learning), pharmacists (temporary registered ones with guidelines set by the Pharmacy Board of Malaysia), nurses, paramedics, and physiotherapists, though practice is limited to certain locations and subject to proving competence through a qualifying examination.

Overall, one finds that there is hardly any appetite among FTA partner countries to commit to mobility of Indian health workers into their markets, except in select occupational categories, then too in a very limited way. Notwithstanding the lack of meaningful progress on mode 4 access for health workers in India's FTAs, in request–offer negotiations, mode 4 facilitation in the health services sector remains a common request by India to its FTA partners. For instance, in the recent Regional Comprehensive Economic Partnership (RCEP) negotiations, one of India's requests across RCEP partner countries was the liberalization of market access for health professionals, including for alternative medical practitioners and yoga trainers. Offers made by RCEP partners, however, did not address these requests, indicating continued unwillingness to negotiate mode 4 in health services.

The same restrictiveness is also visible in India's scheduled mode 4 commitments in the health services sector. As seen in Table 8.9, India has left its commitments unbound, for market access and national treatment, excepting for charitable purposes in some FTAs and contingent on finalizing MRAs with its partners in certain FTAs. Like its partner countries, its commitments are often subject to the horizontal commitments, indicating the absence of health sector-specific liberalization of mode 4 conditions. In the India–ASEAN FTA, India has inscribed conditions relating to information and documentation to support mode 4 applications by health care personnel, minimum wages, and additional requirements for educational and professional qualifications for providers from certain ASEAN member countries.

As seen above, neither India nor its FTA partners have made meaningful commitments on health worker mobility. Although both sides have committed more health subsectors in their FTAs than under the GATS, mode 4 commitments have remained restrictive. However, if we compare the commitments made to India by partners such as Japan where there is a need for health workers versus those made by these same partners to other potential source countries for health workers, such as Indonesia and the Philippines, we find that India has received fewer liberal commitments. Take for instance, the provisions regarding the movement of health workers in the Japan–Vietnam Economic Partnership Agreement (JVEPA) of 2008. There are two commitments by Japan granting entry for one to three years for a natural person of Vietnam who has qualified under Japanese law by passing the nursing examination in Japanese as well as an undertaking to negotiate within two years from entry into force of the agreement the possibility of accepting Vietnamese qualified nurses.

Table 8.9 India's Scheduled Mode 4 Commitments in Health Worker Related Sectors/Subsectors

FTA	Sector/Subsector	Limitations on	
		Market Access (MA)	National Treatment (NT)
India–Singapore CECA	Medical and dental services; Services provided by midwives, nurses, physiotherapists, para-medicals	Unbound pending finalization of MRA	Unbound pending finalization of MRA
	Veterinary services	Unbound#	Unbound#
	Hospital Services	Unbound	Unbound#
India–Korea CEPA	Medical and dental services; Services provided by midwives, nurses, physiotherapists, para-medicals	Unbound#. None for charitable purposes for Medical and Dental.	Unbound#
	Veterinary services	Unbound#	Unbound#
	Hospital Services	Unbound#. None for charitable purposes.	Unbound#
India–Japan CEPA	Medical and dental services; Services provided by midwives, nurses, physiotherapists, para-medicals	Unbound. None for charitable purposes for Medical and Dental services.	Unbound.
	Veterinary Services	Unbound.	Unbound.
	Hospital Services	Unbound. None for charitable purposes.	Unbound.
India–Malaysia CECA	Medical and dental services; Services provided by midwives, nurses, physiotherapists, para-medicals	Unbound. None for charitable purposes for Medical and Dental services.	Unbound.
	Veterinary services	Unbound.	Unbound.
	Hospital services	Unbound. None for charitable purposes.	Unbound.
India–ASEAN FTA	Medical and dental services; Services provided by midwives, nurses, physiotherapists, para-medicals	Unbound. Not committed w.r.t. Philippines.	Unbound. Not committed w.r.t. Philippines.
	Veterinary services	Not committed.	Not committed.
	Hospital services	Unbound#	Unbound#

Source: Based on Schedules of Commitments in India's FTAs with selected partner countries

The provisions are similar in the Japan–Philippines EPA of 2009 and the Indonesia–Japan EPA of 2008.[40] Under these FTAs, Japan has granted entry and temporary stay to natural persons who engage in supplying services as nurses or certified care-workers or related activities, based on a contract with public or private organizations in Japan or on admission to public or private training facilities in Japan, who are selected and presented by the administration of their country of origin. Such access is for the purpose of obtaining a qualification as a nurse/certified care-worker under Japanese law or for the purpose of pursuing a training course including Japanese language training for six months followed by acquiring required knowledge and skills at the designated hospital or caregiving facility, during a renewable one-year period. They can take the examinations up to three times and duration of stay can be extended accordingly. Thus, a simple comparison of Japan's FTA with India and that with other partners suggests that there is scope for India to better leverage its agreements and to secure more market access and less restrictive conditions.

One important aspect of these agreements, however, is the provisions they contain on issues such as mutual recognition of qualifications and regulatory cooperation in general. For instance, the Article on Recognition in the India–Malaysia CECA notes that, "after the entry into force of this Agreement, the Parties shall encourage their relevant authorities or professional bodies in the service sectors such as accounting and auditing, architecture, medical (doctors), dental and nursing to negotiate and conclude, within 12 months or a reasonable period of time from the date of entry into force of this Agreement, any such agreements or arrangements providing mutual recognition of the education or experience obtained, qualification requirements and procedures, and licensing requirements and procedures". Although progress in framing such mutual recognition agreements has been slow due to resistance from regulatory bodies and difficulties in harmonization, this is one area where there is scope to use regulatory cooperation mechanisms built into trade agreements to facilitate and manage health worker mobility in a mutually beneficial manner. For instance, building on the India–Singapore Comprehensive Economic Cooperation Agreement (CECA) which came into force in 2005, India entered into an MRA in nursing services with Singapore. This agreement was signed in 2018 and establishes mutual recognition of education, experience obtained, licensing and certification requirements to facilitate the mobility of registered nurses. It identifies seven recognized training institutions from India and four from Singapore.[41] Applications are accepted from nurses who hold valid professional nursing qualifications from the sending country, provided they have no record of violating technical or ethical standards. The host country will evaluate their qualifications, register, and licence them. It will allow them to practice in the host country and monitor their conduct and practise to ensure standards are maintained. Additional requirements such as submission of personal medical examination reports, competency tests, induction programme, etc. may be additionally required by the regulatory authority in the host country.

In sum, the experience with India's approach to managing mobility of health workers through preferential trade agreements suggests that unless countries are willing to extend the coverage of their sectoral commitments in health services and make more liberal market access commitments for a greater range of health workers, at least for India, they have not been very useful as migration management instruments. However, a comparative analysis with other FTAs suggests that there is scope to leverage these agreements better. This will require a more strategic approach to the request–offer process during services negotiations to ensure that there is more specificity in the way concerns and sensitivities are addressed in mode 4 for health services, failing which the commitments would become largely uniform across categories of health workers and blanket restrictive in nature as is the case currently. This is where an understanding of specific needs in individual categories of health workers, mapping demand–supply gaps, and taking a more targeted approach to occupational groups within the health sector, may be useful. Another area to leverage further is the cooperation chapters of these agreements which can provide the basis to enter into MRAs for selected occupational categories. MRA discussions would be of mutual benefit by helping benchmark to international standards and forcing an upgrading of quality to meet the partner countries' requirements.

One aspect that is not addressed in the schedules for health services is ethics and welfare. Reference to issues such as post entry conditions of work, ethical recruitment practices, and welfare of health workers is completely absent from the mode 4 commitments. These are not inscribed in the additional commitments either. A review of the FTA schedules suggests that there may be scope to address such concerns bilaterally and to make binding additional commitments to honour such obligations. This would go one step further than the bilateral MoUs and international protocols which are largely driven by voluntary obligations while mode 4 commitments made under a trade agreement, would be legally binding, giving them more teeth.

Primary Evidence on Managing Health Worker Mobility

To get a ground level understanding of the thinking behind India's approach to managing health worker mobility and recent initiatives in this regard, discussions were carried out with experts. The latter included central government officials engaged in skilling and certification initiatives in India as well as private agencies at the state level who are engaged in recruitment and deployment processes. The idea was to not only understand some important features of India's health worker related mobility and capacity building strategies but to also get public and private sector perspectives on the scope for using bilateral arrangements for managing such mobility.

The discussions revealed that there is indeed scope to approach this issue through bilateral initiatives and cooperation frameworks with certain destination countries and that many mutual benefits can be derived from such cooperative management.

A key feature that emerged from these discussions on India's recent approach to health worker mobility was the increased focus on skilling and certification and the viewing of international mobility as part of a larger goal of augmenting domestic availability and quality of healthcare workers and of creating employment opportunities through training and pathways for career advancements. Discussions with the NSDC and the Healthcare Skills Council highlighted the government's focus on skilling persons in less visible segments such as allied health professionals and care-workers, who could be trained more quickly. The focus on this occupational category was seen as addressing the objective of improving domestic health care capacity by relieving the burden on nurses and of simultaneously meeting the growing global demand for such providers, especially in the areas of geriatric and home care. The MSDE's partnership MoU with Japan was mentioned wherein 300,000 trained caregivers are to be sent to Japan over the next five years. Training would be provided through a network of 600 training partners (e.g., Apollo Medskills) and 110 training centres which would equip them for working in different host countries. This skilling programme for care-workers has also been linked to healthcare organizations and hospitals for providing hands-on, real life training. The NSDC official noted that the caregiver segment presented a great opportunity as it is not in the WHO's list of critical shortage occupations for India and is also subject to fewer restrictions, being outside the purview of established regulatory authorities, although ethical and welfare considerations would be particularly important in case of such providers.

Respondents highlighted the immense domestic benefits that could be derived from a cooperative and bilaterally managed approach for the caregiver segment. They noted the positive effect it would have in terms of benchmarking Indian standards for this neglected category of health workers, and that it would help raise their numbers, improve domestic quality, and create job opportunities for this less skilled section with wider income and developmental benefits. The focus on certification mechanisms would also lead to our qualifications and training getting accepted by other countries, even if incrementally. Respondents noted that due to such efforts, our standards are increasingly being accepted abroad for such segments and that interest is being expressed by some governments to hire these providers. NSDC is currently discussing mutual recognition of qualifications with several governments and the ILO and has entered into some MoUs with countries. According to one NSDC official, creating recognition for categories like caregivers, home assistants, geriatric aides, would not only facilitate their mobility to other countries but would also give them self-respect and dignity in their jobs within India. It was also highlighted that these initiatives are being seen within the larger national framework of skilling and certification programmes such as the Pradhan Mantri Kaushal Yojana (PMKY), as the aim is to align all similar schemes and avoid duplication and wastage of resources.

Another segment that was highlighted as having scope for mobility was that of alternative health practitioners. In recent FTA negotiations such as RCEP, India has made requests to its FTA partners to grant market access to such providers, including yoga trainers and Ayurveda practitioners. Till date, the lack of a standardized training and certification system has undermined India's ability to secure market access and national treatment for this section of health care practitioners in its trade and other bilateral agreements. In view of the huge opportunities and growing demand for alternative health systems and interest in general well-being, the Indian government, through the Ministry of Ayurveda, Yoga, Naturopathy, Unani, Siddha, Sowa-Rigpa and Homoeopathy (AYUSH) is trying to establish a credible certification scheme for AYUSH and Panchakarma practitioners as well as yoga instructors. There are requests from some countries which will require standardization of training for alternative practitioners in India. Benchmarks have been established and training is to be initiated. There have already been discussions with the Government of Finland to mutually recognize the primary learning and training of trainers for yoga under the Wellness Skills Council. If such recognition is realized, there would be a big opportunity to send certified yoga trainers.

In contrast to segments such as care-workers and alternative health system practitioners, in the case of nursing, the most prominent segment involving mobility, discussions indicated the significance of bilateral agreements and MoUs between state governments and state-authorized recruitment agencies and partner countries to manage nursing mobility. For instance, the Kerala government has bilateral agreements with the Ministries of Health and private hospitals in Saudi Arabia, UAE, Oman, and Qatar. It also has agreements with NHS hospitals in the UK. Similarly, the states of Karnataka, Andhra Pradesh, West Bengal, Tamil Nadu, and Uttar Pradesh also have MoUs with other governments for the movement of nurses. These agreements allow the supply of nurses from India on a service charge basis. These MoUs require the recruitment agency to check educational, experience, and other qualifications, and helps present eligible candidates to the employer overseas. Upon selection, the agency is responsible for all document verifications and checks, ensuring completion of additional tests and requirements by the selected nurses, and overall ensuring that no fraudulent candidate is sent abroad. These agencies work as direct partners under the MoUs or through subsidiary agencies. There are some differences, however, that apply across different destination countries. For instance, the Middle Eastern countries have a separate rule in that recruitment agencies cannot charge more than Rs.30,000 per candidate. In the case of the European countries, there are no restrictions on service charges. In the case of the UK, there are restrictions on recruitment from states such as Andhra Pradesh, Madhya Pradesh, West Bengal, and Odisha, which are identified as having a shortage of nurses (though this restriction only applies if the nurse is working in these states, not if the nurse is practising in another state which does not fall under the shortage state category). Recruited nurses are provided with a 3-year work permit for earning, learning, and returning. Overall, it is evident that in the case of nurse recruitment and mobility, the system is well institutionalized through bilateral arrangements which involve a network of agencies and intermediaries. A majority of these MoUs, however, are not available publicly, making it difficult to understand how well they address the gamut of issues concerning health worker mobility.[42]

According to all respondents, there are several promising potential markets with which India could enter into such cooperation frameworks. These include the Middle East region, the UK, Germany, and Japan. Discussions are underway with the governments of Japan and Germany. Other potential markets are Canada (the province of Quebec has approached the Indian government to meet their needs in the health sector) and Australia. However, as the developed countries are very particular about standards, for bilateral arrangements to be framed with these markets, increased focus would be needed on training, bridging gaps, improving soft skills like communication, benchmarking with their requirements, and evolving credible certification systems that are recognized by partner countries. With the Middle Eastern markets, while alignment with their requirements would remain important, greater focus would need to be put on working conditions and welfare issues.

Overall, all respondents were of the view that MoUs and bilateral labour agreements can play an important role in facilitating the mobility of health workers from India to different countries. Their advantage is that they can be customized to cover different categories of health workers, including less discussed ones such as pharmacists, medical assistants, geriatric caregivers, physiotherapists, and radiologists, among others. Respondents noted that such arrangements are suited to cover a wide range of issues, starting with skilling and certification, mutual acceptance of qualifications, pre-departure and financial training, monitoring of recruitment and deployment practices, welfare, and working conditions, among others. By inscribing provisions that enable a long duration of work overseas (for as long as 7 years in some agreements) along with incentives for return and reapplication in future, these arrangements can facilitate circular mobility, allaying concerns about brain drain while enabling knowledge and skill transfer and upgradation of quality, with gains to both India and receiving countries.

The discussions also revealed some internal and external challenges in framing and utilizing bilateral arrangements. One internal problem highlighted by respondents was the lack of coherence in the government's approach to skilling and issues with institutional coordination. For instance, the Ministry of Skills was authorized to provide skilling in a very limited number of job roles in the health sector (vision technicians, radiology technicians, refractionists, etc.) but not nurses. Moreover, many of its training courses have been deactivated. Only a few of the courses under its purview, such as those for home health aides, general duty assistants, and geriatric care-workers, remain. This limits the Skills Ministry's ability to address a wide range of health workers through skilling and certification initiatives. In addition, the training courses that have been set up under the Ministry are of very short duration (three months) whereas other countries require nine months or more of rigorous training. Hence, even where skilling is being provided, the quality and rigour of the training can be questioned, and it would be difficult to get recognition of Indian qualifications. Hence, if these skilling and certification programmes under the Skills Ministry are to be leveraged to facilitate the mobility of selected categories of health workers, they will need to be better aligned with the requirements of destination countries. This is particularly important in the case of developed countries such as Australia and Germany which at a bare minimum recognize nursing qualifications, thus precluding access for categories such as home health aides and assistants, who do not meet these minimum qualification requirements.

A second challenge pointed out by respondents relates to language and culture which are major barriers in the case of key destination markets such as Germany, France, and Japan. For instance, even though India has entered into a partnership arrangement with Japan, the likelihood of Indian nurses learning the Japanese language and acclimatizing to the Japanese culture is low. This is evident from the fact that in the past three years, not more than 100 Indian care-workers have been sent to Japan under the Technical Training Internship Programme. Destination countries like Japan also have their preference for certain source countries, such as the Philippines and Vietnam. Although the Indian government has targeted sending 300,000 caregivers to Japan by 2022, according to one respondent, it may be difficult to send more than 3,000 such workers to Japan by then. Thus, bilateral arrangements may not be as effective in the case of non-English-speaking countries due to linguistic and cultural factors which inhibit demand from the partner country as well as interest on the part of Indian health workers.

Several other challenges were also highlighted such as the multiplicity of ministries, agencies, regulatory bodies that are involved in the process of health worker mobility and resulting problems of alignment in approach and goals. Added to this is the presence of state and central government involvement at various levels. It was pointed out that there needs to be greater clarity on who does what and commitment to the plans made rather than shifting stance as has happened with some of the skilling initiatives. Long-term investment in building systems and both public and private capacities is thus needed, which countries such as the Philippines have done.

The primary evidence thus confirmed the possibilities for using bilateral cooperation agreements and partnership initiatives more strategically than India has done so far. It emphasized the importance of both public and private sector engagement in facilitating mobility of health workers while balancing ethical, welfare, and larger social objectives. At the same time, it made evident the limitations to using such frameworks for managing health worker mobility. It was thus suggested that engagement with potential partner countries needs to be framed within an umbrella agreement on all the issues that will be addressed. Government-to-government dialogue has to be the entry point. Trade agreements can serve as such an umbrella. Their cooperation chapters can be used to pursue regulatory cooperation on a range of issues, including licensing, visas, skilling, recognition, etc. along with progressive liberalization commitments in mode 4 for health workers under the schedules of commitments. In parallel, B2B and B2G discussions as well as sector and occupation specific strategies can be pursued, for which the overarching framework and the governments can be leveraged whenever needed.

Concluding Thoughts and Future Considerations

With the growing global demand for health workers and challenging source country conditions which incentivize the movement of health care providers to more affluent markets with better pay and working conditions, the need to balance private incentives with the larger public good has never been so great. In a post-COVID world, this pressure will only increase as countries focus more on building healthcare capacity and their workforce. Amidst ageing populations, health worker shortages, and increased thrust on building health systems in receiving countries, the significance of source countries such as India will continue. As human resources for health are a global public good, a coordinated response between major receiving and sending countries is needed to manage the mobility of healthcare workers. This is possible through bilateral and global collaboration frameworks and agreements.

As a major sending country, India's participation in global protocols concerning health worker mobility, its bilateral arrangements with destination countries, and its national approach to developing and managing human resources for health are significant for the global community. The discussion in this chapter has highlighted that India needs policies that enable its health workers to realize their potential to utilize their skills and advance their careers, be it in the domestic or international market while also ensuring that their rights are protected during recruitment and in the workplace, and that domestic capacity is not compromised. This requires well-coordinated and coherent strategies that involve the public and private sector, and which focus on training (including language and cultural training), raising domestic standards, and harmonizing them with those of partners, credential recognition, ethical practices in recruitment, return, and reintegration, with due recognition of overseas work experience and skills acquired, among others.

Wider trade and economic cooperation/partnership agreements have the potential to provide the broader framework within which these initiatives can be undertaken. They also provide the scope to make legally binding commitments to address market access and national treatment conditions in specific subsectors and occupational categories of health services. The cooperation chapters and additional commitment provisions in these agreements can be leveraged for framing bilateral arrangements like MoUs and labour mobility agreements, which are specific to services like health. To date, however, analysis of these agreements in terms of their coverage of health and related mobility provisions and commitments suggests that India has not really used its existing trade agreements to provide such a framework. It has not strategically pursued specific interests, occupational categories, or issues concerning health workers in these agreements. However, the shift in emphasis towards skilling and capacity building and addressing the mobility of health workers within this larger context, coupled with better monitoring and regulation of emigration, is a step in the right direction.

Going forward, in addition to more strategic use of trade and other economic agreements, several other initiatives and issues may be worth considering, some of which are proposed here. First, there is scope to integrate health worker mobility initiatives with education and R&D tie-ups with universities and medical training institutions. The latter would make it easier to benchmark and harmonize standards, enter into apprenticeship and training arrangements with identified institutions, identify specific occupational categories of health workers that are of mutual interest, and address linguistic and cultural differences. These steps could pave the way for bilateral labour mobility agreements and recognition of credentials in health with these countries in future. There would also be positive spill overs for education, training and accreditation systems, and standards in India.

A second area where more strategic thinking is needed is the specific occupational segments where there are prospects to facilitate mobility and how their training and certification can be aligned with the requirements of destination countries. Care-workers and geriatric aides are some such segments where there is some focus already in India. There are other segments such as radiology technicians, physiotherapists, pharmacists, among others, which could be considered using benchmarking and training initiatives to cover these occupations under bilateral arrangements. Exploring mobility prospects in some of these segments will have the added benefit of creating employment opportunities directly after school and also for women.

A third issue which requires much more attention than has received till date is that of return and reintegration of health workers. If the aim is to facilitate circular mobility through bilateral agreements and MoUs and not aggravate brain drain, it will be important to simultaneously improve human resource management practices in the Indian healthcare system so that those returning can translate their work experience abroad through promotions, salary increments, or other forms of recognition. Portability of social security benefits may also be useful to consider in these frameworks, wherever applicable.

A fourth issue which has not been discussed sufficiently in India's cooperation frameworks and agreements is the development of a database and an information sharing system with partners to track demand–supply gaps and possibilities for recruitment and training initiatives. For instance, an online integrated labour market information system can be developed which tracks job opportunities in nursing and allied services abroad in selected partner countries along with providing statistics on labour supply and training numbers in India for at least selected health worker occupations that are of mutual interest. Digital mapping and data management systems can be used to capture data about supply and demand conditions, registration of health professionals, and transition and movement of workers within and outside the countries. Such information, if available on a real time or regularly updated basis, can be used to coordinate bilateral efforts in designing training and exchange programmes for health workers, internships, return and reintegration into national health systems, focused programmes and targeted interventions for specific categories and skill sets where there are actual or projected shortages, and address the pull and push factors. This could also potentially help in bringing some control over the private recruitment process digital efforts would, however, require coordination across multiple agencies and government departments, including the Ministries of Health, Education, professional councils and associations and immigration authorities, and private recruitment agencies and intermediaries. There are examples from certain regions like the East African Community which have developed digital platforms for tracking and monitoring health worker migration, which could serve as examples.

Finally, there is a need for more evidence-based management of health worker mobility. The evidence from India suggests that there isn't a well-articulated, long-term strategy. Rather, policies seem to be driven by demands from different partner countries on one side and labour market dynamics and actors and state-level dynamics on the other. A well-crafted migration management strategy requires both stock taking and review. It requires an understanding of good practices from other countries, analysis of the evidence from existing or earlier agreements that India has entered into, and a review of the features that worked and those which failed. Similarly, the experience with covering mode 4 issues in general and specifically in the case of health services under trade and comprehensive economic cooperation/partnership arrangements, needs to be assessed. Such an evidence-based approach can help inform future mobility arrangements and also strengthen existing ones. However, once again, coordination across multiple stakeholders within and outside government will be critical. To a large extent, the success or failure of mobility partnerships and cooperation frameworks in the health sector and also more generally, will depend on the ability to bring different stakeholders together and to develop a coherent strategy that balances private, national, and international interests.

Notes

1 Paul Kagame, President of the Republic of Rwanda, Africa 2016 Summit.
2 Trines (2018).
3 https://www.who.int/whr/2006/overview/en/
4 Data for 2017; https://data.worldbank.org/indicator/SH.MED.PHYS.ZS
5 Mobility and migration are used interchangeably throughout this chapter.
6 Elliott (2019).
7 Trines (2018).
8 Push and pull factors include higher remuneration in rich countries, better working environment and infrastructure, training and specialization opportunities, incentives offered by host countries and aggressive recruitment drives by rich countries while the push factors include low wages, poor human resource management practices and work environment, political, and economic instability, among others.
9 Walton-Roberts and Rajan (2020).
10 Elliot (2019).
11 Chisholm (2019).
12 Elliot (2019).
13 Chisholm (2019) and Shaffer et al. (2019).
14 Chisholm (2019).
15 It is important to note that foreign-born health professionals are not necessarily reflective of migrating professionals, but these figures are nevertheless indicative.
16 See, WHO (2010a), (2010b), Commonwealth Code of Practice (2002), Department of Health (2004), Melbourne Manifesto (2002).
17 WTO (1994).
18 PAHO has provided technical training to a large number of persons who previously had only in-service hospital training and has qualified them as auxiliary nurses, supported their conversion into nursing technicians and progressively converted auxiliaries and technicians to professional nurses.
19 Yeates and Pillinger (2018).
20 This network has been established through Health Systems Trust (HST) South Africa and University of Namibia, Namibia in cooperation with the Regional Health Secretariat East, Central and Southern Africa (ECSA-HC).
21 Carzaniga et al. (2019).
22 https://www.giz.de/en/worldwide/18715.html
23 https://www.giz.de/en/worldwide/69851.html
24 Carzaniga et al. (2019).
25 Batalova (2020) and Batalova and Fix (2020).
26 Walton-Roberts and Rajan (2020).
27 NORKA refers to Non-Resident Keralite Affairs, ODEPC refers to Overseas Development and Employment Promotion Consultants, OMCAP refers to Overseas Manpower Corporation of Andhra Pradesh, OMCL refers to Overseas Manpower Corporation Limited, TOMCOM refers to Telangana Overseas Manpower Corporation.
28 Chandna (2021).
29 Chandna (2021).
30 The WHO estimates the need to double the number of domestic nurses if India has to bridge its shortfall.
31 Rao et al (2016), https://apps.who.int/gho/data/view.main.HWF10v,and https://apps.who.int/gho/data/view.main.HWF10WHOREGv?lang=en
32 The Emigration Act, 1983 aimed to facilitate recruitment of Indian workers abroad on best possible terms and conditions of employment (Sasikumar and Hussain 2008). It has, however been ineffective in monitoring or regulating the

flow of skilled or highly skilled professionals such as health professionals as these occupations are not covered by the Act.

33 PTI (2020).

34 Buchan et al. (2008).

35 Murthy (2019) and MHLW (2017).

36 https://www.labournet.in/titp-japan/#:~:text=LabourNet%20is%20one %20among%20the,of%20three%20to%20five%20years

37 Dhasmana (2021).

38 https://www.giz.de/en/worldwide/62831.html

39 In services negotiations, countries made sectoral and horizontal (cross-sectoral) commitments. In the case of mode 4, countries have generally made unbound entries, meaning no commitments have been made, and have referred to their horizonal commitments. The entries are either "none" meaning unrestricted, "unbound" meaning no commitment, and partial meaning commitments with limitations and conditions. Market access commitments relate to the extent and nature of entry to be permitted to foreign service suppliers while national treatment commitments refer to the treatment of foreign versus domestic service suppliers following entry into the host market.

40 Carzaniga et al. (2019).

41 INC (2017).

42 Respondents noted that there are violations of terms and conditions which can be obtained through the Ministry of External Affairs in case of the 18 ECR destination countries. The enforcement status of the MoUs in case of other markets may only be possible to gauge in a few years' time once the registration data for nurses becomes available from the E-Migrate system (as nurses going to Europe are now required to mandatorily register under this system).

References

Batalova, J. (2020). "Immigrant Health-Care Workers in the United States", https:// www.migrationpolicy.org/article/immigrant-health-care-workers-united-states -2018#Pre-COVID-19%20Trends%20and%20Projections

Batalova, J., & Michael Fix, M. (2020). "As U.S. Health-Care System Buckles under Pandemic, Immigrant & Refugee Professionals Could Represent a Critical Resource", https://www.migrationpolicy.org/news/us-health-care-system-coronavirus -immigrant-professionals-untapped-resource (accessed January 3, 2021).

Blacklock, C., Heneghan, C., Mant, D., & Ward, A.M. (2012). "Effect of UK Policy on Medical Migration: A Time Series Analysis of Physician Registration Data", *Human Resources for Health*, 10(35), 1–9.

Buchan, J., Baldwin, S., & Munro, M. (2008). "Migration of Health Workers: The UK Perspective to 2006", OECD Health Working Paper No. 38. Organisation for Economic Co-operation and Development (OECD), Paris. https://www .oecd-ilibrary.org/docserver/228550573624.pdf?expires=1613240838&id=id &accname=guest&checksum=97091256356A83C50CA552D2B1FE94A0

Carzaniga, A.G., Dhillon, I.S., Magdeleine, J., & Xu, L. (2019). "International Health Worker Mobility and Trade in Services", WTO Staff Working Paper No. ERSD-2019-13, World Trade Organization (WTO), Geneva.

Chandna, H. (2021). "Ireland to Malta, UAE to Belgium — All Want Indian Nurses, Offer Better Pay and Perks", https://theprint.in/health/ireland-to-malta -uae-to-belgium-all-want-indian-nurses-offer-better-pay-and-perks/612606/ (accessed April 19, 2021).

Chisholm, G. (2019). "Migration and Mobility", Brief for the 2nd Review of Relevance and Effectiveness of the WHO Global Code of Practice on the International Recruitment of Health Personnel. https://www.who.int/docs/default -source/health-workforce/eag2/2nd-review-of-code-relevance-and-effectiveness -evidence-brief-3-thet.pdf?sfvrsn=541bdee3_2

Connell, J. (2010). "Migration of Health Workers in the Asia-Pacific Region", Technical Report Series, University of New South Wales, Human Resources for Health Knowledge Hub of the School of Public Health and Community Medicine.

Department of Health, UK. (2004). "Code of Practice for the Healthcare Professionals", London, United Kingdom (UK). http://www.nursingleadership .org.uk/publications/codeofpractice.pdf

Dhasmana, I. (2021). "Indian Skilled Workers to Get Job Opportunities in 14 Sectors in Japan", https://www.business-standard.com/article/economy-policy/indian -skilled-workers-to-get-job-opportunities-in-14-sectors-in-japan-121010600806 _1.html (accessed January 7, 2021).

Dhillon, I.S., Clark, M.E., & Kapp, R.H. (2010). *A guidebook on bilateral agreements to address health worker migration*, Aspen Institute, Realizing Rights/Global Health & Development.

Elliot, R. (2019). "Health Care Labour Markets and International Health Worker Migration", Brief for the 2nd Review of Relevance and Effectiveness of the WHO Global Code of Practice on the International Recruitment of Health Personnel. https://cdn.who.int/media/docs/default-source/health-workforce/eag2/2nd -review-of-code-relevance-and-effectiveness-evidence-brief-6-healthcare-labour -markets-and-international-health-worker-migration.pdf?sfvrsn=3f354795_2

GMC. (2020). *The state of medical education and practice in the UK.* London: General Medical Council (GMC). https://www.gmc-uk.org/-/media/documents/ somep-2020_pdf-84684244.pdf?la=en&hash=F68243A899E21859AB1D31866 CC54A0119E602

IHME. (2018). *Findings from the global burden of disease study 2017.* Seattle, WA: Institute for Health Metrics and Evaluation (IHME).

INC. (2018). *The comprehensive economic agreement between the Republic of India and the Republic of Singapore mutual recognition agreement on nursing services.* New Delhi: Indian Nursing Council (INC). http://www.indiannursingcouncil.org /uploads/pdf/16001723668534003245f60b14e8d7c1.Pdf

MHLW. (2017). "Memorandum of Cooperation on the Technical Intern Training Program Between the Ministry of Justice, the Ministry of Foreign Affairs and the Ministry of Health, Labour and Welfare of Japan and the Ministry of Skill Development and Entrepreneurship of the Government of India", Tokyo: Ministry of Health, Labour and Welfare (MHLW), Japan. https://www.mhlw .go.jp/file/06-Seisakujouhou-11800000-Shokugyounouryokukaihatsukyoku /0000180846.pdf

MITI. (2011). "Comprehensive Economic Cooperation Agreement Between the Government of Malaysia and the Government of the Republic of India', Kuala Lumpur: Ministry of International Trade and Industry, Malaysia. https://fta.miti .gov.my/miti-fta/resources/Malaysia-India/MICECA.pdf

MITI. (2014). "Agreement on Trade in Services under the Framework Agreement on Comprehensive Economic Cooperation between the Association of Southeast Asian Nations and the Republic of India', Kuala Lumpur: Ministry of International

Trade and Industry, Malaysia. https://fta.miti.gov.my/miti-fta/resources/ASEAN-India/ASEAN-India-Trade_In_Service_Agreement.pdf

MoC. (2005). *Comprehensive economic cooperation agreement between the Republic of India and the Republic of Singapore.* New Delhi: Ministry of Commerce and Industry (MoC), Government of India. https://dot.gov.in/sites/default/files/India%20Singapore%20CECA%2001.08.2005.pdf

MoC. (2009). *Comprehensive economic partnership agreement between the Republic of Korea and the Republic of India.* New Delhi: Ministry of Commerce and Industry (MoC), Government of India. https://dot.gov.in/sites/default/files/India%20Korea%20CEPA%2007.08.2009.pdf

MoFA. (2011).*Comprehensive economic partnership agreement between Japan and the Republic of India.* Tokyo: Ministry of Foreign Affairs of Japan. https://www.mofa.go.jp/region/asia-paci/india/epa201102/pdfs/ijcepa_ba_e.pdf

Murthy, B. (2019). "India – Japan Strengthen Cooperation in Skill Development, Will Bring Scale and Speed to TITP", https://www.nationalskillsnetwork.in/india-japan-strengthen-cooperation-in-skill-development-will-bring-scale-and-speed-to-titp/ (accessed April 27, 2021).

Press Trust of India (PTI). (2020). "Only ECR Passport Holders and Nurses Travelling to 18 Countries need to Obtain Emigration Clearance", https://www.business-standard.com/article/pti-stories/only-ecr-passport-holders-and-nurses-travelling-to-18-countries-need-to-obtain-emigration-clearance-120010301281_1.html (accessed April 19, 2021).

Rao, K.D., Shahrawat, R., & Bhatnagar, A. (2016). "Composition and Distribution of the Health Workforce in India: Estimates based on Data from the National Sample Survey", *WHO South-East Asia Journal of Public Health*, 5(2). http://www.who-seajph.org/temp/WHOSouth-EastAsiaJPublicHealth52133-3673272_101212.pdf

Sasikumar, S.K., & Hussain, Z. (2008). "Managing International Labour Migration from India: Policies and Perspectives", Asia-Pacific Working Paper Series, ILO, International Labour Organization (ILO), Delhi.

Shaffer, F.A., Bakhshi, M.A., Sciasci, N.G., & Álvarez, T. (2019). "Making the WHO Global Code of Practice Actionable for International Healthcare Recruiters", Brief for the 2nd Review of Relevance and Effectiveness of the WHO Global Code of Practice on the International Recruitment of Health Personnel. https://www.who.int/docs/default-source/health-workforce/eag2/2nd-review-of-code-relevance-and-effectiveness-evidence-brief-4-cgfns-and-recruiters-perspective.pdf?sfvrsn=3ecfa2c5_2

Trines, S. (2018). "Mobile Nurses: Trends in International Labour Migration in the Nursing Field", World Education News and Reviews (WENR). https://wenr.wes.org/2018/03/mobile-nurses-trends-in-international-labor-migration-in-the-nursing-field

Walton-Roberts, M., & Irudaya Rajan S. (2020). "Global Demand for Medical Professionals Drives Indians Abroad Despite Acute Domestic Health-Care Worker Shortages", https://www.migrationpolicy.org/article/global-demand-medical-professionals-drives-indians-abroad (accessed January 3, 2021).

WHO. (2010a). "The Global Code of Practice on the International Recruitment of Health Personnel", Sixty-third World Health Assembly, Geneva: World Health Organization (WHO). https://www.who.int/hrh/migration/code/practice/en/

WHO. (2010b). *User's guide to the global code of practice on the international recruitment of health personnel*. Geneva: World Health Organization (WHO). https://apps.who.int/iris/bitstream/handle/10665/70525/WHO_HSS_HRH_HMR_2010.2_eng.pdf;jsessionid=BACA64B1B7FA97907ACD64897ABF8EF7?sequence=1

WHO. (2003). "Commonwealth Code of Practice for the International Recruitment of Health Workers", Pre-World Health Assembly Meeting of Commonwealth Health Ministers, World Health Organization (WHO), Geneva. https://assets.aspeninstitute.org/content/uploads/files/content/images/%7B7BDD970B-53AE-441D-81DB-1B64C37E992A%7D_CommonwealthCodeofPractice.pdf

WHO. (2017). "From Brain Drain to Brain Gain: Migration of Nursing and Midwifery Workforce in the State of Kerala", Report, Geneva: World Health Organization (WHO).

Wonca. (2002). "A Code of Practice for the International Recruitment of Health Care Professionals: The Melbourne Manifesto", 5th World Organization of National Colleges, Academies and Academic Associations of General Practitioners/Family Physicians (Wonca) World Rural Health Conference, Melbourne, Australia. https://ruralhealth.org.au/sites/default/files/other-bodies/other-bodies-02-05-03.pdf

WTO. (1994). "GATS: General Agreement on Trade in Services, Marrakesh Agreement Establishing the World Trade Organization", Annex 1B. Geneva: World Trade Organization (WTO). https://www.wto.org/english/docs_e/legal_e/26-gats.pdf

Yeats, N., & Pillinger, J. (2018). "International Healthcare Worker Migration in Asia Pacific: International Policy Responses", *Asia Pacific Viewpoint*, 59(1), pp. 92–106.

Web Resources (accessed May 14, 2021)

https://apps.who.int/gho/data/view.main.HWF10v

https://apps.who.int/gho/data/view.main.HWF10WHOREGv?lang=en

https://www.giz.de/en/worldwide/18715.html

https://www.giz.de/en/worldwide/62831.html

https://www.giz.de/en/worldwide/69851.html

https://www.labournet.in/titp-japan/#:~:text=LabourNet%20is%20one%20among%20the,of%20three%20to%20five%20years

https://www.nmc.org.uk/about-us/reports-and-accounts/registration-stat

https://www.who.int/whr/2006/overview/en/

OECD Health Workforce Migration Statistics https://stats.oecd.org/Index.aspx?DataSetCode=HEALTH_WFMI (accessed April 27, 2021).

9 The Transmutation of Care and Emotional Labour for a Technologically Advanced Workplace

A Case of Indian Nurse Migration

Neha Adsul

Indian Nurses Crossing Borders

The latest medicines and the newest technologies may have little impact on human health if there are no systems with skilled personnel in place to deliver these health care services. Nurses are and have been the front-line service providers in most health care systems globally (WHO, 2006). A global shortage of nurses now affects both developed and developing countries as the international mobility of nurses has grown significantly in recent decades in response to globalisation and supply–demand dynamics. Drawing cues from recent work on health human resource (HHR), India is an eloquent example of being a nation with the mismatch between health pre-requisites and inadequate HHR even when it continues to experience nursing shortages and a high disease burden (Gill, 2016).

Indian public health institutions face the dual challenge of dealing with an existing shortage of nurses and losing trained nursing personnel to developed countries. Systemic problems like a low social status, public image distortion, poor working conditions, un-stimulating careers, and low salaries are the known push factors that have resulted in the large-scale migration of nurses from India over the past several decades (Kingma, 2008; Kline, 2003; Nair and Webster, 2013). Migration also depends upon the portability of skills, recognition of qualifications, social networks, and active recruitment (Dussault et al., 2009). Mainstream literature on nurse's global migration has been conceptualised through various perspectives, including push-pull, brain-drain, post-colonial ties, and the like.

Against this backdrop, the chapter argues that the labour mobility of Indian nurses is not just an outcome of push-pull processes of migration but also of the techno-social structure, including social networks and training institutions which often reinforce a person's decision to migrate. However, this labour mobility may bring remittances to the country of origin in the absence of initiatives to compensate for the vacuum left by these professionals. Here, a question of significance emerges – What other elements, apart from the traditional push and pull, hold the key to the mobility of nurses from a low human development region to a high development region?

DOI: 10.4324/9781003315124-9

As expressed previously, push and pull forces in a labour market and structural factors that shape nurses' decisions are surely endogenous to the system, but this leaves a huge space for other proxy factors that influence nurse labour market decisions. Presumably, the effects of changes in science and technology tend to be visible in the education and training systems which transform the primary source of labour supply into a workforce that caters to demand labour from an emerging economy. This, in turn, is based on the aforesaid technological change.

Commodifying the Nursing Profession

Developed countries are 'commodifying' by not investing adequate resources in training their health human resources and are looping in the health workforce from resource-poor settings making care-work into a commodity that can be bought and sold in the contemporary global market. This process of importing sufficiently trained health workers to meet their country-specific demand is internationally known as a 'free-rider phenomenon' (Organisation for Economic Co-operation and Development, 2008). Rather than considering the deficit of nurses in their own country as a warning alarm, the recruitment of nurses from developing countries seems to be the 'solution of choice' of the western countries (Kingma, 2006) based on an implicit assumption that migrant nurses were 'essentially available on tap' and that any future skills shortfall nationally could similarly be met from a global skills pool (Brugha et al., 2009).

Despite the on-going debate about how best to manage a nurse's international mobility, nurse migration remains relatively unchecked, uncoordinated, and individualised, such that most resource-poor countries lose their health human resource to developed nations (Brush, 2008). Although there is a lack of comprehensive information, the data available suggests that the emigration of Indian nurses is substantial. Developed nations like the United Kingdom (UK) and the United States of America (USA) are entering into bilateral agreements with India to recruit nurses from India actively. The UK and Kuwait departments of health have an agreement with the government of India primarily to recruit Indian trained nurses and to promote medical tourism (Health Services Union, 2007; Ministry of External Affairs, 2012), whereas the USA has four offices in India which work for gauging the Indian nurse's ability to work in their respective health service delivery system (Health Services Union, 2007; Ministry of External Affairs, 2012; Rao et al., 2011). As per the CARIM/India research report (India Centre for Migration (ICM) New Delhi, 2013), the Indian government maintains the stance of being 'facilitators' for nurse migration against being 'active promoters' of the same. The Commission on Graduates of Foreign Nursing Schools ranked India sixth in the 1990s based on the number of Indian trained nurses applying for the USA visas, and from 2003 onwards, it ranked India second after the Philippines (Matsuno, 2009). As per Kumar and Simi

(2007), India became the principal supplier of nurses to the UK and Ireland, as well as the third-largest source of internationally educated nurses (IEN) in the US and the third- and the fourth-largest supplier of nurses respectively to New Zealand and Canada. India accounted for 10% of IEN in the US in 2008 and 5.3% of the foreign-trained workforce in Canada in 2005 (compared to 30.3% from the Philippines) (Kumar and Simi, 2007). It remains important to assert here that, when such a large number of nurses are on the move, health and healthcare are globally produced.

Partly in response to the increasing overseas opportunities, the numbers of nurse training institutions are increasing in several states of India (Walton-Roberts, 2015; Walton-Roberts et al., 2017; Walton-Roberts and Rajan, 2013, 2020). It remains noteworthy to mention the data recorded till 31 October 2012 on the webpage of the Indian Nursing Council, which reflects that there is a total of 1,578 institutions in India offering a Bachelor of Science (B.Sc.) nursing course out of which 1,485 are private nurse training institutions as against only 9 government training institutions. Out of the total 80,245 B.Sc. nursing seats across India, 75,088 seats are with private colleges, and only 5,157 fall under government nursing institutions. Thus, of the nurse training institutions offering courses in general nursing (B.Sc.), 93.57% are private institutions. In addition to these, the hospitals in the corporate sector also have separate nurse training programmes. At present, the Indian health service delivery system is the most privatised in the world, with the private sector catering to more than 80 percentage of outpatients and 60% of admissions; 71% of health expenditures being out of pocket (Madhukar, 2008; Rao et al., 2011).

The current and emergent Indian health scenario suggests that in India, private capital lies at the centre of health professionals training to better target and capture the emerging health professionals' labour market. Although the migration of nurses is not a new phenomenon, its character seems to have radically changed due to the involvement of private capital, which endorses a 'technological optimism' to compete globally. As asserted by Margaret Walton-Roberts (2015), the health human resource training in the private institutions is always centric to compete in the emerging market, reinforcing the tendency to commodify the health sector, resulting in 'best practices' rooted in a market-oriented spirit. Thus, it is important to scrutinise the surge in migration of nurse labour from India has its roots in the internalisation of technology by training institutions under the relative influence of market forces.

Linking the Philosophy of Science, Technology, and Society to Migration of Nurses – Technological Optimism and Negotiating Nursing Care (?)

The impact of technology on contemporary nursing practice is multifaceted and extensive. Ihde (1990) views technology from two broad perspectives;

utopian and dystopian. The utopian perspective seeks knowledge as a means of gaining power which helps in overcoming human limitation. However, the dystopian perspective views people as being entrapped by technology, and it revolves around the understanding that technology can magnify the objective aspects of human life while reducing subjective qualities. On similar grounds, Sandelowski (1996) leans towards the writings of Ihde (ibid) while analysing technology as an object. She explains her position by stating that it is important to analyse it in such a way to know of the independent force that objects exert through human–machine interactions (how the meaning and hence the importance of these objects/technology changes in a particular context). According to Scarbrough and Corbett (1992), seeing technology as a process helps us recognise the hardware involved and the flows of knowledge associated with that technology. In this way, political factors emerge, such as power and control. By determining the flows of knowledge pertaining to technological usage and by shaping the context for its user, powerful groups, according to Scarbrough and Corbett (ibid), can assert their own interests through the technological process. They usually do this by presenting themselves as experts acting as technical gatekeepers controlling the flow of information.

Barnard (1996) suggests that technology seems to transform the nursing profession and practice in terms of machinery or equipment and the skills nurses develop, the values that they espouse, and how society views nursing. Wilkinson (1992) and Purnell (1998) argue that the healthcare sector is suffering from a 'technological fix' in which the treatment of illness is being left to the mercy of applying appropriate technologies. In this, the nurse is looked at as a 'caring technician' gradually causing a change in the role of nurses from being caregivers to care-takers.

Barnard and Sinclair (2006) assert the balance between technologies and caregiving, especially after the healthcare sector had seen drastic technological advances. Technological advances made it possible to distance a caregiver from the patient, and in this process, the patient's subjectivity experiences faded away, resulting in the objectification of the patient's bodies. If we perpetuate this way of knowing that gives primacy to objective and detached knowledge, the nursing profession will contribute to an impersonal healthcare system in the same way as the biomedical model. Therefore, the aim of care is not immediately to 'fix' the person who is sick but to focus and to see treatment on the whole person, seeing illness as a life-world disturbance and a biological disturbance (Gadamer, 1996).

Sandelowski (2000) argues that technology has been integrated into nursing practice to (re) shape the nursing profession. Thus, the ontological and conceptual boundaries between nursing and technology are becoming increasingly blurred. This is because nurses were never regarded as specialists having various caring skills which supported positive outcomes of the medical treatment as the articulation of the process of 'caregiving' is difficult. Thus, the values of nature, care, women, and empathy, which depict nursing and its importance as a profession in relieving the sick through the human touch, are undermined by technology's veil. This also reflects that only when technology is paired with nature does it occupy a superior position by reference to the ideological system in which nature is 'female' and technology is 'male'. A key feature in Sandelowski's (ibid) writing is the duality or the paradox of technology. Technology has a dual function in demonstrating the role and status of nursing in health care. On the one hand, technology functions to showcase and promote nursing practice while on the other it also renders nurses and their work 'invisible'. What determines whether a technology dehumanises, depersonalises, or objectifies is not technology per se, but rather how individual technologies are used and operate in specific user contexts, the meanings attributed to them, how anyone individual or cultural group defines what is human. The potential of the technique to emphasise efficiency and rationale order (Barnard and Sandelowski, 2001). Emphasising the 'care' aspect of nursing does not mean that technology is extremely detrimental. However, the research reiterates that the human aspect must be preserved and adequately rewarded alongside technical innovations as one increases, so too must the other with the patient in focus. Nurses and women, in general, have been performing the vital work of caregiving; we must demand its recognition and high value and not simply treat it as a gender attribute.

The results presented in this chapter draws on interviews with 29 nurses, 27 were females, and 2 were males. The interviews were conducted at different periods between the year 2016 and 2017. Of the 29 participants, 21 were Christians, whereas the remaining 8 were Hindus. Out of the Christian nurses, 18 nurses belonged to Kerala, and the rest belonged to Maharashtra. The chosen field location was across hospitals in Mumbai. The sample had an equal representation of nurses from public hospitals, missionary hospitals, and private-corporate hospitals. Some nurses like the nursing directors, matrons, and nursing tutors were purposively included in the research. It was believed that their seniority and experience would bring in the added dimension required to justify the research findings. The rest of the nurses were younger nurses, i.e., those who had started working from the year 2000 onwards.

Churning Tech-Savvy Nurses for Export

I begin this section by discussing and understanding the perceptions of senior nurses about the influence of technology and changes in 'caring work relevant to contemporary nursing.'

For most of the senior nurses from the public hospitals, the response to this discussion was that, in their view, caring had to do with establishing a therapeutic relationship with the patients. They felt that caring could not be overlooked even with the advancement of technology as it remains an integral part of determining the treatment outcomes for the patients. They all echoed a similar sentiment that the ethos of nursing called for much emotional work to extend care and compassion to their patients. However, almost all the senior nurses (from the public hospitals) strongly felt that the essence of caring is getting eroded as they felt that the younger generation nurses lack the ability to develop emotional engagements with the patient's and that they contemplate their careers based on the economic opportunities available abroad. This response was similar throughout the group of senior nurses interviewed across all the hospitals. On further probing on areas related to adapting to technological changes and if the technology was changing how nurses viewed the caring work, a senior nurse replied:

> Indeed, now-a-days things have changed from what they were 25-30 years ago ... see I was a GNM and that too I worked all my life here only. Three years ago, I completed my PBB.Sc. I was a sponsored candidate, so I completed it from a private college. In that private college, they have a certain way in which they handle their work ... certain protocols. Talking softly, greeting and everything. They are very young nurses who enroll and with an intention to immediately complete, get training and move (migrate). They have many ventilators there, here also we have, but not many and GNMs cannot use them. They have volumetric syringe pumps, beds which are automatic or very heavy patients are lifted by hoists, they teach them ECG reading, and you know so many small small things including the way you dress and compulsory speaking in English and all that ... here we speak in Marathi and so do the patients. Not that we cannot speak in English but then many of the patients can't. So, they make them completely like MBA's all ready to be shipped. So along with the tag that they get they go abroad...
>
> (Senior Nurse, public hospital)

Some forms of basic technologies that directly assisted the nurse's routine work were considered beneficial, especially by the senior (GH) nurses who linked it to the skewed nurse–patient ratio in the government hospitals. They further stated that such basic technologies are more useful to the nurses in their routine work, as many laborious tasks get done easily, and the nurses can get more time in attending to the patients. However, the idea of touching and caring for the patient's as being a therapeutic activity always underlined the narratives of these nurses. While elaborating on the role of technology in bringing out changes in the caring work of nursing, she said:

> I saw there in that hospital (private hospital from where she finished the PBB.Sc.) they have this thing like sheets, hoists which carries very obese patients from one bed to other and it helps in shifting the patients. Now if we can we have this in the government hospital...this is luxury and its technology too...here we are breaking our backs while carrying patients. So many of our nurses suffer from back pain. Here our

aaiyabai's (female attendant) and ward boys help us in that and sometimes the patient's relatives also do it. I am not complaining as it is
part of the work but there (private hospitals) they don't even touch the
patient's. Here we always show the human side to patients we treat
them with that tender love and care. So our work has not changed.

(Senior Nurse, GH)

The PBB.Sc. (Post Basic BSc)[1] trained senior public hospital nurses seemed to
be well-acquainted with the idea of getting exposed to technological training being associated with overseas migratory prospects. They all were GNM
(General Nursing and Midwifery)[2] nurses, and after being in service for ten
or more years, their training to complete the Bachelor's in Nursing Science
(B.Sc. Nursing) were sponsored by the government. These senior nurses also
mentioned a trend even among the B.Sc. nurses educated in government
hospitals to undergo training from corporate hospitals driven by the desire
to become migration worthy. Expressing their views on how contemporary
nursing (caring work) had changed due to technology, a senior nurse said:

Where do you see young B.Sc. nurses? You tell me ... we don't have
them ... here all our young nurses are GNMs. B.Sc. nursing means
going abroad. Now the nurse's and their parents take loans as the private fees are very high. I saw it during my PBB.Sc ... all these Kerala
girls mostly and now even our Maharashtrian girls are not behind them
... they are all studying by taking borrowing money and parents also do
not hesitate to invest in them because they know that they will get more
returns on that money when their girl goes abroad rather than keeping it in banks! During our times also nurses used to migrate, but they
were mostly girls from Kerala now it's all nothing like region specific...
B.Sc. degree hainna? (You have a B.Sc. degree, isn't it?) chalo! (let's go-
abroad) So obviously getting trained in these hospitals(corporate hospitals) helps them to migrate. These corporate hospital people know the
entire process and they take so much money by assuring them all the
assistance to migrate... I mean they give them transcripts, experience
certificate and all. Just knowing that they are trained from a certain
hospital, with certain kind of machinery they get placed. Exposure ...
exposure to new technology ... they want so that they can migrate.

(Senior Nurse, public hospital)

The narratives of the senior generation public hospital nurses did revolve
around the prioritisation of technological aspects in contemporary nursing
and remain insightful for the fact that, although blurred, they brought to
the forefront the link between the migration of new generation nurses to
the type of institutions (mostly private/corporate) that they get trained in.
The senior nurses interviewed at the mission hospital (MH) very strongly
avowed that technological training had prestige value attached to it as most

of the younger generation nurses were demanding that they be placed in the ICUs during their recruitment interviews itself. The nursing director related it to the fact that the new generation nurses were not joining with a missionary zeal, but this mission hospital was a NABH (National Accreditation Board for Hospitals)[3] approved hospital. She further asserted that, abroad, nurses who have work experience of working in a NABH accredited hospital and have completed some stipulated hours of working as an ICU staff nurse are in great demand. This explains why the new generation (MH) nurses insisted on getting ICU postings. However, she also mentioned that most of the new generation nurses from this mission hospital would migrate to the Gulf countries after acquiring 2–3 years of work experience as a nurse needs a minimum of two years of work experience to work in the Gulf countries. The nursing director (MH) said:

> I see that being technologically exposed and competent increase their chances to migrate. They all demand that they wish to be in the ICU and I exactly know why! They require a certificate at the time of applying for jobs in the Gulf, and there we have to mention clearly as how many hours have these nurses spent in ICU, so that means they require that experience of being trained in ICU. So with ICU comes all these advanced technology as we are an NABH accredited hospital, these nurses are very smart they know that working here they get absorbed there faster. They take experience here and then migrate. So all of them greedily run after the same thing as they must be feeling it gives them chance to migrate, so it's prestigious like that ... Nursing is like a market now you buy nursing services. The ethos is no longer there in these new nurses ... But we don't immediately post them in the ICUs. At the higher management level, we have decided that if and only if a nurse completes at least 1 year in other wards and in rotation posting then only we put them in ICUs else we don't. So by doing this, they[sic] now stay here for 3 years or 4 years because they then are required to make those hours in ICU.
>
> (Nursing Director, mission hospital)

The deputy director of the nursing department of the mission hospital shared many concerns about the issue of huge turnover among the new generation nurses. The new generation nurses trained in the nursing college attached to their mission hospital also did not continue working with them and were migrating overseas in large numbers. As they were unsuccessful in retaining the new generation nurses, this hospital's nursing department started an induction programme for all the newly recruited nurses. During the induction period, which lasted for the initial three months of joining as a nurse, they were treated like interns, although they were paid the full salary and had to take up daily classes. The lectures in the classes were aimed at inculcating the spirit of 'nursing as worship and service to god' amongst the new nurse recruits. The deputy director (MH) strongly felt that the spirit of nursing care is getting eroded among the new generation nurses, and hence, they were planning such training to re-inculcate the lost spirit in the new nurse recruits. Irrespective of putting in all these efforts, this mission hospital continued to deal with the huge turnover of the new generation nurses. The deputy director (MH) blames it on the 'money-minded' new generation nurses who are only in search of migratory opportunities. The deputy director said:

> Clearly speaking even though this is a mission hospital, the new genera-tion nurses do not have any mission in mind to help the poor. When I was a student, almost 40 years ago, we were told that we are in service of humanity, ... in service to God and we felt proud that we were sav-ing the souls! We have a problem of [sic] huge turnover like they (new nurses) stay here for maximum 3–4 years and some even lesser and then they are all moving straight to Gulf. Like I told you, we induct them but nothing ... so obviously they are not faithful to their job but only see it as a chance to earn money as these girls have all become only money minded.
>
> (Deputy Director-Nursing, Mission Hospital)

The nursing director (MH) also had similar views to the deputy director-nursing (MH). The nursing director (MH) also mentioned that they were paying the new nurse recruits a salary of Rs.20,000 per month, which was much higher than the recruits' salaries in the other hospitals across the city. In addition to their salaries, these nurses at the mission hospital had many other added benefits like access to free accommodation, insurance coverage for themselves, and all their meals were provided from the hospital canteen for a meagre payment of only Rs. 2,000 per month. Irrespective of offer-ing all these facilities to the new recruits, the hospital directorial board still struggled to retain the new nurse recruits.

It remains remarkable to note the fact that, as per the narratives of the senior nurses (MH), the new generation nurses from the mission hospital were migrating mostly to the Gulf countries and not to any other developed western countries. This was attributed to the fact that the nurses here were mostly Malayali Christian nurses who had social contacts in the Gulf coun-tries. Gulf countries have easier employment criteria and do not require passing nurse qualifying tests to serve as an easy passage for these new gen-eration nurse migrants. On asking to elaborate on this aspect of the choice of the countries to migrate, a senior nurse tutor (MH) added:

> All of them only go to Gulf, very few here and there like only if their hus-bands are in other countries and these girls have to join them then only. Two important reasons are, first, that they are all mostly Malayali[4] girls who have some or the other relative in Gulf and the other is for working

in Gulf as there they don't have very stringent requirements. They (in Gulf countries) only require two years of work experience, and this is an NABH hospital, so that gives them an advantage, and there are no qualifying tests required for working the Gulf like no IELTS (English language test) or anything which is compulsory in US and all. Also, some of these girls learn to speak proper English after joining here, and in Gulf, that is enough, but in other western countries, you need to clear an English language test with a good score.

(Senior Nurse Tutor, Mission Hospital)

The responses reflect that the new generation nurses' desire to get trained in a technologically intensive setup is rampant, making them overlook the caring work. The senior nurses (MH) shared their thoughts on technology, bringing about a change wherein they felt that present-day nursing care is getting replaced by techno-centric care. The senior nurse tutor's (MH) expressed mixed feelings about the usage of technology in nursing. They felt that some form of technological training overshadows the importance of a humane touch, whereas some other forms of technologies like automatic beds can comfort both the patients and the nurses.

See technology has seeped through nursing, and it has changed the way even nurses look at their profession now. When I was a student, we as nursing students had to give a sponge bath to each other during our practical sessions. So we had this feeling of shame like touching each other so it remained imbibed in us as how a patient will feel when we give a sponge bath to them. We used to soap the patients and talk to them and comfort them. Now the new nurses learn this on a dummy, so it's so mechanical that they don't feel what the patient is going through so there is lack of that emotional connect with the patients. So this dummy can also be called a technology that's detrimental as it lessens the bond between the nurse and patients. Like that, considering automatic beds as technology, they can be very useful for the patients as they can be raised and lowered in height near the head or feet which helps the patient to get on the bed more comfortably. And all this can be done with a button, so it's easier for the nurses also.'

(Senior Nurse Tutor, Mission Hospital)

And;

Technology is helping to manage the patient, but care is not provided by technology as it is the human touch that has a lot of magic. We need to interact with the patient we need to look for the pulse of the patient we cannot just depend upon the pulse oximeter. While looking at the pulse one also needs to engage in talking with the patient, and this is important otherwise even a robot can do this and is the patient going to feel good? Talking, asking about the recovery is all caring as well, isn't it? Now there are digital thermometers that record the temperature changes and then beep once the temperature is recorded, so my job gets done even if I practically don't speak anything with the patient. That is when care is important else it is misuse of technology. The junior nurses get trained in handling technologies, but then they are forgetting these skills. Is it not my responsibility as a nurse that even after the use of the digital thermometer, I should touch the forehead of the patient?

(Senior Nurse Tutor, mission hospital)

In the mission hospital, the senior nurses viewed technology as being of help only in moderation, whereas they also mentioned it playing a major role in dampening the spirit of the nursing profession if not coupled with adequate care. They expressed concern that the new generation nurses considered technology very prestigious, probably because working in technologically intensive units made them migration worthy.

The above discussion highlights that the concerns of the senior generation nurses from the government and the mission hospitals pertaining to the 'caringwork' getting compromised in contemporary nursing stemmed out very strongly. These senior nurses affirmed that the new generation nurses looked at nursing opportunities as the most economically rewarding and a passport to an overseas job. They felt that nursing was evolving from being a vocation to being a job that provided lucrative job opportunities overseas, making these new generation nurses on duty in person, although the spirit to perform the caring work by being emotionally engaged was lacking. The concern that underlined the narratives of most of the senior nurses (from the government hospital and the mission hospital) was that of the caring work being compromised in the case of the new generation nurses whom they felt were more inclined towards gaining experience in handling technologies because it made them migration worthy. Although quite a few of them also returned from overseas and again worked with the mission hospital, the attitude of migration remains quite rampant amongst the new generation nurses.

The interview with the nursing director of the corporate hospital revealed divergent views from those expressed by the senior nurse's (of government and mission hospital) while expressing her opinion towards the concept of care changing in nursing with the changing technology. She refused on the dot that the essence of caring work was compromised in contemporary nursing because of the introduction of technology in nursing work. She appreciated the talent and skills of the nurse's from her institution and further corroborated it by saying that it was only because of the skill set that they acquired through their intensive training that they were all migrating abroad in large numbers. In her case, it seemed that she understood caring work as equivalent to being technologically skilled and took pride in sharing the fact that because the nurses from her institutions were so well oriented towards the latest advances in medical sciences and the technologies associated with it, that they were all getting placed overseas.

> I am not aware of the outside scenario! But my nurses are superbly trained and we at our institute take care that they are globally oriented. We maintain international standards ... like very very strict standards and no wonder our nurse's migrate to the best countries. All our nurse's carry the tag of being trained under us and get well-placed because even the recruiters know that they have undergone intensive training. And our nurses are updated with all the latest knowledge be it the newer machines, the theory and practical's or be it ... anything ... technologically we are very advanced here ... extremely competent ... and we work hard to make them reach there. Once a week we have in-service training sessions or lectures, they are additionally trained rigorously in a course on Critical Care nursing, and all the nurses are supposed to compulsorily go through this training as well. We have **client's** coming in from various parts of the world, and they stay for longer durations ... they are so happy with the nurses that they praise them a lot and write testimonials ... many of them also become friends on Facebook. Patients get attracted to technology only these days and what is wrong in techno-centric nursing care? In fact, it is the need of the hour!
>
> (Nursing Director, corporate hospital)

Only the government hospital senior nurses and the mission hospital nurses seemed to express deep concern about the essence of caring work being compromised, whereas the private hospital senior nurses, including the nursing director, expressed contrasting responses towards this situation. None of them mentioned the importance of engaging emotionally with patients. Although the government and the mission hospital senior nurse interviewees seemed to express great concern over the virtues pertaining to this profession being compromised, invariably relating it to new generation nurses migrating overseas for acquiring economic rewards; the nursing director of the corporate hospital blatantly refused that caring work was getting compromised and seemed to assess the prospects of new generation nursing in being capable of migrating overseas. The nursing director (corporate hospital) referred to the patients as 'clients', which is a quite noteworthy aspect of the narrative. She validated the success of her institution against the fact that they were capable of training nurses who were globally acclaimed.

It was noted through the narrative responses of senior generation nurses across the institutions visited, any detailed discussion pertaining to the varied aspects of the nursing profession would incessantly bring to the forefront the topic of migration of new generation nurses. Although migration was to be discussed at length in the latter part of the interview, the narratives of the senior nurses about nursing prospects always got drawn towards and linked with the phenomenon of overseas migration. Thus, I started seeing a link between nursing profession-engagement with technology and migration. The present study also visualised exploring the role of institutional training structures in influencing migration. As the findings so far constantly reflected upon this issue, I decided to further address the same by digging deeper by looping in the new generation nurses from the corporate hospital. Firstly, I chose the new generation nurses from the corporate hospital to speak up on the issue of migration as I was intrigued by the display of fanatical fixation by the senior nurses from the corporate hospital towards their nurses attaining a globally acclaimed status, second, as revealed through the previous narratives the newer generation nurses were on the move (mostly to the western countries), so I felt that they would be the perfect potential interviewees to elaborate on the entire process associated with contemporary emigration. Also, the revelations from the interview of the nursing director compelled me to delve deeper into understanding the reasons as to why was the word 'client' (which is suggestive of adherence to and propagation of market tendencies) was being used interchangeably with the word 'patient' and what kind and form of training reproduces these migratory tendencies? These questions emerged from the data procured and interpreted in the context so far. However, finding a reasonable explanation was important as these questions coincided with the final and most important objective of the present study, exploring the role of training and exposure to technology in reproducing migratory tendencies.

What Should We 'Care' For? The Patients, Meagre Salaries, or Repaying Loans

The analysis of the interview data of the senior nurses interviewed across the institutions provided grounding of the idea linking technological competency to determine migratory prospects of younger generation nurses. However, the questions mentioned above that emerged from the data, required engagement with the new generation nurses to establish a clear understanding of how acquiring training from certain institutional structures contributes to making the nurses migration worthy.

The new generation nurses from the corporate hospital were very blunt in accepting that they had chosen nursing as a career strategy that enabled them to migrate abroad. The decision to migrate abroad was strongly rooted in the desire to earn more and that nursing was considered a prestigious job (abroad) devoid of any stigma. Most of these nurses complained that nurses in India are not well-paid and many of the younger generation nurses from the corporate hospital mentioned relying on bank loans to support the costs of their nursing education. They also shared a concern regarding their inability to repay the debt anytime soon if they relied on the meagre salaries they earned through the corporate hospitals. The average wage of the younger generation nurse interviewees in the corporate hospital was about ten to fifteen thousand per month. As the nurses mentioned that this was a very well-renowned hospital, they were being paid on the higher side of the general wage scale for nurses working in other private/corporate hospitals. However, they further mentioned that in the rest of the private hospitals, the wages are very low and lack uniformity in the pay scale for nurses across the county. Most of the nurses spoke about nursing being underpaid, further stating it as a compelling reason to change quite a few jobs within a short career span before adjusting to the current job. They also mentioned having contacts in friends and acquaintances working as nurses in various private hospitals across the country and faced similar situations. This could also be why they confidently spoke about the entire country scenario pertaining to meagre wages that nurses are offered in the private healthcare sector. A young nurse expressed her views:

> How many B.Sc. nursing colleges' government colleges are there? There are only private colleges, who charge a lot of money and not just the fees but the accommodation, food everything the hostel expenses are also too much. Most of us here come from private colleges by taking some or the other form of loan. We can't sustain on such less salaries. At least here they pay [sic] minimum like 10,000 (Rs.), and then they increase according to till when you stay. In private clinic where I was working earlier, I was getting accommodation free, but he (the doctor) was only paying me 2,500 (Rs.) can you believe it! Still, I worked there for about 6–8 months and then came here. And after doing all this, there is no respect for nurse's in this country. I had decided to migrate right in the beginning, but some issues came up, and also experience is required of 2 years plus clearing the language test and all.
>
> (Young Nurse, corporate hospital)

The young nurse's from the corporate hospital presented the decision to migrate abroad to acquire a significant return on the investment that they had made in the form of taking loans for undergoing nursing training in private nursing colleges, an investment that they feel has very less financial returns if they were to stay in India.

It is not easy to ascertain the salary scale in private and corporate hospitals as they vary greatly and seem to be fixed by the institutions themselves. Therefore, the private sector salaries seem to be fixed extremely low compared to the salaries in the government hospital or mission hospital. Also, the nurses' salaries varied depending upon the time spent by the nurses in this hospital. When I spoke to the nursing director (corporate hospital) about this issue, she refused to comment on the difference in nurses' pay. However, when I asked the new generation nurse's to comment on the same, they stated that higher pay was given to nurses who would commit to staying with the hospital for a longer time. Also, as the younger nurses were mostly migrating abroad, they did not bother much about this kind of practice of not having a fixed salary. A young nurse from the corporate hospital explained:

> Actually, she (Nursing Director) will not tell you as these are all internal things, and they are there everywhere. All means all nurses migrate from here. So they know that right from the first day itself. They give good salaries to nurses who stay for 10 years or so and they are very few and those senior ones. Among us also some stay for 3–4 years so then they have a little more salary than us, but they stay because they can't clear the IELTS, TOEFL (English language test) or something like that. Some nurses come from some colleges and speak broken English, and they come here to learn English as we compulsorily speak in English here. These kinds of nurses get paid very less, so it all varies. If you are a nurse here, it's very easy to get a job in the US, UK, Canada even today irrespective of the market not being much in the US, our nurses get jobs. Lots of nurses migrate to Ireland and Australia from here. These hospital people know this. So they show our need, and we also see that we get good exposure which helps in migration and they immediately relieve us without asking many questions.
>
> (Young nurse, corporate hospital)

It is noteworthy to mention that the younger generation nurses from the private hospital recalled incidences about their wages with their previous private sector employers and asserted that although they were entitled to receive a salary of Rs.20,000 (as per the order of the Supreme Court when they serve in more than 100-bedded hospitals), they were being paid as low as Rs.2,500–6,000. As previously mentioned, many of the participant nurses mentioned that they were compelled to change several jobs within a very short span of their nursing career owing to the false promises about the payment of high wages made by the private sector employers. The most striking and remarkable aspect of this entire discussion was the nurse's explanation of dealing with the employers' deceit. They mentioned that this kind of deceitful act on the part of the private hospital employers almost always never gets challenged because it remains like an unsaid, agreed-upon understanding between the employer and the nurses that the employers will record the decided upon wages on the hospital registers and in turn the nurses get hands-on experience of getting trained in a highly intensive and technologically advanced private hospital ambience. This sets the stage for the newer nurses to get conditioned and receptive to the international nurse labour market. A pre-requisite for migrating overseas is a certificate mentioning the number of hours the respective nurses have received hands-on training in an intensive care unit. This certificate must be approved by the competent authority, which remains the private hospital employer in which the nurses undergo such training. The nurses who feel exploited with this entire setup choose to resign and leave and are few in number. In contrast, the others continue working under such exploitative conditions, considering it an obvious trade-off to fulfil their dreams of overseas migration towards better salaries and improved professional status. As explained by a young nurse (corporate hospital):

> At least here its better they give minimum 10,000 (Rs.), but I have worked in places where they show that they are paying you more and take our signatures to maintain records. But actually, we get very less salaries. There is no match between anything that they record and the amount that we get. No one says anything as anyway they want experience to migrate and that too from a good hospital. The ones who have a problem leave but such cases are very few … I mean there is no other way, so everyone (new nurses) suffers for about 2–3 years initially and then once they get experience they leave (abroad). This is a renowned hospital, so they don't do that (discrepancies in payments) but anyway it's like if you want to gain experience which actually is the reason as why most of the nurses are here for, and then you have to lose something. In this hospital, as soon as we tell them we are migrating, they are supportive, and without much questioning, they arrange for our experience certificates, and immediately they let us go. It is very common here, … they have a nursing college here, so they are used to their students migrating in batches (huge numbers).'
>
> (Young nurse, corporate hospital)

It is important to note that this corporate hospital had a private B.Sc. nurse training college attached to it, and the students from this college get completely trained in this hospital during their B.Sc. course, internship and later for gaining experience. A young nurse (corporate hospital) asserted they get exposed to certain advanced critical care training in a 'hi-tech' in this hospital environment, improving their migratory prospects. She explained:

> See, this is an NABH accredited hospital and is very renowned, so obviously, we get jobs in other countries very easily. In fact, that is the reason many nurses take education from here and practice here itself. Here we have a certain way of conduct. Everyone knows that we have very good ICU facilities; all nurses have to undergo advanced Critical Care nursing, and the ones in paediatrics have to undergo training in Critical Care Paediatric nursing. Everything is hi-tech here…very client friendly. We have skype sessions with hospitals abroad, and they teach us about what are new things going on there and the kind of expectations they have from us.
>
> (Young nurse, corporate hospital)

The word 'client' from this narrative again captured my attention as it had already intrigued me during the previous interviews conducted with the senior nurses (corporate hospital). On enquiring about the rampant usage and preference given to this specific word 'client' over the word 'patient/s', the new generation nurse explained:

> Oh yes! Patients! All high-profile patients' come here, you see ... all are very rich, and obviously, this is an expensive hospital, but we give good service also in return. It can be explained like..., corporate behaviour perhaps.
>
> (Young nurse, corporate hospital)

On further probing her to elaborate on what she meant by corporate behaviour, she hesitantly replied:

> See here we have different culture. Here we are given permission to use lipstick and basic make-up also. Just that it should not be too bright. And here it's still a little strict, but if you go to other private hospitals like (names other corporate hospitals) ... nurses carry a comb in their pockets. So, I think the kind of patients that come here also determines the hospital culture.
>
> (Young nurse, corporate hospital)

While conducting these interviews, I came across a new generation nurse trained in the B.Sc. nursing college attached to this hospital. She was all set to migrate to Australia in about a month, so I took this opportunity to ask her further about the role of this hospital and technological competency in making her migration worthy. Her words too echoed similarly, emphasising the importance of getting trained in a technologically advanced environment to get a job overseas. Her response also highlights that the nurses from this corporate hospital belong higher in the hierarchical order in the global nurse labour market when she stated that nurses from this hospital mostly migrate to western countries as against Gulf countries. She candidly shared her experience.

> Definitely, if you want to migrate being in this hospital, you will definitely go to a good place like Australia, UK, Ireland and all. Here every week we have nurses going (abroad) and not to like Oman or Gulf or places like that OK, we all go to Australia and all. This is like a lucky place where you come, and then you get a foreign job. We don't go through any agency, and all our seniors tell us everything. We require an experience certificate and our license and mark sheets to migrate. Also, this hospital people are very supportive, and they motivate us to go (migrate). Here we get a lot of experience of working in neonatal ICU, of working with patients on ventilator, CRRTs (Continuous Renal Replacement Therapy), Neuro ICU, Cardiac ICU and in like about 300 bedded hospital and that too like this hospital then that's all you need. They don't ask you further questions during the interviews.

Interviews are conducted in Mumbai, Cochin, Bangalore cities like these and the hospital people come and start the process immediately if they like you. They pay for all our expenses till we reach there and even the accommodation for first 6 months till we settle down.

(Young nurse, corporate hospital)

This nurse also introduced me to one of her batchmates and work colleagues, a new generation nurse, and was all set to move to Ireland in a couple of weeks. This hospital imports equipment from the UK and these nurses get hands-on experience, which was considered important as it helped these nurses immediately start working as a staff nurse abroad. The others who did not carry such an experience and exposure to training had to compulsorily register as interns under a nurse supervisor for 6 months to 1 year, and based on their performance, they promoted and approved as being eligible to work as a staff nurse. I probed her on similar lines, and she revealed:

Most of the apparatus like defibrillators, ventilators, syringe pumps, arterial blood pressure monitors, suction and many others are quite advanced and are imported from the UK. So we are very well advanced and in sync with the apparatus used in the UK. We have these Skype sessions where we get knowledge about all the advancement that happens in the UK. As we are already trained with handling this equipment here, getting entry into UK is easy. They don't have to train us again, and they are constantly in need for nurses. The Nursing Director is very supportive here, so she also lets us go easily.

(Young nurse, corporate hospital)

On asking her to elaborate on the process of migration to Ireland and what made her choose this county she added:

I cleared the IELTS it's valid for Ireland and UK. Additionally, in UK they require you to have CBT (Computer Based Training) that we all are well-acquainted with here. That's the advantage of being here. They train you so well that you don't have to struggle to get placed there (abroad). I chose Ireland because I have contacts with many of our nurses from here who are settled there. So I kind of get support especially in the initial days and here it works like this only. We all go to these places because we have nurses from this hospital going to these places and there is a culture among us to take care of the new nurse when she reaches to that county. I applied for the National Board of Nursing for Ireland, and it's like getting your application registered. Then they mail you a package that has some templates which you have to get them filled from the authorities here. In templates, there is one template in the form of a reference letter from the hospital where you practiced and in what and the details regarding the number of hours. This has to be filled and signed and stamped by the hospital authorities. Then we require the transcripts again a template in the form of a reference letter from the MNC (Maharashtra Nursing Council) stating that this nurse is registered with the MNC. I had to pay 30,000 (Rs.) for this entire package and its valid for a period of 6 months. Then once I filled all this an [sic] emailed it to them, they arranged for a Skype interview for me which I cleared.

(Young nurse, corporate hospital)

These nurses mentioned other nurses who had previously migrated from this hospital and guided them to migrate overseas. This is suggestive of social networks playing an important role in migration. All these nurses who had plans to migrate overseas were mostly from Kerala and were Christians. A very important cultural aspect that stemmed out very strongly from these new generation nurses' narratives was the repeated mentioning of 'earning money to pay towards dowry.' This also stood as an important reason to migrate overseas. The nurse's narratives revealed that a considerable amount of money and other assets must be paid towards dowry in Kerala. These nurses further mentioned that this tradition has deeply penetrated the societal structure, not just limiting to any religion or faith. All of them had paid huge amounts towards fees (range varied from 4.5 to 7 lakh towards the entire course) in private B.Sc. nursing colleges, and some of them mentioned lack of government B.Sc. nursing colleges as a reason to choose private colleges. Also, nowadays, to get enrolled in a government nursing college in Maharashtra, one needs to produce a domicile certificate stating that the concerned person is a Maharashtra domicile for the past 15 years. As the nurse's from other states could not produce such a certificate, private B.Sc. nursing colleges were preferred over government colleges. The discussions also revealed that the new nurses (corporate hospital) immediately dissociated themselves completely from government nurses as this was perceived as a threat to their professional image. The following narrative from a new (corporate hospital) nurse details this discussion as:

See mostly Malayali Christian girl means 90 percent of the times she is either a nurse or a teacher. Culturally we are like this, and there is a culture of migration among us. So it's accepted in our society. Here also 95 percent nurses are Malayali's and all are aware that we are known for our gold and dowry. So many girls pay their own dowry. So we need to earn for that. Additionally, we support the family, and we have some form of loans to repay. We have to go abroad. Here we will never get that kind of money. We have paid so much for our college (B.Sc.) and where are the government colleges? Only one here and that too they require a domicile of Maharashtra so what can we do? And anyway it's good in a way as it's difficult for nurses from government background to migrate as they don't get such advanced trainings.

(Young nurse, corporate hospital)

Finally, on asking the nursing director (corporate hospital) about the overseas migratory interests of these entire new generation nurse's from this hospital she replied:

Yes lots of them go abroad and what is wrong in that? They only come to us and tell us that they want to migrate. It is their right to migrate, and we cannot stop anyone. What do we provide the nurses here (in India)? No respect, salary issues and the nurses here stay in small houses. There (abroad) they immediately buy a house, a car and few years down the line their children get free education in those countries, and if I have to send my child for pursuing post-graduate education, then I have to keep 1 crore (Rs.) ready. So it's better that they leave now when they are unmarried, settle there (abroad) itself and have children there. They can later get married and take their husband's also over there, and they get paid in dollars, so they practically face no problems. I mean what more can one ask for!

(Nursing director, corporate hospital)

On asking the new nurses (corporate hospital) if they would return to India, they refused and again due to the previously discussed factors like low payments and stigma attached to this profession in India. It was also noted through the interviews that nurses in the corporate hospital had nurses' aides who used to clean the patients, their bodily fluids and perform work of giving them bedpans and assisting them in performing any other such physical activities. So, while nurses (corporate hospital) preferred to get trained in ICUs, handling advanced technologies, medicine, computerised record-keeping (more prestigious tasks), all menial tasks catering to the bodily needs of patients were relegated to the nurses' aides.

On similar inquiries, several young nurse interviewees from the mission hospital were interested in working abroad and were planning their training accordingly. However, through their interviews, the choice of a country which these nurses (mission hospital) chose to plan their overseas migration were mostly the ones in the Middle East (the Gulf countries). On asking the reason for this choice of countries to migrate, the response was like the one given by the senior nurses from the mission hospital. They mentioned no qualifying tests for working in these countries, and even a telephonic interview would suffice. Also, nurses from varied backgrounds came here, and many of them were not fluent in speaking English. In the Gulf countries, they could even do with basic English-speaking skills. These nurses migrate to the Gulf mostly because of the easier employment criteria. Also, most of the young generation nurse participants in the mission hospital were

Malayali Christian girls who stated that Kerala has a long history of nursing, and due to comparatively easier passage to the Gulf countries, Malayali's chose to migrate to these places. They stated that each Malayali family in Kerala has at least one member who stays in the Gulf countries. So, their social network plays an important 'pull factor' in influencing their decision to migrate to the Gulf. Explained a new generation (mission hospital) nurse:

> Going there is easy. No exams and all. Only on phone, they will interview. Also being from Kerala means having at least one and in fact many family members or extended family in the Gulf. In Kerala mostly all girls and Christian girls you will find as nurses only. We supply nurses to the entire country, and we have so many that they are there in Gulf as well. This has been traditionally there.
>
> (Young nurse, mission hospital)

Most of the new generation (mission hospital) nurses denied the role of the mission hospital in helping them migrate overseas. On enquiring if the mission hospital helped make them technologically competent to aid their migration, most of them denied such a thing happening. They stated that the younger nurses from the mission hospital migrated out of their free will, especially to earn money to repay their loans and help their families back at home. They also stated that many of them return to India after working abroad for a few years.

> See here (in mission hospital) they honestly don't wish that the nurses leave, and they try hard for that, but new nurses mostly take experience and leave. This is an NABH accredited hospital so getting trained here and having ICU experience is enough to go to any Gulf county. It might be difficult in other countries because of stringent entry level exams, but in Gulf it's alright.
>
> (Young nurse, mission hospital)

And:

> I have taken a loan from my aunt who is a nurse. Yes, I have taken it for my education. So it was decided that I go to her in Muscat and work there and repay the loan. Then I am free to return. I will come and work here only. Here there is a lot of honesty. We care a lot for patients, and we are taught good values here. Here everyone is God-fearing, so everyone behaves well. Patients from all religion come to us and before every surgery that is conducted, we pray with the patient. So the patient also feels very good. They also care a lot for us also. Sisters live like one big family. They provide us food in minimal rates, so obviously, it shows that they care for our health. In other hospitals, nobody cares for nurse's health. Accommodation is also free here. They understand we

have difficulties back at home and hence we migrate. Also, all nurses are from Kerala, so I feel nice that there are people around me from my place.

(Young nurse, mission hospital)

The young generation mission hospital nurses shared mixed feelings towards dowry-payments when probed if their migration overseas was contemplated based on their requirement to pay towards the dowries. Some of them accepted that their plan to migrate was also to earn money towards their dowries; however, others considered earning money for repaying their educational loans, building houses for their families, and supporting siblings' education as the main reasons to migrate overseas. These new generations (mission hospital) nurses seemed to be migrating to shoulder their family responsibilities and expressed a desire to return once their monetary needs were fulfilled. None of them expressed any resentment towards their salaries or mentioned any status issues that the nursing profession faces in India.

In this mission hospital, I also got an opportunity to interact with two male nurses. Both were Christians from Kerala. They were posted in the ICU and were very soon set to migrate overseas. One of them was migrating to the Gulf, and the other was migrating to South Africa. According to him, the one who was migrating to South Africa had more than 8 years of experience working in the ICU; he was waiting for a 'good opportunity' to migrate. Irrespective of being a nurse, he asserted that he was not interested in playing any role even remotely related to performing any caring activity. He took pride in associating himself with performing only clinical work to be a surgical assistant to the surgeons while they conduct surgeries. He held a fixed posting with the ICU. He insisted that people recognise him as a 'medical-surgical assistant to the surgeon' and not as a 'male nurse.' On asking him what makes him feel so dissociated from the caring working in nursing and as to why he insists that people recognise him differently from being a nurse, he replied:

Coming into nursing was pre-planned as I had a lot of my aunts in nursing. We are two brothers and no sister. My elder brother chose nursing; as actually, he was not very clear about what studies to take. So he thought anyway nursing is alright. We see nurses all around in Kerala. There are many men also have started taking nursing now and only because they can migrate abroad. Otherwise, who will choose a field so dominated by women ... I have many friends who did pharmacy and engineering depending upon their condition (socioeconomic status), but then I am more in demand in abroad than them. It's so funny!... I chose to be a nurse when I started seeing working opportunities abroad. I learnt from my brother when he discussed with me that doing nursing means an easy passage abroad. In no other profession can you migrate so easily with only a basic graduation. My brother went to the Gulf as my aunty was a head nurse by then. I am now leaving to South Africa. I was managing the paperwork and all and was waiting for a high paying opportunity. I do keep myself away from attending directly to patients because it does not pay you well. Even patients behave weirdly when you are a man and touching them, they want a female only to do such things then, be it! If you are into medical-surgical ICU, you are so much in demand abroad, and you get paid well. Anyway, I don't like to be called a nurse I tell my friends even to call me a surgical assistant. If they make fun of me, then I remind them that I have better job opportunities abroad that they do even MBAs don't get jobs easily abroad, but I can then obviously they shut up!

(Male surgical nurse, mission hospital)

Working in an ICU setup propels you towards migrating abroad was reflected in the views expressed by these male nurses. The determination to work in an ICU is linked to getting jobs easily in overseas countries. The other male nurse who was migrating to Gulf also shared the 'shock and horror' with which his family responded when he shared his decision to take up nursing as a career.

I remember very well of telling my sister first. She is elder to me, much elder and she was doing law. She panicked I don't know why and then she immediately told my mother and yes, we had nurse's in the family like distant relatives and all but no one directly related. You won't believe, my family went into shock you know that horror mode! ... I didn't realise for long as what did I do so wrong? My mother started keeping a close watch on me any like all my activities and all. I kept quiet and ignored. Then one day a very close friend of mine came to me as my mother had been to his house and was crying because she felt that something was terribly wrong with me and then he asked me about, you won't believe! .... my sexual orientation...you know ... can you believe it! Then the reverse shock came to me! He (friend) asked me as what type of man will like do nursing? People think like this. Then I was like determined that I will show to them that this is my choice and it's a profession like any other one, in fact, it's a noble one, and I took it up (nursing). They resisted initially, but later now they know there is nothing like that as I am happily married now. Now I tease my sister sometimes that I get so many opportunities being a nurse it would have been better if she would have been a nurse than a lawyer.

(Male nurse ICU, mission hospital)

The above narrative from the male nurse participants brings forth traditional professional stereotypes, which pressure people to play societal sanctioned gender-appropriate professional roles. It reflects the prejudices of the societal outlook towards their fixation with 'nursing' being synonymous with 'women.' That irrespective of being a male nurse, the urgency of the need to dissociate oneself from the caring-role is reflected very strongly from one of the narratives belonging to the male nurse.

It was not easy to find new generation B.Sc. trained nurses in the public hospital. Almost all young nurses were trained GNMs. The ones who were B.Sc. nurses were always posted with the ICU and were extremely busy. However, after repeated request, I got a chance to engage with both the young B.Sc. nurses from the public hospital. Both belonged to the state of Maharashtra and were Hindus. They agreed to be interviewed only on the condition that I would have to adjust to the interruption in the interview as they felt that they could not sit and engage in a conversation with me on account of their busy schedule. I also was asked to limit my queries and was made to interview both at one go itself. So, I immediately rushed to asking them to share their views about the role of training acquired through a particular institution (hospital) in making them technologically competent and, in their view, if technological competency has any links to overseas migration of nurses.

While replying to this, both knew the process of overseas migration. Both spoke about specific exams required to be cleared to migrate to western countries. One of them had planned to migrate overseas, but due to the lack of family support, she had given up on the idea of migration. Also, the feeling of having a secure and permanent public sector job made her stay back. She also clarifies that being technologically competent is always seen as 'prestigious' by the new generation of nurses. It helps them get better jobs. She further added that present-day nursing has undergone a change and believed being technologically competent helps the nurse eliminate the stigma attached to doing a menial job. She expressed:

> I got this job and being a government job, I also thought of the security it provided so I gave up on that going abroad dream. Having knowledge of technology is useful only, and it is seen as prestigious, and it's especially true when you are migrating. Those countries are very advanced, and they prefer well-trained nurses. They (in abroad) will not take you only till you are aware of the latest development in the field. Now here in government hospital, this is overlooked but you know if you can use even a stethoscope and check the patients then you are looked at differently.
>
> (Young nurse, public hospital)

On asking her to elaborate on what she meant by 'looked at differently' she added:

> See now, for example, many a times when I am at home; patient's from the neighbourhood come to me and ask for medicines so before that I make it a point to use a stethoscope and check them. So, I consider this

also as technology that the present-day nurse's use. And that makes them feel better. That image of a nurse only handling bed-pans goes away and especially when you say that you are an ICU nurse, then again people look differently as against saying that I am just a nurse.

(Young nurse, public hospital)

The other B.Sc. nurse was also nodding her head in affirmation and further corroborated it by adding:

I totally agree and actually that stigma that people still hold you know… that suddenly disappears… You can see it in their (patient's) eyes and talk.

(Young nurse, public hospital)

This nurse was also contemplating pursuing M.Sc. nursing, which would help her get the job of a nurse tutor in a nursing college. She was aware that she would have to leave the current job to pursue her higher studies. However, she procrastinated on this plan due to a lack of surety of getting a nursing tutor job in a government nursing college.

On further asking if getting trained in any specific institutions had any links to overseas migration, both believed it was easier for the nurse's trained in the private B.Sc. nurse training colleges attached to corporate hospitals to migrate overseas. They felt that private hospitals always followed protocols very closely adherent to those followed in hospitals abroad. Also, the nursing students get trained in a particular manner right from the beginning of their postings in the wards, which conditions them better to migrate. They also mentioned private nursing education as a 'business' where 'nurses are manufactured for export.'

Nurses also deliberately choose these corporate type hospitals and colleges. Mostly these nurses work in their hospital only. This is like a business. You come to us and learn here, get a degree, get experience certificate, and migrate. All these new nurses are manufactured for export! They charge a lot of money towards fees, and then these nurse's get assured that they will get to go abroad. So many of these private colleges mention it on their website itself like come and join us, get trained in well-equipped hospitals and so many of our nurses have migrated like that. This is an open business.

(Young nurse, public hospital)

During the fieldwork, I also managed to get about ten minutes of interview time from the Deputy Registrar of the Maharashtra Nursing Council, who urged me to keep the questions short and focused. When asked about the private nurse training institutions and current migration scenario of Indian nurses, she assertively stated:

Who brought in the private players and is there any accountability that is asked from the private hospitals? Is it not a shame for the entire nation if nurse's today have to be on the streets in Kerala just for demanding salaries and that too as less as merely 20,000 rupees?! Isn't it a reflection of how the medical lobby is just not concerned of their most important counterpart? Why will they (nurses) not migrate when such is the situation? I agree that a lot of nurse's are leaving this country and very soon we will face a huge crisis of nursing workforce. It is so ridiculous I tell you, even long after the English left, we are still making our public hospital nurse's carry a masala-dosa (with reference to the nurse's cap) on their heads! We fought so much for it to be removed from being a part of the uniform but all in vain! So nobody gives attention to what happens to the nurse's in general. The cost of the doctor, the cost of these useless advanced medical equipment's gets factored in the bills of innocent patients in the private hospitals, isn't it? What does a private hospital nurse get? Then what is wrong in learning skills and migrating?

(Deputy Registrar, Maharashtra Nursing Council)

(Re) Shaping the Nursing Profession to Fit the Global Market 'Calling'

The study reflects that most of the young nurses interviewed across the institutions prefer to undergo training in Intensive Care Units (ICUs), symbolising medical-technical labour. This suggests a process of transmutation that the contemporary nursing profession is undergoing along with a thrust on techno-centrism. This process demands a certain purging of menial work associated with nursing, which is considered easily dispensable. The new generation nurses recognise the importance of professionalising nursing services and making it respectable by seeking training that identifies with technical knowledge, science, and reasoning by leaving the distasteful part of their jobs to nurses' aides. These nurses prefer to undertake technology-intensive work, which helps them delink from the traditional association of nursing work with feminine, stigmatised, and menial work.

From this research, it remains evident that private/corporate institutions nursing education and training growth are oriented towards the global market, and this is evidenced by younger nurses' intentions to seek overseas opportunities and the increasing imbalance between B.Sc. nursing educational costs and the domestic salaries, especially in India's private health service delivery system. It is further corroborated from the corporate hospital managerial authorities' responses, who take pride in the fact that most new generation nurses gain work experience from their hospital land with overseas employment opportunities. The same response was echoed by the younger generation corporate hospital nurses, who clearly emphasised the importance of training in techno-intensive hospitals to compete in the global nurse labour market. The feeling of becoming globally competent because of the exposure to hands-on experience on advanced technological skills stemmed from the new generation nurses from the corporate hospital.

The study also brings out an important finding that there is a tendency among corporate/private hospitals to exploit nurse labour by making them work on dismal salaries. The nurses mentioned paying about Rs.4.5–7 lakh to complete the entire B.Sc. course, whereas there is no uniformity in the remuneration they receive from the private/corporate hospital. Many new generation nurses mentioned relying on bank loans and loans from relatives to pay towards their B.Sc. nursing course fees. However, nurses claimed that they remain underpaid, with the payments varying from Rs.10,000 to 15,000 in the corporate hospital considered under study. These findings stand true with the article published in *The Times of India (TOI)* dated 23 September 2016, titled 'Now, equal pay for private and state-run hospital nurses, recommends committee set up by the Indian Nursing Council' (Chappia, 2016) wherein the article mentions lack of uniformity in payment to nurses across the country, especially in the private health service delivery setups. Thus, compared to the junior nursing wage rates in India, it is evident that the private nursing programmes' costs reinforce the motivation to seek overseas employment. From the findings, it is also clear that this corporate hospital imports equipment is from the UK due to which new generation nurses prefer to work in this hospital to get trained in handling such equipment in India itself so that chances of getting placed in the UK get easier as they are already acquainted with most of the equipment and the procedures as per the hospital standards in the UK and other developed countries as well.

Additionally, many nurses who are not fluent in English come to this hospital to be proficient in the English language as the nurses are compulsorily made to speak in English in this hospital. This is considered important by the nurses intending to migrate to developed nations as it's mandatory for them to clear the English language proficiency tests to migrate and practise in those nations. The study results revealed that meagre salaries and unavailability of a uniform payment mechanism in the corporate/private hospitals are considered an acceptable trade-off for getting trained in a tech-intensive corporate hospital ambience to procure an experience certificate from the corporate hospital managerial authorities. This certificate is documented evidence of the number of hours the respective nurse has spent in an ICU which is extremely important as an experience in an ICU setup and is a known gate pass to lucrative overseas job opportunities. These findings suggest a business model wherein the nurses are made to work on less salary, and the nurses also agree to get hands-on experience of getting trained in a techno-intensive hospital setup that remains a peculiarity of the corporate hospital.

These findings add to the findings of Kingma (2006), wherein in the context of nurse migration, the author mentions that some institutions have indeed become high-end technical schools that are fashioning their future worker products for export to markets, tailoring their courses and skills to suit a particular market niche. On similar lines, Johnson (2014), in her study titled, 'A suitable job? A qualitative study of becoming a nurse in the context of a globalising profession in India' and Walton-Roberts (2015) in 'International migration of health professionals and the marketisation and privatisation of health education in India: From push-pull to global political economy,' specifically mentions that mostly the nurses trained in private hospitals in India tend to migrate overseas. Thus, the present study builds on these studies and extends the understanding of migration of the new generation nurses by building a structural explanation intertwined in changes that emanate from science and technology in healthcare organisations, institutional structures, and the socially embedded nurse labour market in India. Given this, the present research also strongly contradicts the findings documented by (Bland and Woolbridge, 2011; Brugha et al., 2009; Johnson et al., 2014; Thomas, 2006), wherein they mention that the opportunity to learn new health-related technologies and their usage in countries abroad played a significant role than financial incentives in influencing the decision of nurses to migrate to developed countries. The present study brings to the forefront and states that corporate hospital nurse training resonates with the marketisation and privatisation throughout the country, wherein marketised tendencies are given a scope to be reproduced through nurse training. These nurses do not migrate to learn technological skills. Rather, they do so to use these private/corporate hospitals' already learnt skills for a greater pay-off abroad. The primary push factors, such as the poor status of nursing in India, which contrasts its more respected status elsewhere and meagre salaries, play a substantial role in overseas migratory decision-making among new generation nurses.

As reflected in the literature review, the four southern Indian states are home to 63% of India's nursing colleges, of which 95% are private. The private sector in India is responsible for producing 95% of nurses (Rao et al., 2011; Reynolds et al., 2013). Acquiring education and training from private institutions is recognised to mould the nurses to reinforce market-responsive ethos, which reshapes the health sector (Walton-Roberts, 2015). This can be corroborated based upon the interview responses of the corporate hospital nurses, many of whom used the word 'clients' to refer to their patients. The new generation nurses interviewees from the corporate hospital mentioned nurses trained in intensive care of being in high demand abroad.

Further, this was corroborated by the senior nurses from the corporate hospital who boasted that the nurses trained in their hospital were all migrating for overseas jobs in developed countries. This means that the nurses get trained here in a particular manner suited for meeting the stringent employment needs in the developed countries. Thus, market demands penetrate the nursing education and training structures with out-migration becoming the means of resource extraction in paying high fees towards nursing education and later working on meagre salaries to gain intensive techno training with the hope of getting overseas employment opportunities for the nurses aspiring to migrate.

With this backdrop, this research posits that change in science and technology generates a path of outcomes impacting the human capital formation (in the study, the nurse labour market). Building upon the theory of science, technology, and society and contextualising this argument in the case of the nursing labour market, the findings of the study are suggestive of the fact that technological changes in healthcare following the product innovations in biomedical sciences necessitate healthcare organisations (especially the for-profit ones) to invest in new artefacts to compete in the market. To minimise the sunken costs,[5] the specificity of technology usage might deepen throughout the organisational culture so that the new technological artefact gets internalised in every bit of healthcare service provided through a particular institution. This can be corroborated with the study's findings wherein the nurses from the corporate/private hospitals mention that after they join the hospital as a staff nurse, they are compulsorily made to undergo ICU and ICCU training lasting for one year. Thus, the private entities/organisations adhere to the utopian perspective, which seeks and builds knowledge for gaining power, which revolves around the understanding of technology, reducing subjective qualities. Thus, as Scarbrough and Corbett (1992) asserted, determining the flows of knowledge pertaining to technologies and shaping the context for its powerful user groups assert their interest through the technological process. In the present research context, the corporate hospitals internalise the importance of these artefacts to minimise their sunken costs and express power and control over the knowledge produced. They present themselves as experts acting as technical gatekeepers controlling the flow of information. Thus, the expensive course fees for B.Sc. nursing and the meagre salaries paid to the nurses during their training before they migrate for job opportunities overseas reflects the position of power possessed by the corporate/private hospitals as they control the flow of technological pieces of training required by the nurses to get employment overseas which is suggestive of the transmutation of nurse migration following the techno-intensive training. The above discussion asserts and supports Barnard's (1996) view that technology indeed transforms the nursing profession in terms of practice and the machinery used, the skills that nurses develop, and the values they espouse the responses of new generation nurses. Similarly, it also supports Lupton's (2012)argument that the dominant approach of contemporary technologically based curative therapies that are capital intensive and hospital based legitimate and facilitate capitalist economic growth. The obsession of the young generation nurses to learn technological skills can be explained based on market tendencies pushed through the corporate/private institutional training structures.

This appears like a series of dependent patterned events wherein a cascading phenomenon is observed on the one hand influenced by undervaluing nursing care in the country's context by stigmatising it. It remains an underpaid occupation (commonly documented 'push factors' in nurse migration). On the other hand, the private nurse education and training institutions recognise the social stigma underlying this profession, moulding the nursing labour that emanates from the overseas employer's expectations by making them comply with and consent to the market-driven ruling mechanism creating nurses who are technophiles. However, the research findings also reflect that the young generation mission hospital nurses intend to migrate overseas. However, there is a marked difference in the choice of destination country among the mission hospital new generation nurses compared to the new generation nurses from the corporate hospital who boast of migrating to developed nations. The new generation mission hospital nurses mostly migrate to the Gulf countries wherein the employability requirements are not very stringent and can sustain basic English-speaking skills. The corporate hospital nurses who pay huge amounts towards fees and get enrolled in the degree programme, get trained in such techno-intensive set-up to compete for nursing jobs in the western countries. None of the younger nurses (even the ones from Kerala) from the corporate hospital mentioned having an ambition to seek a job in the Gulf countries. This is indicative of the fact that the corporate/ private institutions have created a pyramidal hierarchical nurse training structure wherein nurses trained from their institutions retain the topmost position and are capable to compete in the global west and the rest stand at lower rungs in this structure. The ones who stand at the lower rung (the mission hospital trained nurses), are also Malayali girls who have a strong social network and chose the Gulf countries to emigrate stating reasons like paying money towards dowries, easier passage wherein less money is required to pay towards the emigration process and their poor socioeconomic status.

Also, many of the mission hospital trained younger nurses mentioned their intent to return to India after making enough money to meet their family requirements. This was corroborated by the senior generation nurses in the mission hospital, who also asserted that the hospital's managerial body always dissuaded new generation nurses from migrating overseas, further stating that most of these young nurses migrated to the Gulf always returned after a few years. Thus, brain-drain, which implies a loss to the source country of vital skills and professional knowledge, stands relevant only when linked with permanent nurse migration. If migrant nurses return to their home country, they can again be a national resource if their acquired knowledge and experience are put to good use. The state should attempt to improve nurses' working conditions and wages by giving more serious attention to retention strategies that work in various government and private hospitals. As asserted by Brown and Connell (2004), most nurses are reluctant to leave their home countries and be willing to stay if offered a living wage. This is essential to have a sustainable domestic workforce that effectively delivers equitable care. It calls for action by the state to intervene and bring about a delicate balance between the human and labour rights of the individual and a collective concern towards the health of its citizens.

Overseas network (especially in the Gulf countries) was particularly important to new generation mission hospital nurses from Kerala, many of whom were keen to join friends and family members already working there. Here, migration seems to be culturally imbibed wherein the Malayali community has very strong social ties and networks with the Malayali's who are in the Gulf. Many female migrants from Kerala tend to be skilled nurses, and researchers estimate that 90% of migrant nurses across India and the Gulf are from Kerala (Nair and Percot, 2010; Percot and Rajan, 2007). This finding also stands true with the study findings of Reddy (2015), who mentions that nurses in Kerala continue to pay large dowries by adhering to the culturally imbibed tradition, which also needs to be considered as an important social factor that makes them contemplate their decision to migrate overseas for better remuneration. This suggests the possibility of better economic rewards through employment as a powerful factor that motivated many new generation nurses, which reveals infiltration of and resonance with market ethos, regardless of institutional ethos and seeking employment abroad.

Barnard and Sinclair (2006) assert the balance between technologies and caregiving, especially after the healthcare sector had seen drastic technological advances. As reflected from the senior nurses narratives belonging to the public hospital and mission hospital, various technologically advanced equipment used in contemporary nursing has made it possible to distance a patient's caregiver. The senior generation nurses from the mission hospital and the government hospital expressed concerns that in the process of techno-intensive training, the new generation nurses are overlooking the patients' subjectivity experiences. Thus, often aided by technological thrust and socialisation, human capital formation assumes significant centrality, especially in translating tremors of change in science and technology manifested through knowledge mix to high magnitude changes in the labour markets. Consequently, if we perpetuate this way of knowing that gives primacy to objective and detached knowledge, nursing labour will contribute to an impersonal healthcare system in much the same way as the biomedical model.

There remains a serious threat that the international orientation of nurse training structures in India can transform our health system into what can be best described as 'leaky-kettle' wherein more and more human resources are trained such that it does not meet the public health needs of our country's population but rather to export them. Even if privatisation is inevitable, it has been controlled and regulated by governments that can keep up with these changes (Chandain Drager et al., 2002). If the government cannot provide healthcare on its own, it needs to regulate and steward the work of others. This will require a substantial shift in policy thinking with adequate regulation of private nursing education and training to discipline this sector to fight the 'war over retention of skills' to achieve better health outcomes. This, coupled with inadequate retention strategies, will certainly fail to 'plug the holes that cause the drain' from the overseas migration of Indian nurses.

Notes

1. Post Basic BSc Nursing (PBBSc) is a two-year duration undergraduate course in nursing wherein candidates are provided a holistic mixture of classroom lectures and hands-on training in clinical nursing. GNM nurses get enrolled for this course to get a degree in nursing. Many a times, such nurses are sponsored by the state after completion of at least 10 years in service as a GNM nurse.
2. General Nursing and Midwifery (GNM) is a three-year and six-month diploma course designed for aspirants who want to pursue a career in clinical nursing.
3. National Accreditation Board for Hospitals and Healthcare Providers (NABH) is a constituent board of Quality Council of India (QCI), set up to establish and operate accreditation programme for healthcare organizations.
4. Malayalis, are Malayalam-speaking people chiefly inhabiting the Indian state of Kerala.
5. Sunken cost, it is a cost that an entity/organisation has incurred, which it can no longer recover.

References

Barnard, A. (1996). Technology and nursing: An anatomy of definition. *International Journal of Nursing Studies*, *33*(4), 433–441. https://doi.org/10.1016/0020-7489(95)00069-0

Barnard, A., & Sandelowski, M. (2001). Technology and humane nursing care: (Ir)reconcilable or invented difference? *Journal of Advanced Nursing*, *34*(3), 367–375. https://doi.org/10.1046/j.1365-2648.2001.01768.x

Barnard, A. G., & Sinclair, M. (2006). Spectators & spectacles: Nurses, midwives and visuality. *Journal of Advanced Nursing*, *55*(5), 578–586. https://doi.org/10.1111/j.1365-2648.2006.03947.x

Bland, M., & Woolbridge, M. (2011). From India to New Zealand-A challenging but rewarding passage. *Kai Tiaki: Nursing New Zealand*, *17*(10), 21.

Brown, R. P. C., & Connell, J. (2004). The migration of doctors and nurses from South Pacific Island Nations. *Social Science & Medicine*, *58*(11), 2193–2210. https://doi.org/10.1016/j.socscimed.2003.08.020

Brugha, R., McGee, H., & Humphries, N. (2009). "I won't be staying here for long": A qualitative study on the retention of migrant nurses in Ireland. *Human Resources for Health*, *7*(1), 1–12. https://doi.org/10.1186/1478-4491-7-68

Brush, B. L. (2008). Global nurse migration today. *Journal of Nursing Scholarship*, *40*(1), 20–25. https://doi.org/10.1111/j.1547-5069.2007.00201.x

Chappia, H. (2016, September 23). *Hospital nurses: Now, equal pay for private and state-run hospital nurses, recommends committee set up by the Indian Nursing Council - Times of India*. Times of India. http://timesofindia.indiatimes.com/city/mumbai/Now-equal-pay-for-private-and-state-run-hospital-nurses-recommends-committee-set-up-by-the-Indian-Nursing-Council/articleshow/54471610.cms

Drager, N., Vieira, C., & Organization, P. A. H., Development, P. A. H. O. D. of H. and H., Organization), P. P. and H. P. (Pan A. H., & Unit, W. H. O. O. of the D.-G. S. (2002). *Trade in health services: Global, regional, and country perspectives*. Pan American Health Organization, Program on Public Policy and Health, Division of Health and Human Development.

Dussault, G., Fronteira, I., & Cabral, J. (2009). Migration of health personnel in the WHO European Region. WHO Europe, 1–45.

Gadamer, H. G. (1996). *The enigma of health*. Palo Alto, CA: Stanford University Press.

Gill, R. (2016). Scarcity of nurses in India: A myth or reality? *Journal of Health Management, 18*(4), 509–522.

Health Services Union. (2007). *Discussion paper ethical recruitment & employment of overseas trained health workers*. https://hsu.net.au/publications/discussethicalr ecruit.html

Ihde, D. (1990). *Technology and the lifeworld: From garden to earth*. Indiana University Press, Bloomington, Indiana.

India Centre for Migration (ICM) New Delhi. (2013). *Carim India-developing a knowledge base for policymaking on India-EU migration: Proceedings of the national consultation workshop on facilitating safe and legal migration and prevention of irregular migration*, 6 and 7 September 2012. https://cadmus .eui.eu/bitstream/handle/1814/29480/CARIM-India-2013-18.pdf?sequence=1 &isAllowed=y

Johnson, S. E., Green, J., & Maben, J. (2014). A suitable job?: A qualitative study of becoming a nurse in the context of a globalizing profession in India. *International Journal of Nursing Studies, 51*(5), 734–743. https://doi.org/10.1016/j.ijnurstu .2013.09.009

Kingma, M. (2006). *Nurses on the move: Migration and the global health care economy*. Ithaca, New York: Cornell University Press.

Kingma, M. (2008). Nurse migration and the global health care economy. *Policy, Politics, and Nursing Practice, 9*(4), 328–333. https://doi.org/10.1177 /1527154408327920

Kline, D. S. (2003). Push and pull factors in international nurse migration. *Journal of Nursing Scholarship, 35*(2), 107–111. https://doi.org/10.1111/j.1547-5069 .2003.00107.x

Lupton, D. (2012). *Medicine as culture: Illness, disease and the body*. SAGE Publications.

Madhukar, C. V. (2008, August 20). *India together: Missing: A "healthy" debate – 21 August 2008*. http://www.indiatogether.org/hlthdbt-opinions

Matsuno, A. (2009). *Nurse migration: The Asian perspective*. https://doi.org/10 .1111/j.1475-6773.2007.00711.x

Ministry of External Affairs. (2012, April 12). *India-Kuwait relations*. https://mea .gov.in/Portal/ForeignRelation/Mission_s_Brief_-_Kuwait.pdf

Nair, M., & Webster, P. (2013). Health professionals' migration in emerging market economies: Patterns, causes and possible solutions. *Journal of Public Health (United Kingdom), 35*(1), 157–163. https://doi.org/10.1093/pubmed/ fds087

Nair, S. (2012). *Moving with the times: Gender, status and migration of nurses in India*. Taylor & Francis, Routledge India. https://books.google.co.in/books?id =CWsHEAAAQBAJ

Nair, S. R., & Percot, M. (2010). Transcending boundaries: Indian nurses in internal and international migration. *Esocialsciences.Com*, Working Papers. https:// www.researchgate.net/publication/46476400_Transcending_Boundaries_Indian _Nurses_in_Internal_and_International_Migration

Organisation for Economic Co-operation and Development. (2008). *The looming crisis in the health workforce: How can OECD countries respond?* Organisation for Economic Co-operation and Development.

Percot, M., & Rajan, S. I. (2007). Female emigration from India: Case study of nurses. *Economic and Political Weekly, 42*(4), 318–325.

Pranav, K., & Simi, T. B. (2007). *Barriers to movement of healthcare professionals a case study of India.* Retrieved March 18, 2021, from http://www.cuts-citee.org /pdf/RREPORT07-03.pdf

Purnell, M. J. (1998). Who really makes the bed? Uncovering technologic dissonance in nursing. *Holistic Nursing Practice, 12*(4), 12–22. https://doi.org/10.1097 /00004650-199807000-00004

Rao, M., Rao, K. D., Kumar, S., Chatterjee, M., & Sundararaman, T. (2011). Human resources for health in India. *www.Thelancet.Com, 377,* 587–598. https://doi.org/10.1016/S0140

Reddy, S. K. (2015). *Nursing and empire: Gendered labor and migration from India to the United States.* University of North Carolina Press Chapel Hill ,NC.

Reynolds, J., Wisaijohn, T., Pudpong, N., Watthayu, N., Dalliston, A., Suphanchaimat, R., Putthasri, W., & Sawaengdee, K. (2013). A literature review: The role of the private sector in the production of nurses in India, Kenya, South Africa and Thailand. In *Human Resources for Health* (Vol. 11, Issue 1, p. 14). BioMed Central. https://doi.org/10.1186/1478-4491-11-14

Sandelowski, M. (1996). Tools of the trade: Analyzing technology as object in nursing. *Scholarly Inquiry for Nursing Practice, 10*(1), 5–16.

Sandelowski, M. (2000). *Devices & desires: Gender, technology, and American nursing.* University of North Carolina Press. https://books.google.co.in/books?id =SAGHlA3xfR8C

Scarbrough, H., & Corbett, J. M. (1992). *Technology and organization: Power, meaning and design.* Routledge, London: Taylor & Francis Group.

Thomas, P. (2006). The international migration of Indian nurses. *International Nursing Review, 53*(4), 277–283. https://doi.org/10.1111/j.1466-7657.2006 .00494.x

Walton-Roberts, M. (2015). International migration of health professionals and the marketization and privatization of health education in India: From push-pull to global political economy. *Social Science and Medicine, 124,* 374–382. https://doi .org/10.1016/j.socscimed.2014.10.004

Walton-Roberts, M., & Rajan, S. I. (2013). Nurse emigration from Kerala: 'Brain circulation' or 'trap'. In S. I. Rajan (Ed.), *India migration report 2013: Global financial crisis, migration and remittances* (pp. 206–223). New Delhi: Routledge.

Walton-Roberts, M., and Rajan, S. I. (2020). Global demand for medical professionals drives Indian abroad despite acute domestic health-care worker shortages. *Migration Information Source.* Retrieved January 23, 2020, from https://www.migrationpolicy.org/article/global-demand-medical-professionals -drives-indians-abroad

Walton-Roberts, M., Runnels, V., Rajan, S. I., Sood, A., Nair, S., Thomas, P., Packer, C., Mackenzie, A., Murphy, G. T., Labonté, R., & Bourgeault, I. L. (2017). Causes, consequences, and policy responses to the migration of health workers: Key findings from India. *Human Resources for Health, 15*(1), 28.

WHO. (2006). *Scaling up health workforce production: A concept paper towards the implementation of world health assembly resolution WHA59. 23.* Geneva: World Health Organization. https://www.who.int/hrh/documents/scalingup _concept_paper.pdf

Wilkinson, P. (1992). The influence of high technology care on patients, their relatives and nurses. *Intensive and Critical Care Nursing, 8*(4), 194–198. https:// doi.org/10.1016/0964-3397(92)90049-P

10 India and the Global Provision of Health Professionals

Recent Developments and Potential Policy Responses

*Margaret Walton-Roberts and
S. Irudaya Rajan*

Introduction

The COVID-19 pandemic has exposed the vulnerabilities of the health system with the sudden upsurge in demand for acute health-care services globally. It is well established that globally the health-care sector faces an emerging shortage of personnel, leaving health systems vulnerable to the demands of a global pandemic (Britnell, 2019). In India, it is estimated that there are 3.3 qualified allopathic doctors and 3.1 nurses and midwives per 10,000 populations—well below the World Health Organization (WHO) benchmark of 22.8 doctors, nurses, and midwives per 10,000. Such shortages exist in spite of India producing the largest pool of trained health-care personnel in the world. India has been the world's largest source for immigrant physicians since the country gained independence in 1947. As of 2017, 69,000 Indian-trained physicians were working in the United States, United Kingdom, Canada, and Australia, according to the Organization for Economic Cooperation and Development (OECD), which is equivalent to 6.6 percent of the number of doctors registered with the Medical Council of India (MCI). The country, which boasts the world's highest number of medical schools, also has become a leading source for nurses (typically trailing only the Philippines). Nearly 56,000 Indian-trained nurses work in the same four countries, equal to about 3 percent of the registered nurses in India (Adkoli, 2006; Anand, 2016; Baker, 2019; Brahmapurkar et al., 2018; Chhapia, 2019). The allure of working abroad is strong for both physicians and nurses; researchers estimate that anywhere between 20 and 50 percent of Indian health-care workers intend on seeking employment overseas for a range of reasons (Walton-Roberts et al., 2017).

Several countries have facilitated Indian health-worker migration in recent years. The United Kingdom, for example, introduced fast-tracked visas for medical professionals in November 2019 and offered free visa extensions for health workers during the COVID-19 pandemic. The fast-tracked visa would aim to address shortages in the UK's National Health Service (NHS) and the extension will facilitate their battle against the pandemic (Economic

DOI: 10.4324/9781003315124-10

Times, 2019; Garner et al., 2015; Global Health Observatory, 2019; Hohn et al., 2016). As of 2017, more than 15,000 doctors in the NHS had received their primary medical qualification[1] in India, and Indians represented the top non-British nationality for NHS staff as of early 2019.[2]

Even as Indian medical professionals are drawn internationally by affirmative policies and perceived better opportunities, less than optimal conditions at home also drive their decision to leave. Among the factors: the central government's lack of investment in health-care, limited residency spots available for graduate doctors, frustration linked to bureaucratic bottlenecks in appointing senior medical professionals, and the perceived importance of building professional status through international residencies and training opportunities (Walton-Roberts et al., 2017).

Against this global pull, the Indian government has undertaken a number of policies to limit the emigration of doctors and nurses, though these have been more ad hoc in nature and not part of a fully realized strategy. Based on these changes, it seems fair to say that the Indian government has realized the downside of sizable outmigration of health-care professionals; yet the effectiveness of its policies remains questionable (Humphries et al., 2012; Kaushik et al., 2008; Kumar and Pal, 2018; Mullan, 2006).

The global migration of doctors and nurses has generated considerable debate regarding the impact of this process on both sending and receiving nations' health-care systems. In India, issues of "brain drain" and the need for an adequate stock of medical professionals inform media and policy debates (Nair and Rajan, 2017; Potnuru, 2017; Rao et al., 2011, 2016; Rajan et al., 2019). These issues are cast into further relief in the context of India's critical shortfall of domestic health-care workers. Overall, looking at all skilled health-care personnel, the ratio in India was 28.52 professionals per 10,000 residents in 2016, compared to the 52.82 globally (WHO, 2017b).

This chapter analyzes India's role in the global provision of health professionals by exploring international migration patterns and processes, considering the established and emerging patterns of migration, and presenting the relevant Indian policy responses. While these issues affect a range of health occupations, the chapter focuses, in particular, on doctors and nurses.

The Indian Health-Care Context

The health-care sector in India—which is the world's second most populous country with more than 1.35 billion residents—has been expanding since the post-independence period. This has particularly been the case in the 1990s' post-liberalization era, which saw private capital leading the expansion of the health-care sector. The number of registered medical colleges has soared, from 86 in 1965 to 539 in 2019; annually, more than 67,200 students begin bachelor of medicine and bachelor of surgery (MBBS) programs. Current projections suggest there will be 1,493,385 registered doctors in India in 2024, which would meet the WHO-recommended ratio of one doctor per 1,000 individuals. Despite such promising projections, the concentration of health services and medical professionals in urban areas in the face of a wide urban–rural gap remains a challenge, especially in a country where two-thirds of the population still live in rural areas (Reddy and Qadeer, 2010; Scroll, 2018; Sharma et al., 2016; Shetty, 2010; Sood, 2008).

The MCI is the main regulatory body for the western, allopathic form of medical treatment (the use of medications or surgery to suppress or treat disease). The more traditional medicines, including ayurveda, yoga and naturopathy, unani, siddha, and homeopathy (AYUSH), are regulated by the ministry of AYUSH. In order to be recognized as legal practitioners, all allopathic or ayurvedic doctors must be registered with these institutions; however, researchers suggest that as many as 25 percent of Indians receive medical treatment from unlicensed providers, especially in rural areas. India's health-care workforce includes allopathic doctors (31 percent); nurses and midwives (30 percent); pharmacists (11 percent); practitioners of AYUSH (9 percent); ophthalmic assistants, radiographers, and technicians (9 percent); and others (10 percent). Despite the public concern regarding corruption in MCI—which is caused in part by the extreme gap between the supply and demand for medical education—the central government's efforts to reform this sector have been slow (Rao, 2014).

Nursing and midwifery are regulated by the Indian Nursing Council and the respective state nursing councils. Nurses complete either a three-and-a-half-year diploma in general nursing and midwifery or a four-year bachelor's degree and are registered with the council. The number of nursing colleges increased from 30 in 2000 to 1,996 in 2020, with the majority, 1833, being private institutions.[3] New calculations based on National Sample Survey (NSS) and registration data indicate that in 2015 there were more than 1.6 million nurses registered in India, or about 4.2 nurses per 10,000 people (Times of India, 2016, 2017; Thomas, 2006; Thompson and Walton-Roberts, 2018; Varghese et al., 2018). The nursing profession in India has long been neglected, positioned as subservient in the medical hierarchy (Percot and Rajan, 2007). Salary and working conditions are generally poor, especially in the growing private hospital sector, with limited opportunities for continued professional development. Factors including career progression, professional status, and income are among the reasons nurses seek opportunities overseas.

International Migration of Indian Medical Professionals

Popular destinations for Indian health professionals include the United States, United Kingdom, Australia, Canada, and the Gulf Cooperation Council (GCC) countries (Table 10.1).

Table 10.1 Top Five Countries of Destination for India-Trained Doctors, 2014–19

Country	2014	2015	2016	2017	2018	2019
United States	46,447	46,137	45,830	—	—	—
United Kingdom	17,011	15,119	15,517	15,685	15,870	17,737
Australia	4,481	4,821	5,037	5,182	5,336	—
Canada	1,998	2,036	2,088	2,150	2,163	—
New Zealand	468	480	479	489	490	—

Source: OECD Statistics, Health Workforce Migration, "Foreign-Trained Physicians by Country of Origin – Stock," accessed April 23, 2021. Data for Physician stock is missing for U.S during 2017–19; Australia, Canada and New Zealand during 2018–19.

English is the language of instruction for most Indian health training institutions, facilitating overseas migration for graduates. While India has the majority share of internationally trained doctors in the United States and the United Kingdom, the share of Internationally Educated Health Professionals (IEHPs) in these two countries saw a decline between 2000 and 2014 due to increased domestic production of graduates and the effects of the global financial crisis. International migration continued to increase for other destinations—including other OECD countries (Walton-Roberts, 2012, 2015; Walton-Roberts and Rajan, 2013; WHO 2017b).

Furthermore, 57 percent of nurses migrating from the Indian state of Kerala resided in the Gulf countries in 2016 (with Saudi Arabia the top destination). Saudi Arabia's health-care system is heavily reliant on IEHPs, with Saudi nationals comprising just 32 percent of physicians and 38 percent of nurses in the country as of 2018. Other countries with a significant share of Indian-trained nurses include the United States (6 percent of the overall nursing workforce in 2016), Canada (5.5 percent), and a smaller share in Australia, Germany, Ireland, Italy, Maldives, and Singapore (2–3 percent). Ireland, for instance, is an example of an emerging market for Indian-trained nurses, with 35 percent of nurse recruitment into the country between 2000 and 2010 coming from non-European Union sources.

Training Patterns Often Determine Migrants' Destinations

As mentioned earlier, the post-liberalization era has seen private investment dominate health education expansion in India. Several health corporations, such as Apollo Hospital chain and Fortis Group, are involved in training, and are funded through private capital from non-resident Indians (NRIs) or returning migrants. Indian corporate health groups value international training and experience; indeed, many have international partnerships that facilitate health-worker exchanges, and they leverage their internationalism to promote medical tourism to India. Additionally, international agencies (such as Joint Commission International for hospitals, United States Medical Licensing

Examination for doctors, and National Council Licensure Examination testing centers for nursing) see India as an important growth market, and their presence adds to the internationalized environment that encourages Indian health professionals to consider international migration options.

The number of health training institutes grew throughout the country with the aid of private investment: an estimated 95 percent of Indian nursing institutes are private, and just more than half of all medical college positions are in the private sector. These institutes have emerged in part to service the increased interest by health-care professionals in response to international migration opportunities. The private market has also pushed some, especially nurses, in to a vicious debt trap. Private training institutes generally cost more than the government ones, and these costs eventually become an important migration driver, since domestic salaries are too low to cover educational debts (Walton-Roberts and Rajan, 2013). The high cost of migration—which includes fees paid to local recruiting agents—is ultimately outweighed by the prospective salaries and benefits earned abroad. Using purchasing power parity, researchers have found that in the US nursing and physician salaries are 80 percent and 57 percent higher than comparative Indian salaries (George and Rhodes, 2017).

The competitiveness of medical education and the potential rewards from international opportunities are driving would-be health-care professionals unable to enter Indian programs of study to opt for degrees in Russia, China, and Eastern European countries. According to the Indian Ministry of External Affairs, in 2018, approximately 18,000 Indian students were enrolled in Chinese universities and around 11,000 in Russian universities—mostly in medical programs. To practice in India, these students must pass the foreign medical graduate examination (FMGE), which the majority fail. Further research is needed to reveal if this offshoring of Indian medical students will become part of an international multi-step migration pathway rather than just a route back to India.

However, with looming worries of subsequent waves of the pandemic, there is an overhanging demand for the health professionals all over the world. Patterns of health-worker mobility have become increasingly complex. Intra-regional, South–South, and North–South movement and further complicated return and step-by-step movement had emerged along with the long-established movement from the Global South to the Global North (WHO, 2017a).

The Dawn of Policies to Control and Limit Migration

The Indian government has advanced a number of policies to regulate and limit the emigration of health workers in recent years. Yet, these seem to be mostly a patchwork of bureaucratic reforms instead of a centralized policy framework designed to balance the country's health-care worker needs with policies to better facilitate emigration.

Limiting Doctor and Nurse Migration

In order to limit the migration of doctors, the Ministry of Health and Family Welfare decided in 2011 to stop issuing a No Obligation to Return to India (NORI) certificate, which is necessary for medical graduates who wish to apply for a J-1 visa to the United States. The ministry explicitly cited an acute shortage of doctors, due to large-scale emigration, in making the announcement. In response, Maharashtra Association of Resident Doctors (MARD) challenged the decision in the Bombay High Court, which termed the policy unfair but left it in place.

Nurse emigration has been subject to bureaucratic restrictions, including nursing institutions' imposition of bonds on students if they fail to meet a term of service in the country; these policies proved unpopular with regulators. In April 2015, the government also included nurses in the Emigration Check Required (ECR) category, citing corruption and nurse exploitation as a result of non-transparency in the recruitment process. The Emigration Clearance (EC) system, applied to workers going to 18 countries, requires clearance from the Protector of Emigrants office, which is situated in New Delhi. This regulatory process previously only applied to low-skilled domestic and construction workers, or those who lack a tenth grade (matriculation) certificate. This policy requires nurse recruitment be channeled through six state-related employment agencies (see Table 10.3) and nurses may only work on international contracts approved by government authorities.

Imposition of the emigration clearance process on nurses represents a heavy regulatory hand. Rather than addressing the issue of corruption among migrant recruitment intermediaries, the state has chosen to constrain the mobility of nurses through a series of regulatory hurdles in the form of recruitment and emigration clearance, which has increased the cost of migration. After the imposition of this regulation, the numbers of ECR nurse migrants fell, though they have since increased (see Table 10.2). The majority (4,460) of these ECR nurses in 2018 headed to Saudi Arabia. This

Table 10.2 Emigration of Nurses by State under Emigration Check Required (ECR), May 2015–November 2018

State	2016	2017	2018	2019
Kerala	4,111	3,611	6,085	8,453
Tamil Nadu	330	242	560	994
Karnataka	110	70	129	278
Maharashtra	67	58	112	179
Telangana	71	43	95	113
Delhi	37	25	54	61
Andhra Pradesh	57	17	52	75
Total	4,858	4,123	7,174	10,207

Source: Data obtained by the authors in 2018 through the Right to Information Act.

Table 10.3 Indian State-Run Agencies through Which International Nurse Recruitment Is Allowed

Agency	State
NORKA-Roots	Kerala
Overseas Development and Employment Promotion Consultants (ODEPC)	Kerala
Overseas Manpower Corporation Limited (OMCL)	Tamil Nadu
Telangana Overseas Manpower Company (TOMCOM)	Telangana
Overseas Manpower Company of Andhra Pradesh (OMCAP)	Andhra Pradesh
UP Financial Corporation	Uttar Pradesh

Source: Ministry of External Affairs, Government of India, office order dated September 9, 2016.

concentration in specific markets poses a threat if international relations or economic conditions shift.

Nurses going through the emigration clearance stream must process their applications through six state-run agencies, five of which are in the south and one in the north.

While one of the purposes of including nurses in the ECR category was to also regulate recruiting fees, fees charged by recruiting agents have not reduced noticeably, putting into question the whole rationale for this policy.

Beyond the imposition of bureaucratic requirements and other efforts to limit nurse migration, some policymakers are seeking more proactive ways of stemming departure. The state of Kerala, which is the source of most Indian nurses going abroad (Oda et al., 2018) in 2018 mandated that those working in private hospitals be paid a minimum wage of Rs. 20,000 a month (equivalent to US $282). This move can be seen as a way to bridge the gap in wages that is one factor enticing nurses to seek overseas employment.

Monitoring Emigration

The government is also taking steps to centralize the Emigration Clearance process, with the Ministry of External Affairs in 2019 proposing legislation that would bring all intending emigrants—including students—under its purview. The draft bill, which would overhaul the 1983 Emigration Act, would also make the emigration clearance system far more streamlined and regulate recruitment intermediaries, who are currently outside the purview of the Emigration Act and are seen as the main source of exploitation for prospective nurse migrants.

Limited Policy Impact?

Overall, these various policy changes may have limited influence on health-worker emigration. Limiting the provision of NORI for US-bound physicians and the ECR imposition on nurses suggest a more active government stance on health-worker migration. But, this is being achieved through bureaucratic reform—not systematic change to the underlying employment situation in the country of origin that could make remaining a more desirable outcome for health-care workers.

The Indian government has made clear its view that medical tourism presents an economic opportunity. For example, the Ministry of Tourism website states: "India holds advantage as a medical tourism destination due to the following factors: Most of the doctors and surgeons at Indian hospitals are trained or have worked at some time in the leading medical institutions in the U.S., Europe, or other developed nations." There is a certain irony in this, however, considering government efforts to restrict international mobility. While medical tourism is playing an increasingly important role in India, it is not yet documented how this will intersect with the dynamics of health-care worker migration. However, the COVID-19 pandemic is also providing opportunities for policy reform. The Uttar Pradesh state government, for instance, made it mandatory for government doctors pursuing post graduate courses to serve in the state for at least 10 years or pay compensation.[4]

The Way Forward

Even as it is possible to track the migration of Indian health-care professionals through the available data from the destination countries, much remains unknown about the scope of this overall migration pattern. Domestic data on the migration of Indian health workers are extremely fragmented, making it difficult to assess the exact nature and dimensions of this migration flow (Rajan and Sumeetha, 2019; Rajan, 2020). What is certain, though, is that amid aging populations and health-care worker shortages globally, the migration of Indian health-care professionals will continue.

The global nature of the current pandemic will promote the need for better policies to address health workforce shortages and promote collaboration between sending, receiving, and transit countries involved in the circuits of health-worker mobility. As a result, policies need to be developed in India and destination countries that will protect the rights of professionals during recruitment and in the workplace, and allow them to fully utilize their skills. Barriers to credential recognition, workplace discrimination, professional deskilling, and austerity-informed restructuring in the health labor force area constant challenge that need to be addressed through adequate policy initiatives. Greater bilateral and global collaboration is needed to address these problems. As India maintains its leading position as a source for health-care workers to the world, monitoring and regulating emigration will be equally as important as protecting the rights of Indian workers overseas.

Note: Originally published as Walton-Roberts, M. and S. Irudaya Rajan (2020) "Global Demand for Medical Professionals Drives Indians Abroad Despite Acute Domestic Health-Care Worker Shortages." Migration Policy Institute (MPI). Obtained permission and slightly modified for this publication. https://www.migrationpolicy.org/article/global-demand-medical-professionals-drives-indians-abroad.

Notes

1 https://www.bbc.com/news/world-48205445
2 https://digital.nhs.uk/binaries/content/assets/website-assets/supplementary-information/supplementary-info-2020/hchs-doctors-and-those-with-country-of-qualification-india_ah3455.xlsx
3 https://pib.gov.in/PressReleasePage.aspx?PRID=1658280
4 https://www.newindianexpress.com/nation/2020/dec/13/uttar-pradesh%E2%80%8B-govt-doctors-should-serve-in-dept-for-10-years-official-2235641.html#:~:text=LUCKNOW%3A%20Government%20doctors%20in%20Uttar,issued%20on%20April%203%2C%202017

Sources

Adkoli, B. V. 2006. Migration of Health Workers: Perspectives from Bangladesh, India, Nepal, Pakistan, and Sri Lanka. *Regional Health Forum* 10(1): 49–58.

Anand, Sudhir, and Victoria Fan. 2016. The Health Workforce in India. Human Resources for Health Observer Series No. 16, World Health Organization, Geneva.

Baker, Carl. 2019. NHS Staff from Overseas: Statistics. House of Commons Briefing Paper, No. 7783, July 8, 2019.

Brahmapurkar, Kishor, Parashramji Sanjay P. Zodpey, Yogesh D. Sabde, and Vaishali K. Brahmapurkar. 2018. The Need to Focus on Medical Education in Rural Districts of India. *The National Medical Journal of India* 31(3): 164.

Britnell, Michael. 2019. *Human: Solving the global workforce crisis in healthcare.* Oxford: Oxford University Press.

Chhapia, Hemali. 2019. China Gets More Indian Students than Britain. *The Times of India*, January 7, 2018.

Economic Times. 2019. UK Home Secretary Promises New Fast-Track Visa for Doctors from Countries Like India. *The Economic Times*, November 8, 2019.

Garner, Shelby L., Shelley F. Conroy, and Susan Gerding Bader. 2015. Nurse Migration from India: A Literature Review. *International Journal of Nursing Studies* 52(12): 1879–1890.

George, Gavin, and Bruce Rhodes. 2017. Is there a Financial Incentive to Immigrate? Examining the Health Worker Salary Gap between India and Popular Destination Countries. *Human Resources for Health* 15(74): 1–10.

Global Health Observatory. 2019. Nursing and Midwifery Personnel. Updated March 14, 2019.

Hohn, Marcia D., James C. Witte, Justin P. Lowry, and José Ramón Fernández-Pena. 2016. *Immigrants in health care: Keeping Americans healthy through care and innovation.* Fairfax, VA: George Mason University Institute for Immigration Research.

Humphries, Niamh, Ruairi Brugha, and Hannah McGee. 2012. Nurse Migration and Health Workforce Planning: Ireland as Illustrative of International Challenges. *Health Policy* 107(1): 44–53.

Kaushik, Manas, Abhishek Jaiswal, Naseem Shah, and Ajay Mahal. 2008. High-End Physician Migration from India. *Bulletin of the World Health Organization* 86: 40–45.

Kumar, Raman, and Ranabir Pal. 2018. India Achieves WHO Recommended Doctor Population Ratio: A Call for Paradigm Shift in Public Health Discourse! *Journal of Family Medicine and Primary Care* 7(5): 841.

Medical Council of India. n.d. List of College Teaching MBBS. Accessed January 17, 2020.

Ministry of Health, Kingdom of Saudi Arabia. 2019. Health Manpower in KSA. Updated July 10, 2019.

Ministry of Human Resource Development, Department of Higher Education, Government of India. 2019. Scholarships and Education Loan. Updated January 22, 2019.

Ministry of Overseas Indian Affairs, Government of India. 2015. F. No. 01-11012/10/2013-EP, April 8, 2015.

Mullan, Fitzhugh. 2006. Doctors for the World: Indian Physician Emigration. *Health Affairs* 25(2): 380–393.

Nair, S., and S. I. Rajan. 2017. Nursing Education in India: Changing Facets and Emerging Trends. *Economic and Political Weekly* 52(24): 38–42.

Oda, H., Y. Tsujita, and S. I. Rajan. 2018. An analysis of factors influencing the international migration of Indian nurses. *Journal of International Migration and Integration* 19(3): 607–624.

Organization for Economic Cooperation and Development (OECD) Statistics. n.d. Health Work force Migration, Foreign-Trained Doctors by Country of Origin–Stock. Accessed January 16, 2020.

Percot, Marie, and S. Irudaya Rajan. 2007. Female Emigration from India: Case Study of Nurses. *Economic and Political Weekly* 42(2): 318–325.

Potnuru, Basant. 2017. Aggregate Availability of Doctors in India: 2014–2030. *Indian Journal of Public Health* 61(3): 182.

Rajan, S. I. 2020. Migrants at a Crossroads: COVID-19 and Challenges to Migration. *Migration and Development* 9(3): 323–330.

Rajan, S. I., Varun Aggarwal, and Priyansha Singh. 2019. Draft Migration Bill 2019: The Missing Link. *Economic and Political Weekly* LIV(30): 19–22.

Rajan, S. I., and M. Sumeetha (Eds.). 2019. *Hand book on internal migration*. Delhi: Sage.

Rao, Krishna D. 2014. *Situation analysis of the health workforce in India*, Human Resources Technical Paper 1. New Delhi: Public Health Foundation of India.

Rao, Mohan, Krishna D. Rao, A. K. Shiva Kumar, Mirai Chatterjee, and Thiagarajan Sundararaman. 2011. Human Resources for Health in India. *The Lancet* 377(9765): 587–598.

Rao, Krishna D., Renu Shahrawat, and Aarushi Bhatnagar. 2016. Composition and Distribution of the Health Workforce in India: Estimates Based on Data from the National Sample Survey. *WHO South-East Asia Journal of Public Health* 5(2): 133.

Reddy, Sunita, and Imrana Qadeer. 2010. Medical Tourism in India: Progress or Predicament? *Economic and Political Weekly* 45(20): 69–75.

Scroll. 2018. After Months of Protests, Kerala Government Revises Nurses' Minimum Monthly Salaries to Rs 20,000. *Scroll*, April 24, 2018.

Sharma, Anjali, Sanjay Zodpey, and Bipin Batra. 2016. India's Foreign Medical Graduates: An Opportunity to Correct India's Physician Shortage. *Education for Health* 29(1): 42.

Shetty, Priya. 2010. Medical Tourism Booms in India, But at What Cost? *The Lancet* 376(9742): 671–672.

Sood, Rita. 2008. Medical Education in India. *Medical Teacher* 30(6): 585–591.

Times of India. 2016. 80 Percent Drop in Graduates Clearing MCI Screening Test. *The Times of India*, May 24, 2016.

———. 2017. Government Denies Visa Nod to Doctor Seeking to do Research in U.S. *The Times of India*, July 18, 2017.

Thomas, Philomina. 2006. The International Migration of Indian Nurses. *International Nursing Review* 53(4): 277–283.

Thompson, Maddy, and Margaret Walton-Roberts. 2018. International Nurse Migration from India and the Philippines: The Challenge of Meeting the Sustainable Development Goals in Training, Orderly Migration, and Health-Care Worker Retention. *Journal of Ethnic and Migration Studies* 45(14): 1–17.

Varghese, Joe, Anneline Blankenhorn, Prasanna Saligram, John Porter, and Kabir Sheikh. 2018. Setting the Agenda for Nurse Leadership in India: What is Missing. *International Journal for Equity in Health* 17(1): 98.

Walton-Roberts, Margaret, and S. I. Rajan. 2013. Nurse Emigration from Kerala: 'Brain Circulation' or 'Trap'? Chapter 13. In S. Irudaya Rajan (Ed.), *India migration report: Socail costs of migration* (pp. 206–223). New Delhi: Routledge.

Walton-Roberts, Margaret. 2012. Contextualizing the Global Nursing Care Chain: International Migration and the Status of Nursing in Kerala, India. *Global Networks* 12(2): 175–194.

———. 2015. International Migration of Health Professionals and the Marketization and Privatization of Health Education in India: From Push–Pull to Global Political Economy. *Social Science & Medicine* 124: 374–382.

Walton-Roberts, Margaret, Vivien Runnels, S. Irudaya Rajan, Atul Sood, Sreelekha Nair, Philomina Thomas, Corinne Packer, Adrian MacKenzie, Gail Tomblin Murphy, Ronald Labonté, and Ivy Lynn Bourgeault. 2017. Causes, Consequences, and Policy Responses to the Migration of Health Workers: Key Findings from India. *Human Resources for Health* 15(1): 28.

World Health Organization (WHO). 2017a. A Dynamic Understanding of Health Worker Migration. WHO Brochure, Geneva.

———. 2017b. *From brain drain to brain gain: Migration of medical doctors from Kerala.* New Delhi: WHO.

———. 2017c. *From brain drain to brain gain: Migration of nursing and midwifery workforce in the State of Kerala.* New Delhi: WHO.

11 Aspirations of Health Professionals in India for Migration Abroad

A Pre-COVID and COVID-Time Comparison of Nurses

Binod Khadria and Shekhar Tokas

Introduction: COVID-19, Health Workers and International Migration

The number of international migrants reached 281 million in 2020, which was an increase of more than 100 million since the year 2000 (up from 173 million) (Khadria and Mishra, 2021; UNDESA, 2020). The prime reasons for this increase have been labour migration, family migration (OECD, 2020), refugees and asylum seekers (UNHCR, 2020), student migration leading to settlement, etc. (UNESCO, 2018). The COVID-19 pandemic and the consequent worldwide lockdowns severely impacted the growth in the number of international migrants. The lockdown of national borders disrupted the number of international migrants to fall by around two million by mid-2020, i.e., 27% less than the growth expected since mid-2019 (UN DESA, 2021, p. 1). In March 2020, India also closed its international borders, leading to a two-fold impact on migratory flows: on the one hand, there was a frantic rush among large sections of Indian migrants abroad to come back home, triggering return migration. On the other, it impacted the international mobility aspirations of millions in India for out-migration itself for work and education abroad.

The Human Resources for Health (HRH), i.e., the health workers have, in such a context, also faced disruptions and discontinuities in their plans and aspirations while looking for opportunities with regard to international mobility for education, training, job opportunities, etc. The health workers are the lifeline of healthcare systems without whom the latter would cease to exist. These health workers are the 'people engaged in actions whose primary intent is to enhance health' (WHO, 2006, p. 1). The pandemic has brought forward the primacy of HRH comprising doctors to nurses to midwives to pharmacists to pathologists to ward boys to janitors and a whole range of other support staff nicknamed 'COVID warriors' and 'frontline workers'. Given the close relationship between health and international migration (Khadria, 2012, 2020a; Wickramage et al., 2018; IOM, 2019), it is important to recognise that any progress in overcoming this pandemic would be difficult without the sharing of HRH among nations.

DOI: 10.4324/9781003315124-11

The developed nations such as the United States, United Kingdom, member states of the European Union, etc. have pledged help in terms of what we might call 'Physical Resources for Health' (PRH) i.e., ranging from ventilators to oxygen cylinders and concentrators to life-saving drugs to vaccines and so on.[1] What can become a vital complement to this is a global rights-based equitable HRH sharing by declaring STEM (Science, Technology, Engineering and Mathematics) professionals including the HRH as the sixth among the Global Commons[2] that Khadria has been advocating for over a decade now (Khadria, 2012). Even at the beginning of the COVID-19 pandemic, he renewed his call to strategise this through the formation of a 'UN Health-keeping Force' comprising migrant HRH of different nationals – along the lines of a 'UN Peace-keeping Force' that consists of transnational soldiers – specifically for dealing with epidemics like Ebola, not to speak of the present COVID pandemic (Khadria, 2020a).

An important mode through which such global resource-sharing of HRH could become possible is international migration. The recent legislations by two major players in international migration, i.e., India as the origin and the USA as the destination, respectively on the 'preservation' and 'freer mobility' of specific human capital, viz., foreign doctors, nurses, and other healthcare workers during the COVID–19 pandemic are a testimony to this (Khadria, 1999, pp. 19–31; 2020a).[3] Importantly, it also highlights the grim reality of global imbalance and shortage in the supply of skilled health professionals (Buchan et al., 2006; Khadria, 2012, 2020a). The importance of health resource and its global shortage has been well recognised time and again (WHO, 2006, 2016; Khadria, 2007, 2010). A recent analysis conducted by the Global Health Workforce Alliance and WHO estimates a projected shortfall of 18 million health workers by 2030 affecting countries around the world (WHO, 2016, p. 12). Though the production of new health workers is well recognised to boost the flow in the supply chain of HRH, it involves huge cost including the vital input of time. Production of new STEM professionals, particularly high-skilled health-knowledge workers such as medical scientists, doctors and nurses, and optimisation in distribution of the existing ones are the two ways to fill the knowledge and skill gaps in the supply of healthcare around the world – the first in the longer run and the second in the short run (Machlup, 1962; Khadria, 1999, 2020a). Given the present pandemic and the consequent worsening fiscal situation worldwide, investments in health education and training have become more challenging at both the individual and country levels. Under the circumstances, optimisation in the distribution of existing stocks of health-knowledge workers (HRH) would be the only short-run strategy to be possible through international migration.

The relationship between international migration and health is a dynamic one (WHO, 2006, 2014, 2016; Khadria, 2010, 2012; Wickramage et al., 2018; IOM, 2019). International migration of health workers can have both positive and negative effects. On the one hand, migration of health professionals can lead to improved health, improvement in acquisition of skills, better career options, higher standards of living and less polluted and safe environment for the migrants. Moreover, at the macro level, it can solve the problem of supply shortages of health workers in the destination countries (WMR, 2005; Buchan and Perfilieva, 2006; Khadria, 2012; WHO, 2014). On the other hand, 'migration can lead to greater exposure to health risks, such as those migrant workers working in conditions of precarious employment with limited access to affordable health care' (IOM, 2019, p. 209). Additionally, the negative impact of migration of health workers on the source countries in the form of shortage of healthcare workers and precarious health systems has been at the centre of the brain drain debate for decades (Khadria, 1999, 2012). Overall, international migration has major impacts on both the people and the places of the migrants' at origin and destination countries and it is almost impossible to examine the health sector without including the dimension of international migration (WHO, 2014).

Unfortunately, international migration and health is a relationship that has remained an under-researched area for long (Khadria, 2012). More recently, the World Migration Report 2020(IOM, 2019) too has highlighted this fact:

> Globally, various research initiatives are underway to assist in developing improved understanding of – and responses to – migration and health, with a focus on the implementation of evidence-informed interventions to improve the health and well-being of both migrants and communities affected by migration. While this field of research is growing, efforts to improve understanding of migration and health, and examples of migration and health programming, remain limited.
>
> (IOM, 2019, p. 225)

'Research is needed to generate evidence-informed and context-specific interventions to address migration and health, which will, in turn, support UHC (Universal Health Coverage)' (IOM, 2019, p. 227). Therefore, the need for investment to build the research capacity in this field to improve understanding of different dimensions of health and migration (Khadria, 2012; Wickramage et al., 2018).

Importantly, Khadria (2012) had categorised the dimensions of international migration and health into two: (a) migrants' Health: the health of individual migrants; and (b) migration of Health workers.[4] He tried to theorise the interlinkages between migration of health workers and health of international migrants, the two discourses that existed independently of each other until then. Even then, the two sub-fields of research have followed trajectories exclusive of each other, the first getting most of the attention and the second short shrifts.[5]

Given this background and the COVID-19 context, this study has primarily focused upon the relatively neglected but extremely important second dimension of international migration and health, i.e., migration of health workers, particularly of nurses, as an important category of HRH. The main objective of this chapter is to explore how COVID-19 has impacted their mobility aspirations. This has been addressed through a comparative static study of two samples of nurses in India separated by almost two decades. The second section of the study provides the relevance of theoretical approaches on motivations or mobility aspirations of health workers. This is followed by the third section on the conceptualisation of motivations at the micro level. The fourth section is on the method adopted in the study. The fifth section presents the results of the two primary surveys. The chapter concludes with brief remarks on the findings.

Relevance of Theoretical Approaches to International Migration of Health Workers

Although a large number of theories have emerged following Ravenstein's celebrated 'Laws of Migration' (Ravenstein, 1885), and later after Lee's economic 'push-pull' model (1966), none has been accepted in toto by the scholars in explaining all types of migration (Massey et al., 1993; De Haas, 2010), health workers' migration being one of them. In the existing literature, theorisation of health-worker migration and nurse migration per se has been advocated by many in different ways (Khadria, 2007, 2012; Greco, 2010; Dywili et al., 2013; WHO, 2014, 2016; Walton-Roberts, 2014; Walton-Roberts et al., 2017). Largely, mobility motivations of health workers 'resemble the broader sets of motivations that encourage other migrants' (Cabanda, 2017). We review below the relevance of various theoretical approaches to the migration of health workers.

The Neo-classical Approach

The neo-classical economic theory argues that migration takes place due to wage differentials affecting the supply of and demand for labour. Not only wage differentials but differences in employment conditions and economic opportunities between countries are also important factors leading to migration (Harris & Todaro, 1970; Massey et al., 1998; Castles & Miller, 2009). Application of this approach to the mobility of health workers has been explained as an element of highly skilled migration for higher wages and better employment opportunities (Khadria, 1999, 2001, 2007, 2012; Greco, 2010). It is the most well-known application to the study of migration in general, and of nurse mobility in particular (Kline 2003; Greco, 2010).

The Push-Pull Approach

The 'push-pull' model of theorising migration, as developed by Lee (1966), counterposes the factors in home countries to those in the destination countries in terms of motivating people to migrate from the former to the latter (Kline, 2003; Greco, 2010; Freeman et al., 2011; Dywili et al., 2013). In this model, pull factors are the favourable conditions and opportunities in a destination country that attract people, and push factors are the negative circumstances that force people to leave a home country (Lee, 1966). Among the factors pulling health migrants as highly skilled migrants to destination countries, the most important ones are higher salaries, better education and job opportunities, better quality education for children, facilitation by recruitment agencies, etc. (Buchan and Perfilieva, 2006; Khadria, 2005, 2007, 2009; 2012; Dywili et al., 2013; Poppe et al., 2014; Walton-Roberts, 2012; Walton-Roberts et al., 2017). On the other hand, the 'push' factors also play an important role in the ultimate migration decision, viz., lower wages, lack of professional development, poor working conditions, lack of government investment in health and well-being of migrants and their families, etc. (Greco, 2010; Freeman et al., 2011; Dywili et al., 2013; Walton-Roberts, 2014; Walton-Roberts et al., 2017). However, juxtaposing the two sets of factors opposite each other often fails to explain why some health workers choose to stay in the areas experiencing high levels of emigration. Overall, the macroeconomic logic of the push-pull model addressing geopolitical drivers of migration has been criticised because it underplays the variety of micro-level decisions in the formation of migrants' choices (De Haas, 2011; Prescott and Nichter, 2014).

The Human Capital Investment Approach

Early conceptualisation of human capital is attributed to Adam Smith[6] (1776) and Alfred Marshall[7] (1890). The term human capital was first used by Pigou (1928) but proper theorisation was done in the 1960s after the influential work of Mincer (1958), Schultz (1961 1962) and Becker (1964). Human capital, as a concept, gained reputation in economics and got recognised as a field of intellectual and empirical enquiry primarily due to the inability of traditional economics to explain the 'residual' proportion of growth in the American economy. This residual was attributed to the 'technological change' and 'investment in man', and more specifically to education and health (Schultz, 1961, 1963), which ultimately led to the beginning of human capital theorisation. Prior to Schultz's work on human capital, the emphasis of literature on economic development was on the accumulation of physical capital. Schultz (1963) helped shift the attention to investments in education, health, migration and on-the-job training.

Human capital theory states that investment in education, health, on-the-job training and migration enhances competencies of individuals, resulting in the accumulation of skills and better health, which in turn increase an individual's productivity, and thus, monetary earnings (Becker, 1964). The formation of human capital is a long-term exercise and a time-consuming endeavour which requires not only monetary investment (Becker, 1975) but also quality time on a variety of activities such as education (Weisbrod, 1966; Cohn and Geske, 1990), health (Shultz, 1961, 1963), on-the-job training and apprenticeships (Mincer, 1974; Becker, 1975), job market information (Becker, 1975) and migration (Schultz, 1963; Wykstra, 1969). Thus, emphasis on investment in education, health, on-the-job training and migration in order to derive economic benefits is of prime importance in human capital theory (Mincer, 1958; Schultz, 1961, 1963; Becker, 1964).

Investment in health (Shultz, 1961, 1963), as separate components of human capital formation for development of a country, has been well emphasised since the 1960s. It is usually seen in terms of providing benefits of higher productivity, longer life, better standard of living, stress-free life and, thereby in the long-run, have effects on monetary earnings also (WHO, 2006, 2014, 2016; WEF, 2013, 2015). However, investment in migration by health workers for education and on-job-training for long-term economic and non-economic benefits is still a less-explored approach. In the context of migration of health workers, scholars have analysed how the investment cost of educating and training health workers affects the home country and benefits the destination country (Mills et al., 2011; Aluttis et al., 2014). In contrast, return migration of health workers, knowledge sharing with the home country and remittances sent by migrants are seen as return to investments (Khadria, 2007, 2012). The investment approach to migration of health workers is well understood but less researched and applied (Khadria, 2012; WHO, 2014, 2016; IOM, 2019).

The Brain Drain Approach

The historical structuralist theory (Portes & Walton, 1981) which emerged in the 1970s hypothesises the 'unequal distribution of economic and political power in the world economy' (Castles & Miller, 2009). Wallerstein (1974) deconstructed this theoretical framework to be comprising a core, a semi-periphery and the peripheral countries. He looked at migration to be the outcome of an interaction between the core and peripheral countries, resulting in advantage to the former. In this context, brain drain refers to the exodus of the best and the brightest people from the periphery to the core countries, perpetuating the underdevelopment process which benefits the latter at the cost of the former (Massey et al., 1993).

Historically, 'brain drain', as a concept, was used to explain the migration of skilled professionals to developed nations (Khadria, 1999, 2001). Parallels were drawn by applying the brain drain discourse to the migration of skilled health workers towards the 'west' i.e., the developed nations (Khadria, 2007, 2012; OECD, 2007). By the turn of the century, the movement of health professionals was criticised for its negative impacts on the healthcare systems of developing countries. The supply shortages of health workers in the developed countries necessitated the recruitment of health workers from other parts of the world. This had consequences for home countries in terms of 'brain drain' i.e., the loss of highly trained health workers and or the resources spent on the education and health that lead to higher average productivity (Khadria, 1999, 2007, 2012; WHO, 2006, 2014, 2016; Willis-Shattuck et al., 2008). As an antidote to brain drain, there has been the concept of 'brain circulation' and how it can benefit the home country. It is argued that health-worker migration to developed countries is beneficial for developing countries as health workers are able to build their expertise through on-the-job training and foreign education. Through the remittances that they send home and the acquired skills and expertise that they bring with them when they return home, the migrant health workers contribute to building healthcare capacities in the home countries (Hagander et al., 2013; Buchan, 2015). Ironically, this has been termed as the 'brain gain' derived by the origin countries (Khadria, 2020b).

Other Approaches

The contemporary research on HRH has also used several other approaches to study health-worker migration. Some of these include post-colonial approach, globalisation of healthcare systems, network studies, global political economy, etc. The post-colonial approach gives deeper understanding of how the colonial systems control the flow of migration of health workers to the erstwhile colonial rulers for their benefit (Walton-Roberts, 2014). It is evident from the fact that trained Indian nurses from Kerala are specifically routed to the English-speaking colonial master – the United Kingdom. However,

> the historical territorialisation [that] post-colonial approaches impose on our understanding of contemporary HHR [Health Human Resources] migratory circuits can also limit our analysis, since in the case of India the UK no longer dominates health professional migration flows, rather the USA, the Middle East and other neighbouring Asian regions have become key markets for migrants.
>
> (Walton-Roberts, 2014, p. 376).

Many consider that international migration of HRH is a result of globalisation. Similar view is held by the World Systems Theory, attributing migration to economic globalisation and penetration of capitalist market mechanisms. This is supposed to have created a workforce globally mobile enough in search of better jobs (Massey et al., 1993). Migration of health workers from this standpoint seems to be not only demand-driven but also a response to the supply shortages in the western countries. Thus, countries in the modern-day context turn to aggressive recruitment campaigns to supply HRH (Khadria, 2007). For example, England (2015) opines that the shortage of nurses in the United States is the result of neo-liberal reforms in the healthcare systems. These reforms were accompanied by 'cost containment' and 'cost-effectiveness' measures which led to cutbacks in healthcare jobs and, therefore, the closure of nurse-training programmes. This resulted in the shortage of nurses in the US and, therefore, the exponential growth in the private sector nurse-recruiting agencies. Another extension of this is the network approach that examines the interpersonal relations and the links that facilitate migration of HRH, and the recruitment agencies largely thrive on these networks (Khadria, 2007, 2012). Finally, Walton-Roberts (2014), proposes a global political economy perspective arguing that migration of HRH is not merely the result of rational decisions taken by health professionals to maximise their economic welfare; rather it is the global political economy factors that shape the HRH migratory flows embedded within wider power and resource allocation structures.

Conceptualising Motivations at the Micro Level

Despite the enormous value and contribution of the macro-level theories, some of which are discussed above, towards describing international flows of migrants, they have been critiqued for their inability to theorise how macro factors influence micro-level behaviour, particularly of the individual migrants (Massey et al., 1993; De Haas, 2011; Khadria, 2020c). The most credible approach available to understand the micro-level mobility aspiration of migrants is the neo-classical migration theory. At the micro level, neo-classical framework considers migrants as rational individuals maximising their income by investing in migration on the basis of a cost-benefit analysis. Parallels can be drawn from the neo-classical micro theory approach to explain the migration of health workers. Health workers decide to invest in migration for better job opportunities, education abroad, on-the-job training, etc. If the expected private rate of return derived through the higher wages (primarily expected economic earnings) in the destination country is greater than the private costs incurred on migration (education and job search, fees paid to education and recruitment agencies, language tests, visa, travelling cost, etc.), migration will take place subject to adherence to the immigration laws.

A majority of literature and empirical research related to migration of health workers considers motivations to be driven primarily by economic gains.[8] In contrast, some have argued that although financial factors play an important role in migration, for many it is not the main driving force (Khadria, 2007; Poppe et al., 2014; Garner et al., 2015; Suciu et al., 2017; Walton-Roberts et al., 2017). Becker (1998, p. 139) says that 'Unlike Marxian analysis, the economic approach I refer to does not assume that individuals are motivated solely by selfishness or material gains. It is a method of analysis, not an assumption about particular motivations'. In his initial theorisation of human capital also, Becker (1975) talked about the non-monetary aspect of investing in human capital. He says that real earnings are the sum of monetary earnings and the monetary equivalent of psychic earnings. Since many persons appear to believe that the term 'investment in human capital' must be restricted to monetary costs and returns, let me emphasise that essentially the whole analysis applies independently of the division of real earnings into monetary and psychic components.

(Becker, 1975, p. 46)

Emphasis on non-monetary benefits also becomes clear when Becker states that

human capital analysis starts with the assumption that individuals decide on their education, training, medical care and other additions to knowledge and health by weighing the benefits and costs. Benefits include cultural and other non-monetary gains along with improvement in earnings and occupation, whereas costs usually depend mainly on forgone value of the time spent on these investments.

(Becker, 1993).

Presence of non-monetary benefits from investing in human capital is also well recognised by Schultz's comment on human capital. He states, 'It is human because it is embodied in man, and it is capital because it is a source of future satisfaction, or of future earnings, or of both' (Schultz, 1971, p. 48).

De Haas (2011) opines that the macro-level explanations of migration do not necessarily apply on the micro level and even if migration occurs because of 'abstract macro concepts', it is difficult to determine the causality of macro factors with micro decisions. However, Majumdar (1983, p. 68) had not only anticipated but also deconstructed this dilemma succinctly in explaining that, 'one must allow for difference between the logic of the macroeconomic state of expectations in the market, and the equally valid logic of individuals' micro-level expectations'. Therefore, what is needed is a more comprehensive framework of migration that allows for the differences of macro and micro levels to co-exist.

In the present context of the COVID-19 pandemic, therefore, the primacy of economic aspirations of individual migrants for out-migration are no longer sacrosanct. The micro-level approach discussed above provides the appropriate framework to understand the mobility aspirations of health workers in general, and nurses in particular. However, it is the transnational macro-level global pandemic that has disrupted the micro-level mobility aspirations in the case of nurses as discussed later. This we have tried to establish through the comparative static evidence from two contrasting micro-level small sample surveys separated widely apart in time, one distortion free from any epidemic or pandemic and the other totally engulfed by the COVID-19 pandemic.

Methods of the Two Sample Surveys

As discussed above, mobility aspirations of migrants are very complex in nature. Therefore, for a holistic understanding of mobility aspirations of nurses, we conducted interviews through two small sample surveys of comparative static nature – one in 2002 (Khadria, 2004) and the other in March 2021. In both the surveys, a mix of purposive and snowball sampling was followed to have some variation in aspirations. Initially, a few target respondents were identified and located and were asked to provide the names of other members of the target population and so on. Purposive sampling was also important to include cases that are otherwise not reflected in random sampling. The comparative analyses largely in terms of what impacts mobility aspirations of nurses across time provide some understanding of the complex motivations of the nurses.

Description of the Field and Sample Population

The first sample survey was carried out in Delhi in 2002 on the nurses' out-migration (Khadria, 2004). The entire sample of this survey was drawn from one public sector medical institution in New Delhi, i.e., Kalawati Saran Children's Hospital. Of the 40 nurses in the sample, approximately half i.e., 18 nurses were from Kerala, and one-fourth i.e., 10 nurses were from New Delhi. The other 12 respondent nurses came from eight different states – three from Haryana, three from Uttar Pradesh, two from Tamil Nadu, two from Maharashtra and one each from Himachal Pradesh and Bihar. The Lady Hardinge Medical College, to which the Kalawati Saran Children's Hospital was affiliated was said to have provided the training for the largest number in the sample i.e., 10 nurses. Kerala University and Indira Gandhi National Open University at New Delhi, having provided training to four nurses each came next in the rank.

The second sample survey was conducted in the month of March 2021. Interviews were conducted telephonically with the nurses working in a private hospital affiliated to a private university in the Delhi NCR region. In total, 13 nurses were interviewed to first look back and reflect on their 'pre-COVID' mobility aspirations (as if they were in pre-March 2020 period), and then as if a year later in real time during the ongoing pandemic defined as 'COVID-time' (March 2021). Of these 13 nurses, 2 were associate professors, 7 were assistant professors and 4 were tutors. All 13 respondents had both teaching and clinical duties.

The Mobility Aspirations of Nurses – A Comparative Case Study of COVID ('Pre-COVID' and 'COVID-Time') vis-à-vis Normal Times

Decisions to migrate are very complex and are influenced by several economic, social and cultural factors. The present two surveys reveal that nurses have a broad spectrum of mobility aspirations which varies across time. The study finds the following as the prominent factors impacting mobility aspirations: better training opportunities, obtaining a specific kind of training, better employment opportunities and higher salary, better working conditions, social recognition for the nursing profession, etc. These aspirations usually help aspiring migrants make faster progress in the medical profession; but in a pandemic, it is 'personal and family safety' which figures above all. This is elaborated and discussed below.

Postponing the Plan to Migrate: Supremacy of Personal and Family Safety

In normal times, people tend to migrate with minimum fluctuations in the rate of mobility from an origin to a destination, whether within the country or outside. In a crisis, however, whether natural or man-made, that can affect mobility aspirations, the usual expectation is to have a jump in the rate of this mobility as larger numbers of people would tend to look for safer habitats and move towards them as quickly as possible. Normally, this would have been also expected in the present crisis of COVID-19 pandemic as was evident in the case of internal migration of unskilled and semi-skilled labour in India that shook the nation as soon as the national lockdown was announced in March 2020 (Khadria, 2020d). Contrarily, our finding is that this is not the case with nurses, belonging to a high-skill profession, tending to migrate internationally; rather, their aspirations to move quickly seemed to have faded away with the growing realisation that in the pandemic, there were no alternative safer habitats within reach anywhere in the world. Significantly, this has been the finding of our evidence on how counterintuitively the mobility aspirations can behave.

The data from the primary surveys conducted show that under normal times, economic factors influence the mobility aspirations of nurses the most. However, the COVID-time data reflect that 'personal and family safety' involving a life-and-death-question has come to the forefront as the primary factor influencing mobility aspirations of the nurses, overtaking all other factors. Table 11.1 suggests that 9 out of 13 nurses in the COVID-time, i.e., 69% nurses responded that they have postponed their plans to migrate, for at least a year, due to personal and family safety in the context of COVID-19 pandemic. These nurses decided to rather invest their time and money in extending their education or experience within India for at least a year. In contrast, the normal-time sample survey of 2002 (Khadria, 2004) had none of the nurses having such particular 'personal and family safety' concern as the primary factor firing one's mobility aspirations.

Better Employment Opportunities and Training

Table 11.1 compares the aspirations behind the intended out-migration of nurses in the two periods. With respect to sample survey 1 conducted

Table 11.1 Mobility Aspirations for Out-Migration of Nurses in India: 2002 and 2021

Mobility Aspirations of Nurses	Aspiration, 2002	Rank (Aspiration, 2002)	Aspiration, Pre-COVID	Rank (Aspiration, Pre-COVID)	Aspiration, In-COVID	Rank (Aspiration, In-COVID)
Better Training Opportunities	31 (77.5%)	1	9 (69%)	2	0	0
Obtaining a Specific Kind of Training	31 (77.5%)	1	4 (31%)	5	6 (46%)	4
Progress Faster in Medical Profession	25 (62.5%)	3	2 (15%)	6	7 (54%)	3
Better Employment Opportunities/Higher Salary	19 (47.5%)	4	13 (100%)	1	1 (7%)	6
Permanent Settlement in Host Country	13 (32.5%)	5	0	0	1 (7%)	6
Research Assignments	6 (15%)	6	0	0	0	0
Better Working Conditions	NA	NA	5 (38%)	4	10 (77%)	1
Social Recognition for Nursing Profession	NA	NA	6 (46%)	3	5 (38%)	5
Postponed for Now (Personal and Family Safety)	NA	NA	0	0	9 (69%)	2
N=Total Number of Respondents	40		13		13	

Note 1: Wherever there are same rank(s), the next rank is not assigned, e.g., in column 'Rank (Aspiration 2002)' rank 3 follows rank 1, and in column 'Rank (In-COVID)' rank 8 follows rank 6.

Note 2: In both the surveys, nurses were asked to give their top three determinants of mobility aspirations for out-migration. The percentage given for each determinant is a cumulative figure of those nurses who chose it among their top three determinants.

Source: Compiled from Khadria (2004) and the primary survey conducted by the authors in March 2021.

in 2002, out of 40 respondent nurses, 31 mentioned that 'better training opportunities' was the main purpose for going abroad, i.e., 77.5% nurses. But equally important was 'obtaining a specific kind of training', i.e., again 77.5% nurses ranked it as their top determinant of mobility aspiration. Similarly, for the pre-COVID aspirations (March 2020), 13 out of 13 nurses (100%) ranked 'better employment opportunities' as their top mobility aspiration, followed by 'better training opportunities' for 9 out of 13 nurses (69%). In sharp contrast, in the COVID time (March 2021), only 1 nurse ranked 'better employment opportunities' as the top determinant and none of the nurses ranked 'better training opportunities' among their top three determinants. Rather, 6 out of 13 nurses (46%) chose 'obtaining a specific kind of training' i.e., in psychiatry, as their top determinant. These nurses felt that there was and will be an increased demand for psychiatric nursing in developed nations like the United States, the United Kingdom and Europe due to pandemic-driven mental health issues. It is important to note here that although higher ranking to 'obtaining a specific kind of training' already existed in pre-COVID, but when compared to the ranking of 'obtaining better training opportunities' in the COVID-time, it is found remarkably higher in the latter case.

Professional Development

Sample survey 1 conducted in 2002 (Table 11.1) shows that 25 nurses out of 40, i.e., 62.5% nurses wanted to move overseas 'to progress faster in (their) medical career'. These nurses were of the view that a fair selection for medical career was not possible in India because of the complexities of constitutional reservation policies and caste-based policies adversely affecting the job market. Moreover, they shared their concern about stagnation in the career due to out-dated medical facilities. They elaborated that nursing education and training facilities were substandard in India and the compensation packages were unattractive (Khadria, 2004). Counterintuitively, in the 2021 sample of nurses, faster progression in medical career was the least preferred mobility aspirations in the pre-COVID time, i.e., only 2 nurses out of 13 (15%) chose this as a determinant. In sharp contrast, in the COVID-time, faster progression in medical career jumped up to be the third-most important determinant of mobility aspirations, i.e., 7 out of 13 nurses (54%) chose this. The prominent reason for this was the change in expectations that there would be a sudden upward shift in the demand function for highly skilled nurses in the immediate-to-near future. These nurses strongly felt that pursuing further higher studies, viz., PhD or doctoral level specific training in foreign countries would become very critical in their profession. Nurses in both the 2002 and 2021 (March 2020) sample surveys reflected that there was a lack of opportunities in India if a nurse wanted to continue quality higher education. Moreover, they both revealed that the nurses felt that there was a lack of opportunities for learning new technologies or acquiring specialties then as well as now and hence going abroad was of critical value. However, these aspirations reversed drastically in the COVID-time (March 2021).

Better Working Conditions

Better working conditions include organisational culture that promotes professionalism and better working environment, lower workload, extra pay for extra work, safety at workplace, etc. In the pre-COVID time, 5 out of 13 nurses (38%) said that the 'better working conditions' was an important factor for them. In comparison, in the COVID-time, 'better working conditions' has replaced the 'better employment opportunities' as the top determinant. 10 out of 13 nurses (77%) ranked better working conditions as their top mobility aspirations. The obvious reason reflected upon by the nurses has been that COVID-19 has not only increased the burden of workload, but most importantly jacked up the safety risks. Pandemic has put more pressure on the health system leading to lack of resources, both physical (medicine and equipment) and human (shortage of nurses and other staff). This shortage of both physical and human resources has increased the burden of work and created unsafe working conditions for the nurses. In effect, this has led to a worsening of the already high patient–nurse ratio, pushing up the per capita working hours and work load of nurses. It is important to note that the one potent reason for this has been the unique nature of work that the nurses do. In addition, social distancing protocols of COVID-19 have led to a smaller number of nurses on the work floor per unit of time – physical presence being unsubstitutable by video consultation that the doctors can at times resort to.

Social Recognition for Nursing Profession

Lack of social recognition for nursing profession is also an important factor that drives the nurses to migrate out of the country. Nurses tend to migrate citing reasons such as enhancement of their status in societies abroad. In both pre-COVID and COVID-time, low social recognition for nursing profession in India has been cited as one of the important mobility aspirations for nurses. In pre-COVID time, lower 'social recognition for nursing profession' was among the top three determinants for mobility aspirations. 6 out of 13 nurses ranked it as the third-most important determinant influencing their mobility aspirations. In comparison, in COVID-time, there was a slight decline, with 5 out of 13 nurses marking this as an important determinant of their mobility aspirations. This was perhaps because it did not matter as much during a life-threatening crisis like COVID-19.

Conclusion

In the normal times, mobility aspirations of nurses in India have been largely dominated by economic factors like better employment opportunities reflected in higher salary, better training opportunities and obtaining a specific kind of training. The present study finds that: first, the primacy of economic aspirations for out-migration is no longer sacrosanct. The theoretical micro-level neo-classical approach is an appropriate framework to understand the mobility aspirations of health workers in general and nurses in particular. However, our comparative static evidence from two contrasting micro-level small sample surveys, separated widely apart in time, one distortion free from any epidemic or pandemic and the other totally engulfed by the COVID-19 pandemic, shows that the transnational macro factors like COVID-19 global pandemic can severely disrupt the micro-level neo-classical mobility aspirations of the nurses in India. Second, in the COVID-time, 'personal and family safety' involving a life-or-death question has come to the forefront as the primary factor influencing mobility aspirations of the nurses. Third, it has shifted the focus from economic aspirations for mobility abroad to personal and social factors like better working conditions and social recognition of the nursing profession.

These findings are related to the classic question of setting and resetting the priorities between protecting life and securing livelihoods. In the context of COVID-19-driven lockdowns, initially the priority of the governments around the world was only about saving life from death. Subsequently, with the prolongation of lockdowns, when the economic in activities also started threatening the very existence of masses due to deprivation and starvation, saving livelihood surfaced to be an equally important priority.[9] What followed was the reprioritisation of 'life-first' when the positivity rate of corona virus infection surged and death rates surmounted. In the context of health workers and specifically nurses, it is our hunch that they perhaps foresee that they and their families can survive worst conditions of livelihood (by being driven into poor and substandard living and working conditions) by digging deep into their savings and assets that the middle classes normally accumulate. But if there was no life left, then the question of surviving on savings and assets would not arise. This would perhaps add more fuel to the ongoing debate between the quantitative utility maximisation rationale and the qualitative behavioural approach to individual economic decision making where the latter has been already overtaking the former since the award of the 2017 Nobel Prize in economics.[10]

Notes

1 Unfortunately, the lengthy pathway to the WTO endorsement to the proposed patent waiver on COVID vaccines to countries like India by the US under the Biden regime highlights the roadblocks to resource-sharing strategies in the development of HRH, which includes knowledge sharing by countries. This enhances the apprehension about the pandemic continuing uncontained in the near future (see, https://www.ndtv.com/world-news/germany-says-patent-protection-must-remain-2436630).

2 The other five Global Commons are the High Oceans, Atmosphere, Outer Space, Antarctica and the Internet.
3 The two legislations are, first, an amendment to a 123-year-old Epidemic Diseases Act mandating deterrent punishment for any physical harm caused to healthcare workers in India, and the second, the exception allowed to the entry of foreign doctors, nurses, researchers and other healthcare workers in the US from the travel ban imposed through the evocation of Section 212 (f) of the 1952 Immigration and Nationality Act by the presidential executive order under the Trump regime, blocking the entry of people deemed 'detrimental' to the country's interests (Khadria, 2020a).
4 Focusing primarily on the first, the WMR 2020 categorises this relationship between migration and health into four dimensions: '(a) the health of individual migrants ("migrant health"); (b) the ways in which migration can affect the health of populations ("public health"); (c) healthcare systems responses; and (d) the global governance of migration and health' (IOM, 2019, p. 209).
5 Vearey et al. (2019) have devoted only a short single-para section in their chapter on 'Migration and Health' in the WMR 2020 (IOM, 2019, p. 223).
6 Adam Smith included all acquired and useful abilities of the inhabitants of a country as part of capital. He considered acquired and useful abilities of the labour as predominant force of economic progress. His definition of capital also included human capital, which consists 'of the acquired and useful abilities of all the inhabitants of members of the society. The acquisition of such talents, by the maintenance of the acquirer during his education, study, or apprenticeship, always costs a real expense, which is a capital, fixed or realized, as it were, in his person' (Smith, 1776, p. 227).
7 The importance given to investment in human beings is very well reflected in the statement from the book *Principles of Economics* (1890/2013) in which Marshall opines that 'the most valuable of all capital is that invested in human beings' (p. 596).
8 Tokas (2017) had carried out a similar survey to study the motivations of foreign students in India in and around three university campuses in Delhi. His findings were that whereas overseas students from developing countries came to India with their primary motivations of economics gains, those from the developed countries were motivated primarily by non-economic factors, viz., socio-cultural-spiritual enrichment, travel to experience the diversity of India, non-formal learning of ashrams, yoga, Indian cuisine and music, etc. (Chapter 5).
9 This is where countries are faced with the dilemma of whether to distinguish between citizens and migrants and within migrants between legal/regular/ documented and illegal/irregular/undocumented immigrants. See, for example, Khadria (2020b).

References

Aluttis, C., Bishaw, T., and Frank, M. W. (2014), "The Workforce for Health in a Globalized Context—Global Shortages and International Migration", *Global Health Action*, Vol. 7, No.1, pp. 1–7.

Becker, G. (1964), *Human Capital*. New York: National Bureau of Economic Research.

Becker, G. (1993), "Nobel Lecture: The Economic Way of Looking at Behaviour", *The Journal of Political Economy*, Vol. 101, No. 3, pp. 385–409.

Becker, G. (1996), *Accounting for Tastes*. Cambridge, MA: Harvard University Press.

Becker, G. (1998), *Accounting for Tastes*. Cambridge, MA: Harvard University Press.

Becker, G. (2004), "The Concise Encyclopedia of Economics: Human Capital", *Library of Economics and Liberty*. https://www.econlib.org/library/Enc1/HumanCapital.html

Becker, G. S. (1975), "Investment in Human Capital: Effects on Earnings", In G. S. Becker (Ed.), *Human Capital: A Theoretical and Empirical Analysis, with Special Reference to Education*, Second Edition (pp. 13–14). Cambridge: NBER.

Buchan, J. (2015), "Health Worker Migration in Context", In E. Kuhlmann, R. H. Blank, I. L. Bourgeault, and C. Wendt (Eds.), *The Palgrave International Handbook of Healthcare Policy and Governance* (pp. 341–355). London: Palgrave Macmillan.

Buchan, J., and Perfilieva, G. (2006), *Health Worker Migration in the European Region: Country Case Studies and Policy Implications*. Copenhagen: World Health Organization.

Cabanda, E. (2017), "Identifying the Role of the Sending State in the Emigration of Health Professionals: A Review of the Empirical Literature", *Migration and Development*, Vol. 6, No. 2, pp. 215–231.

Castles, S., and Miller, M. J. (2009), *The Age of Migration*. Basingstoke and London: Macmillan.

Cohn, E., and Geske, T. G. (1990), *The Economics of Education*. Oxford, UK: Pergamon Press.

De Haas, H. (2010), "Migration Transitions: A Theoretical and Empirical Inquiry into the Developmental Drivers of International Migration", IMI Working Paper No. 24, (DEMIG Project Paper 1), University of Oxford: International Migration Institute.

De Haas, H. (2011), "The Determinants of International Migration: Conceptualizing Policy, Origin and Destination Effects", Working paper, paper no. 32, University of Oxford: IMI.

Dywili, S., Bonner, A., and O'Brien, L. (2013), "Why Do Nurses Migrate?—A Review of Recent Literature", *Journal of Nursing Management*, Vol. 21, No. 3, pp. 511–520.

England, K. (2015), "Nurses across Borders: Global Migration of Registered Nurses to the US", *Gender, Place & Culture*, Vol. 22, No. 1, pp. 143–156.

Freeman, M., Baumann, A., Blythe, J., Fisher, A., and Akhtar-Danesh, N. (2011), "Migration: A Concept Analysis from a Nursing Perspective", *Journal of Advanced Nursing*, Vol. 68, No. 5, pp. 1176–1186.

Garner, S. L., Conroy, S. F., and Bader, S. G. (2015), "Nurse Migration from India: A Literature Review", *International Journal of Nursing Studies*, Vol. 52, No. 12, pp. 1879–1890.

Greco, G. (2010), "International Migration of Health Professionals: Towards a Multidimensional Framework for Analysis and Policy Response", In R. S. Shah (Ed.), *The International Migration of Health Workers* (pp. 9–24). London: Palgrave Macmillan.

Hagander, L. E., Hughes, C. D., Nash, K., Ganjawalla, K., Linden, A., Martins, Y., Casey, K., and Meara, J. G. (2013), "Surgeon Migration between Developing Countries and the United States: Train, Retain, and Gain from Brain Drain", *World Journal of Surgery*, Vol. 37, No. 1, pp. 14–23.

Harris, J. R., and Todaro, M. P. (1970). "Migration, Unemployment and Development: A Two-Sector Analysis", *The American Economic Review*, Vol. 60, No. 1, pp. 126–142. http://www.jstor.org/stable/1807860.

Hull, E. (2010), "International Migration, 'Domestic Struggles' and Status Aspiration among Nurses in South Africa", *Journal of Southern African Studies*, Vol. 36, No. 4, pp. 851–867.

IOM. (2019), *World Migration Report 2020*, (M. McAuliffe, and B. Khadria, eds.). Geneva: International Organisation for Migration.

Khadria, B. (1999), *The Migration of Knowledge Workers: Second-Generation Effects of India's Brain Drain*. New Delhi: Sage Publications.

Khadria, B. (2001), "Shifting Paradigms of Globalization: The Twenty-First Century Transition Towards Generics in Skilled Migration from India", *International Migration*, Vol. 39, No. 5, Special issue 1, pp.45–71.

Khadria, B. (2004), "Migration of Highly Skilled Indians:Case Studies of IT and the Health Professionals", OECD Science, Technology and Industry Working Papers, 2004/6, OECD Publishing.

Khadria, B. (2005), "Exporting Health Workers to Overseas Markets", In *International Dialogue on Migration No. 6: Health and Migration: Bridging the Gap*, pp. 79–80. Geneva: IOM.

Khadria, B. (2007), "International Nurse Recruitment in India", *Health Services Research*, Vol. 42, No. 3p2, pp. 1429–1436.

Khadria, B. (2009), *The Future of International Migration to OECD Countries. Regional Note South Asia*. Paris: Organisation for Economic Co-operation and Development (OECD).

Khadria, B. (2010), "The Future of Migration and Health Policies", background paper prepared for the World Migration Report 2010, IOM, Geneva.

Khadria, B. (2012). "Migration of Health Workers and Health of International Migrants: Framework for Bridging Some Knowledge Disjoints between Brain Drain and Brawn Drain", *International Journal of Public Policy*, Vol. 8. https://doi.org/10.1504/IJPP.2012.048717.

Khadria, B. (2020a), "STEMming Brain Drain in COVID-19 Era", *Down to Earth*, 04 May, New Delhi.

Khadria, B. (2020b), "Between the "Hubs" and "Hinterlands" of Migration in South Asia: The Bangladesh-India Corridor", *International Journal of South Asian Studies*, Tokyo, Vol. 10, pp. 1–10.

Khadria, B. (2020c), "Migrants and Borders: My Wishlist in a Post-COVID-19 World", *Geography & You*, Special Issue on Rethink-Reboot-Remake: Covid-19 Impacts, pp. 4–7.

Khadria, B. (2020d), "COVID-19: Why are the Migrant Workers so Desperate to Move Out?" *Down to Earth*, 15 April, New Delhi.

Khadria, B., and Mishra, R. (2021), "Migration in Asia and its Subregions: Data Challenges and Coping Strategies for 2021", *Migration Policy Practice: Special Issue on Global Mobility 2021*, Vol. XI, No. 1, pp. 14–20.

Kline, D. S. (2003), "Push and Pull Factors in International Nurse Migration", *Journal of Nursing Scholarship*, Vol. 35, No. 2, pp. 107–111.

Lee, E. (1966), "A Theory of Migration", *Demography*, Vol. 3, No. 1, pp. 47–67.

Li, H., Wenbo, N., and Junxin, L. (2014), "The Benefits and Caveats of International Nurse Migration", *International Journal of Nursing Sciences*, Vol. 1, No. 3, pp. 314–317.

Machlup, F. (1962), *The Production and Distribution of Knowledge in the United States*. Princeton, NJ: Princeton University Press.

Majumdar, T. (1983), *Investment in Education and Social Choice*. Cambridge: Cambridge University Press.

Marshall, A. (1890), *Principles of Economics (Palgrave Classics in Economics)*. New York: Macmillan Publishers. Reprinted 2013.

Massey, D., Arango, J., Hugo, G., Koaouci, A., Pellegrino, A., and Taylor, J. (1998). *Worlds in Motion: Understanding International Migration at the End of the Millennium*. New York: Oxford University Press.

Massey, D. S. (1999), "International Migration at the Dawn of the Twenty-First Century: The Role of the State", *Population and Development Review*, Vol. 25, No. 2, pp. 303–322.

Massey, D. S., Arango, J.., Hugo, O., Kouaduci, A., Pellagrino, A., and Taylor, E. (1993), "Theories of International Migration: A Review and Appraisal", *Population and Development Review*, Vol. 19, No. 3, pp. 431–466.

Massey, D. S., Arango, J., Hugo, G., Kouaouci, A. K., Pellegrino, A., and Je, T. (1994), "An Evaluation of International Migration Theory: The North American Case", *Population and Development Review*, Vol. 20, pp. 699–751.

Mills, E. J., Kanters, S., Hagopian, A., Bansback, N., Nachega, J., Alberton, M., Au-Yeung, C. G., Mtambo, A., Bourgeault, I. L., Luboga, S., Hogg, R. S., and Ford, N. (2011), "The Financial Cost of Doctors Emigrating from Sub-Saharan Africa: Human Capital Analysis", *British Medical Journal*, Vol. 343: d7031.

Mincer, J. (1958), "Investment in Human Capital and Personal Income Distribution", *The Journal of Political Economy*, Vol. 66, No. 4, pp. 281–302.

Mincer, J. (1974). *Schooling, Experience and Earnings*. New York: National Bureau of Economic Research.

NDTV. (2021), "On Covid Vaccines, Germany Says Patent Protection "Must Remain": Rich Nations have Faced Accusations of Hoarding Shots While Poor Countries Struggle to Get Inoculation Programs Off the Ground", reported by Agence France-Presse, 07th May. Available from https://www.ndtv.com/world -news/germany-says-patent-protection-must-remain-2436630

Organisation for Economic Co-operation and Development. (2007), "Immigrant Health Workers in OECD Countries in the Broader Context of Highly Skilled Migration", *International Migration Outlook: SOPEMI 2007*, Part III, pp. 161–228.

Organisation for Economic Co-operation and Development. (2020), *International Migration Outlook 2020*. Paris: OECD Publishing.

Pigou, A. C. (1928), "An Analysis of Supply", *The Economic Journal*, Vol. 38, No. 150, pp. 238–257.

Poppe, A., Jirovsky, E., Blacklock, C., Laxmikanth, P., Moosa, S., De Maeseneer, J., Kutalek, R., and Peersman, W. (2014), "Why Sub-Saharan African Health Workers Migrate to European Countries that do not Actively Recruit: A Qualitative Study Post-Migration", *Global Health Action*, Vol. 7, No. 1, pp. 240–271.

Portes, A., and Walton, J. (1981), *Labor. Class, and the International System*. New York: Acedemic Press.

Potnuru, B., and Khadria, B. (2018), "Have the "London dreams" of Indian Doctors Come to an End?", In I. Rajan (Ed.), *India Migration Report 2018: Migrants in Europe* (pp. 175–191). India, London: Routledge India.

Prescott, M., and Nichter, M. (2014), "Transnational Nurse Migration: Future Directions for Medical Anthropological Research", *Social Science &Medicine*, Vol. 107, pp. 113–123.

Ravenstein, E. G. (1885), "The Laws of Migration", *Journal of the Royal Statistical Society*, Vol. 48, No. 2, pp. 167–227.

Schultz, T. W. (1961), "Investment in Human Capital", *The American Economic Review*, Vol. 51, No. 1, pp. 1–17.

Schultz, T. W. (1962), "Reflections on Investment in Man", *Journal of Political Economy*, Vol. 70, No. 5, pp. 1–8.

Schultz, T. W. (1963). *The Economic Value of Education*. New York: Columbia University Press.

Schultz, T. W. (1971), *Investment in Human Capital: The Role of Education and Research*. New York: The Free Press.

Smith, A. (1776), *An Inquiry into the Nature and Causes of the Wealth of Nations*. Penguin Classics Paperback Edition 1982, New Delhi.

Suciu, Ş. M., Popescu, C. A., Ciumageanu, M. D., and Buzoianu, A. D. (2017), "Physician Migration at its Roots: A Study on the Emigration Preferences and Plans among Medical Students in Romania", *Human Resources for Health*, Vol. 15, No. 1, p. 6.

Tokas, S. (2017), "International Students in India: A Study of their Motivations and Mobility Experiences", unpublished PhD thesis, Jawaharlal Nehru University, New Delhi, India.

United Nations. (2019), *International Migration Report 2019*, (ST/ESA/SER.A/438), Department of Economic and Social Affairs, Population Division, New York.

United Nations Department of Economic and Social Affairs, Population Division. (2020), *International Migration 2020 Highlights*. New York: United Nations Publication.

United Nations Educational, Scientific and Cultural Organization. (2018), *National Monitoring: Inbound Internationally Mobile Students by Continent of Origin*. Paris: UNESCO.

United Nations High Commissioner for Refugees. (2020), *Global Trends: Forced Displacement 2019*. Geneva. Office of the United Nations High Commissioner for Refugees (UNHCR).

Vearey, J., Hui, C., and Wickramage, K. (2019), "Migration and Health", In M. McAuliffe, and B. Khadria (Eds.), *World Migration Report 2020, Chapter 7* (pp. 209–228). Geneva: IOM.

Wallerstein, I. (1974), "The Rise and Future Demise of the World Capitalist System: Concepts for Comparative Analysis", *Comparative Studies in Society and History*, Vol. 16, No. 4, pp. 387–415.

Walton-Roberts, M. (2012), "Contextualizing the Global Nursing Care Chain: International Migration and the Status of Nursing in Kerala, India", *Global Network*, Vol. 12, No. 2, pp. 175–194.

Walton-Roberts, M. (2014), "International Migration of Health Professionals and the Marketization and Privatization of Health Education in India: From Push–Pull to Global Political Economy", *Social Science & Medicine*,Vol. 124, pp. 374–382.

Walton-Roberts, M. et al. (2017), "Causes, Consequences, and Policy Responses to the Migration of Health Workers: Key Findings from India", *Human Resources for Health*, Vol. 15, p. 28.

WEF. (2013), *The Human Capital Report 2013*. Geneva: World Economic Forum.

WEF. (2015), *The Human Capital Report 2015*. Geneva: World Economic Forum.

Weisbrod, B. A. (1966), "Investing in Human Capital", *The Journal of Human Resources*, Vol. 1, No. 1, pp. 5–21.

WHO. (2006), *World Health Report 2006: Working Together for Health*. Geneva: World Health Organisation.

WHO. (2014), *Migration of Health Workers: Who Code of Practice and the Global Economic Crisis*. Geneva: World Health Organisation.

WHO. (2016), *Global Strategy on Human Resources for Health: Workforce 2030*. Geneva: World Health Organisation.

Wickramage, K., Vearey, J., Zwi, A. B., Robinson, C., and Knipper, M. (2018), "Migration and Health: A Global Public Health Research Priority", *BMC Public Health*, Vol. 18, No. 987.

Willis-Shattuck, M., Bidwell, P., Thomas, S., Wyness, L., Blaauw, D., and Ditlopo, P. (2008), "Motivation and Retention of Health Workers in Developing Countries: A Systematic Review", *BMC Health Services Research*, Vol. 8, No. 1, pp. 247.

Wykstra, R. A. (1969), "Economic Development and Human Capital Formation", *The Journal of Developing Areas*, Vol. 3, No. 4, pp. 527–538.

12 South–South Migration

Southern Interpretations of a Northern Discourse

Themrise Khan

Introduction

It is hard to recall when I was first introduced to the term "Global South".[1] Perhaps, it was during the early days of my career as a development practitioner in Pakistan in the late 1990s. Or, perhaps, it was during my Master's degree at the beginning of this century in the UK. But to suddenly realize, indeed, to be told that I and others like myself had been slotted into a geography nearly half the size of the earth, simply by virtue of our developmental and financially humble origins, was an irony that was not lost on me.

Subsequently, this term and its more powerful counterpart, the "Global North", have become indelible in the context of discussions on inequality and power structures around the world. I too, as a development practitioner and migration researcher, have used both terms liberally over the years to juxtapose my research into development, inequality and migration against a more "global" context.

But, by dividing the globe across its horizontal axis, into two halves – upper and lower – scholars, academics and practitioners, have also divided their understanding of these two worlds. The upper half is consistently defined as on the path to progress and wealth, while the lower half is on an inevitable downward trajectory of inequality and disparity. And never the twain shall meet.

This framing has had a marked impact on not only how countries view each other across this divide, but also on how socio-economic and political relationships are defined amongst them.[2] None is more contentious than migration.

Migration has traditionally been viewed in both academic and intellectual literature as a movement from the "marginalized" South to the "prosperous" North.[3] Literature that is widely authored by those in the North. Legal migration pathways have historically led, and continue to lead, from Asia, Africa and Latin America, to Europe, North America and Australia. But, they also contend with being managed and controlled by the latter states. Not just conceptually, but also administratively, legally and politically. Even today, the North gets to decide who migrates, where and how.

DOI: 10.4324/9781003315124-12

But human movement does not simply move in one direction. It is multi-dimensional and multi-directional. As a result, people not only move between these two perceived halves but also within them.

South–South migration, a term ironically also coined by the North, is one of the biggest misnomers when it comes to research into issues of global migration and mobility.[4] The idea that people not only migrate from the North to the South, but also from the South to the South, is one that Northern scholars and academics discovered in the late 1990s/early 2000s.[5] Since then, it has been a subject of constant investigation, and one that Northern scholars continue to define and dissect.

While South to North migration and mobility at least retain the North in its conceptual and practical application, South–South migration is solely contained within one sphere. Why then, is the study and conceptualization of this still viewed from a largely Northern standpoint? And subsequently, how does this impact the ability of countries in the South to define, manage and benefit from such migration?

This chapter will draw on some of my personal perspectives on migration and mobility within the South as both a Southern practitioner and researcher in migration and development, but also as a migrant myself. Albeit, one who belongs to the more traditional South–North corridor. It will look at some of the more traditional Northern literature available on South–South migration, interpreting it in a Southern context, to identify a series of "perception deficits"[6] in how Northern literature perceives South–South migration. Indeed, how it perpetuates the stereotypes of the South–South migrant, and how this could be detrimental to the study of the South, by the South, for the South.

An Obsession with Terminology

The obsession with terminology over how to categorize and define countries according to their wealth and productive capacity, has long since dictated the Global North's approach towards their policies and practices in several areas of human, economic and social development.[7]

Migration and human mobility too, have been subject to this, via the focus on maintaining borders between countries and deciding who gets to move, where and how.

As a Southern development practitioner, these myopic views of the world have done much to influence my own view of the world as a researcher and also of how the world views migration as a whole. The words "migrant" or "immigrant", which I myself am, have brought with them images of an outsider, which continue to haunt us generations beyond, of families moving between oceans and continents and a home left behind.[8] More importantly, for a better home elsewhere. Because the underlying assumption of such migration is that anywhere in the North, is certainly better than anywhere in the South.

In the context of South–South migration, however, this terminology does not appear frequently, or even sporadically in the literature. Instead, South–South migrants are referred to as "labour migrants", "temporary workers" or even "guest workers". Families in this context, are "left-behind", as the South–South migrant is a singular entity in search of livelihood and sustenance for his/her household.

This is the *first* of the perception deficits by which Northern literature delineates South–South migration from other migration patterns – that such migration is *singular* in nature.

Strangely enough though, despite the North's preoccupation with terminology, there is no "academic" definition of South–South migration per se. Simply put, it involves the movement of persons from one country in the South to another. In a policy context, it involves the transfer of human capital within such countries primarily on the pretext of employment (labour emigration). While this pretext also applies to South–North migration, in the context of South–South mobility, it precludes an assumption that since most countries of the South are less developed, the purpose of such migration can only be temporary. The migration governance regimes which control the South–South movement, also adhere to measures that assure these are only temporary migrants, and not permanent.

South–South migration can also include, however, a search for safety from conflict or persecution (refugees/asylum seekers/displaced persons). This pretext is not identified so in the literature, as these are invariably forced migrants and do not fall under the traditional definition of South–South migration, which is largely voluntary. However, as will be discussed later in this paper, this is one of the nuances that is easily ignored in the Northern-centric view on migration.

The majority of the literature on South–South migration flows, therefore, focuses clearly on the South as a labour market for those, it is assumed, who cannot reach the North, either due to weak financial capacity or sheer distance between geographies. While this assumption can be easily challenged, it nevertheless creates an oppositional framework whereby South–South migration is economic, temporary and restricted.

Restricted because migrants from the South to the South, live precarious lives that depend on destination countries to support them. Walzer (1983), for instance, conceptualizes the foreign "guest worker" programme, one of the prominent mechanisms through which Southern migrants access overseas employment, as the destination state attracting foreign workers by making their entry easier, but only for a certain period after which they must return. They are limited to certain employers, housed in worker's colonies and their labour-market mobility is restricted. Most importantly, and perhaps a defining feature, they are denied the right to bring family and settle permanently by the destination state.

This is the *second* of our perception deficits – that such migration can only be of a *temporary* nature.

These characteristics are important from the point of view of Southern practitioners like myself. They reinforce the notion that the perceived difference between the various forms of migration is based on wealth, skill and income, rather than the freedom of movement for all. This marked difference in viewing South–South migration as being set apart from South–North migration, therefore, has more to do with economic production than with constitutional human rights.

Why is the North so minutely obsessed with differentiating migrants based on where they come from and how much they can earn?

The South as a Metaphor for All That Was

It is no secret that the preoccupation of the North with everything that is South, is an outcome of the vast European colonial legacy that was undone across the world, in some countries as early as only a few decades ago. Hot on the heels of the post-colonial development theory of the 1960s and 1970s, development in countries of the Global South, has been seen as the *raison d'être* of more powerful Northern countries, as a way to exert control over their "lost colonies" under the watchful guise of altruism and aid.

The dominant narrative in migration today is also largely focused on the impact of migration from the South *on* the North. This narrative is dominated by Northern academics and practitioners and does not necessarily give academics in the South the space to define the issue independently. Even the migration theory espoused by the likes of North American academics such as Michael Walzer, Michael Todaro and Joseph Carens, frames international migration as the free movement of labour from the South to address the needs of the North.

South–South migration, however, has been a lesser-known casualty of this post-colonial legacy. While migration from the South to the North follows the path of the formerly colonized making their way to their former colonizers, South–South migration, does exactly the opposite. It traces the path of the formerly colonized making their way to other states, many of whom were also formerly colonized.

This should ideally be the fork where the discussion on migration diverges from the current Northern-focused thinking on mobility. After all, the migration route is clearly headed in a different direction, which has nothing to do with the North and is now legally independent. But Northern literature continues to (at times indirectly) frame South–South migration as a form of post-colonial oppression, so that the former colonizers must have some role to play in creating order and equality in these newly independent but Southern states. This is illustrated by attempts made by many Northern institutions to study South–South migration (some in collaboration with the South).[9]

This is the *third* perception deficit Northern literature creates around the South – that such migration is largely influenced by post-colonialism.

Some Northern writers have argued that patriarchy, white supremacy and global capitalism are all systems of oppression that shape migration flows and immigrant incorporation (Golash-Boza et al., 2019, 2). This is more dominant in the discussion on South–North migration and the tensions that exist between post-colonial states and their former wards.

Critical race theory, the antithesis to the post-colonial theory which largely controls the narrative on migration, development and inequality, could strengthen the Southern position of South–South migration and reduce this disparity, as it sees race as a strength as opposed to a disadvantage.[10] One of its key founders, Derrick Bell has claimed in one of his seminal pieces, that critical race theory turns marginalization into an advantageous and concrete advocacy on behalf of those oppressed by race and other related factors such as gender, economic class, and sexual orientation (Bell, 1995, 902).

Applying critical race theory to South–South migration, would therefore benefit its understanding as former colonies now creating their own path to economic success and human development. But instead, the literature on particularly the economic benefits of South–South migration, juxtapose how the North could create a win-win situation for itself if South–South migration were further encouraged.[11] The former colonizers could still stand to gain from their former colonies.

This has made South–South migration almost like a malleable plaything in the hands of Northern researchers, who fashion its impact out of the frameworks they set for it themselves. Their "identification" and "measurement" as one UK-funded project on South–South migration has put it, is also up to Northern researchers, who relentlessly plough into the depths of Africa and Asia to understand "how 'growth dividends' from migration can be shared more equitably between the wealthier and poorer in society".[12] Must South–South migration also be seen largely as a "project" of the North, in trying to assert its "re"-independence over the South?

Similarly, decolonization is fast becoming a prominent buzzword amongst academics and practitioners in many fields of social sciences and humanities. The impetus stems from a need to divorce the murky past of many former Western colonizers from their counterparts in the developing world. But the fact that the decision to "decolonize" has also been decided upon by the former colonizers, is a troubling sign in itself.[13]

So why is South–South migration such a fascinating form of research for the North?

Why South–South Migration? Questioning the North's Rationale

A recent article in the *New York Times* on the beginning of the "great climate migration", uses modelled projections to show that by 2070, 19 per cent of the world will be uninhabitable due to climate change.[14] "Where will everyone go?", it asks. It frames climate as the great disruptor pushing people from the South to safety. Pushing them further to Northern countries

– as in not cooler climes, but to the rich Western nations – who should "allow" more migrants to cross their borders.

It is arguments such as these that cut through the Northern-centricity of literature on who migrants from the South really are; those that are plagued with inequalities, both natural and human-created and who have no way out but to leave. And that the North must be their saviour. It negates, for instance, arguments (made by Northern intellectuals yet again), that climate migrants are not necessarily permanent, nor do they have the resources to migrate very far, even if they do.[15]

Many Northern researchers use a similar stance to justify the importance of South–South migration as a vital area of study in migration and mobility. This includes claims that "over the last decades, new migration patterns have emerged in the Global South that have not been fully analyzed so far. This includes 'new' patterns not only intra-regionally but also inter-regionally" (De Lombaerde and Gup, 2014, 105). Studying South–South migration apparently also allows, "us [*as in Northern researchers*], to re-consider and/or question the meaning and relevance of other related social concepts and variables ... that often emerged in a Northern context and were then a-critically transposed into other contexts" (ibid, 107).

Others claim, that paying more attention to migration in the South is one way "to change how we [*again, the North*], understand and talk about migration, while trying to extricate ourselves from the dichotomies of South and North, rich and poor, black and white, which continue to dominate [*the Northern*] imagination" (Awad and Natarajan, 2020, 55).

But perhaps the most forceful and prominent argument made by many in the North in favour of South–South migration, is the large scale of remittances it generates via labour migrants, and the subsequent impact of that on the "migration-development" nexus (Hujo and Piper, 2007, 20–21; Ratha and Shaw, 2007, 4).

Indeed, one of the oft-quoted studies in the international development community concludes, that in the African context, South–South migration "makes distinctive contributions to human development in terms of income, human capital and that the analysis of migration in poorer regions of the world and its relationship with human development requires much more data than is currently available" (Bakewell, 2009, Abstract).

So, the impetus to study South–South migration is purely economic, even in human development terms by singling out the South–South migrant as an economic commodity to be traded between "poorer" Southern nations.

This is the *fourth* deficit that emerges from the Northern literature – that this migration is a purely *economic* commodity.

Most of the literature that studies the impact of a returning labour migrant on his/her household, is seen in the context of the economic up lift-ment of family and social and economic indicators, than as someone who may have sacrificed more than was required to support his/her family and gained, perhaps not enough in return.

Migrants from the South to the North, have been portrayed as long-suffering,[16] economically productive,[17] and even criminally dangerous[18] in their representations by Northern governments and the media. Indeed, my own representation as a regular high-skilled migrant from Pakistan to North America, has been characterized as a racial invasion into the white territory, to "steal jobs" from white settlers, despite evidence to the contrary.[19] Anti-immigrant sentiment notwithstanding.

But those who navigate only the Southern routes should be more acceptable for Northern economies because they do not "invade" Northern territory to settle permanently. Rather, they do not invade Northern territory at all. So, the threat perception of migration in this context is negligible for the North. It's win-win for all apparently. Except for the migrants.

So why must we pander to a Northern contextualization of South–South migration, that both creates and reinforces the stereotypes of Southern migrants?

South–South Migration as a Southern Issue

The OECD claims that the world's 82 million South–South migrants form about 36 per cent of the total stock of migrants worldwide.[20] These migrants trek across a series of geographic corridors which traverse the globe from East to West and vice versa. The major regions within these corridors include Latin America, Africa, South Asia and South–East Asia. This includes migration *within* these various regions, as opposed to only *between* them.

As one can observe, the geographical scale of these migration pathways is extensive. The assumption in most literature that those in the South prefer to migrate to countries that are closer to them, or those they share a border with (such as within regions), does not necessarily hold when African migrants move as far as South–East Asia and Southern America, or when South–East Asians move to the Gulf States. And that too, temporarily. This is one of the many nuances that the Northern literature ignores when it studies South–South migration pathways – the Southern contexts of movement.[21]

This is the *fifth* deficit – that such migration ignores the important *Southern context*.

The viewpoints of why, how and when people migrate between these regions, are based on country context – Southern country context. Anglo- and Euro-centric analyses of these contexts tend to sidestep many of the nuances that such contexts provide. For instance, my work of observing the dearth of female labour migration from Pakistan to the Gulf States (vis-à-vis other South Asian countries) showed that women across most income levels would rather stay in Pakistan to work if they had the opportunity to do so. While in other South Asian countries such as Bangladesh and Sri Lanka, which had far higher levels of female emigration to the Middle East, female labour emigration, though problematic, was largely encouraged and supported by women as well as the state. So the region itself possesses great variation.

A Northern view of South–South migration also conveniently downplays the vital inclusion of migration and mobility within countries of the South. This includes seasonal migration for employment, particularly in agriculture and rural–urban migration for employment and livelihoods. It also includes internally displaced populations within countries due to civil and/or military conflict. Examples of military action against insurgents in Northern Pakistan, or displacement of populations in India due to the construction of large dams, are important aspects of intra-country forced migration.

Likewise, refugees and asylum seekers also do not come into the ambit of South–South migration, despite the fact that such movement has and continues to primarily take place between countries of the South. Jordan, Kenya, Uganda and Turkey, are host to some of the world's largest refugee populations from war-torn countries like Syria, Congo, Afghanistan, Somalia and Sudan, among others.

The emphasis on the relationship between migration and development is also one that has received enormous attention in Northern literature. But, it primarily focuses on South–North migration and the propensity of more people emigrating (both permanently and temporarily) as "poorer" countries get "richer".[22] It does not focus on the impact South–South migration could have on any of these factors, only reinforcing the disparity that South–South migration can only be temporary with no pathway or aspiration to permanent emigration, whether to more prosperous Southern countries or further proceeding to the North via.[23]

These arguments also fail to see that in Africa, for instance, despite the fact that migration represents an important livelihood strategy for poor households, the link between migration and poverty is often viewed more negatively. Much of the literature across much of the continent assumes that it is poverty that forces poor people to migrate, rather than migration being a potential route out of poverty (Black et al., 2006, 1).

So why can't any of these stereotypes about South–South migration be refuted by the South?

The South Must Take Responsibility – For the South

The *sixth* and final perception deficit this chapter identifies is perhaps the most important. The South as a subject of study by the South and its own institutions is a rare occurrence in the literature. Its relative absence vis-à-vis Northern literature, only reinforces some of the actual *truths* that lie within some of our perception deficits.

For instance, there is clear indication of hierarchical power structures existing between migrant origin and destination countries within the South, where the latter are in control of migration governance and resources. New terms such as the "Asian factor" are beginning to play an increasingly significant role in South–South migration flows (De Lombaerde and Gup, 2014, 105), as more powerful countries such as the Gulf States, Korea, Singapore and China become new destinations in the South for lesser developed countries in South Asia and Africa. For example, considered a "minority within a minority", African migrants and refugees are frequently discriminated against by the Chinese, on the basis of language and are even denied job opportunities solely based on the colour of their skin (Khattab and Mehmood, 2018, 4). Similarly, South Asian labourers and African caregivers and domestic housekeepers to the oil-rich Gulf States and Saudi Arabia, are consistently abused and humiliated, with no social or job security, because of their poorer origins, widely documented in the literature.[24] The South–South migrant remains a victim.

But what is the greatest matter of concern to me as a Southern researcher, is that there has been little resistance from the South towards the Anglo/Euro-centric framing of South–South migration, particularly in recent years, as interest in the subject has been growing exponentially. From a Northern standpoint, perhaps the piece of resistance that stands out the most, is historian Adam McKewon's 2004 article which raises the issue of "Euro-centrism", or "North Atlantic centrism" in much of the migration literature over the last century or so,[25] highlighting the significance of non-European patterns of migration in shaping global economies (Mohapatra, 2007, 115).

Supporters of McKewon claim that Euro-centric perspectives divide global migration flows by granting individual choice and economic incentives to migrants of European origins while denying the same to non-European migrants. (Mohapatra, 2007, 114). But there has been little from the South itself to both further emphasize this point, as well as study it from a Southern migrant's perspective by the South.

While there is an emerging body of academic work which acknowledges the Anglo/Euro-centricity of migration, it is still not being led by researchers from the South.[26] Instead, it is more focused on looking at migration within and between countries of the South, as opposed to ensuring that literature on migration from the South is produced by Southern scholars themselves.[27]

Campillo-Carrete (2013), has similarly identified in her review of the literature on South–South migration, that the term itself throws up a multitude of references online, but upon closer inspection, most of the results have nothing to do with migration per se. Indeed, my own search on the term has revealed thousands of hits. But upon closer inspection, the top 20–30 hits focus on just the earning and remitting power of migration, thus reinforcing the Northern view of South–South migration being simply about economic commodification of temporary labour.

This is reinforced, for instance, by a study of the literature on South–South migration for domestic work that shows that there is little discussion of the reasons for such migration and the impact that it has on migrant households in origin countries. The literature is dominated by the shortcomings of legal frameworks for regulating working conditions and recruitment practices to avoid exploitation, and only a few papers discuss worker agency, which treat migrant domestic workers as victims (Deshinkar and Zietlin, 2015, 169).

There is clearly a dearth of analysis, as well as intellectual space from a Southern perspective which not only creates an imbalance between the quantity of research available on South–South migration, but also the perceptions such research creates about its subject.

So where do we go from here?

Where Do We Go From Here?

One of the biggest contradictions in research on migration and mobility that I see as a Southern researcher, is that none of the research on migration as a whole, focuses on the North as an *origin* country.[28] If people can migrate from the South to the South and from the South to the North, why can they not move from North to South or North to North?

Barring any conversation on this, this essay identifies six perception deficits observed in the Northern literature on South–South migration as being (i) singular, (ii) temporary, (iii) post-colonial in its formation, (iv) a purely economic commodity, (v) ignoring important Southern context and (vi) the need for the South to take responsibility. This final deficit is one that is not reflected in the literature but *should* be.

These perception deficits reinforce stereotypes of migrants and their pathways in the following ways:

i) Singular: South–South migration allows only one person per household to migrate because it is contractual, temporary and expensive – and the migrant is usually poor.

ii) Temporary: South–South migration is controlled by destination countries who do not want migrants to establish permanency in their countries – because the migrant is an outsider.

iii) Post-colonial in its formation: South–South migration is a way to develop former colonies from which the North can equally benefit.

iv) A purely economic commodity: South–South migration is purely for purposes of employment which is controlled by destination countries who view the migrant as a short-term gain for their economies.

v) Ignoring important Southern context: South–South migration does not need to take into account nuances such as conflict, displacement or geographies – because the transaction is purely economic.

vi) The need for the South to take responsibility: South–South migration literature is largely dominated by Northern research which does not give space to Southern points of view.

Anyone can prove me wrong on any of these counts using the existing evidence of which there is no paucity, that says to the contrary. But that is not the objective of this chapter. These perception deficits are not meant to challenge the data on South–South migration by the North. Instead, they are meant to challenge the *perceptions* of the North on how their analysis views the South as a whole, either by using this data or by other forms of critical analysis.

Indeed, there is no evidence in either data or literature that proves that South–South migration can be only these things or just one of them. Migrants can migrate in groups for employment, even from one household. They do not necessarily have to be poor. Their pathways to emigration do not have to be temporary and their families do not have to be left behind. They do not have to migrate just for employment and if so, that employment does not have to be temporary. And it certainly doesn't have to be for the benefit of former colonies, but rather independent nations. And it can and should include several different scenarios that take place between Southern nations.

While this may sound pedantic and simplistic, the reality is that if South–South migration were viewed and studied by the South, it would produce very different viewpoints such as those above. There would still be strong contradictions given the Global South is not a singular, static entity either. But they would be juxtaposed within a context that would consider far more than just economic growth and remittances. Given the Global South's dearth of resources to encourage academic and policy research, sending countries have few tools with which to create a counter-narrative or self-narrative on South–South migration. But this is exactly why these narratives above need to be challenged and questioned with greater authority from the South.

At a time when migrants and asylum-seekers from conflict-ridden countries of the South are being repelled back to those countries by the European North without even a thought for their lives or safety, for South–South migration to be dominated by Anglo/Euro-centric perceptions, is nothing short of both an opportunity lost to build on migration dividends, as well as narrow the gap between the globe's upper and lower halves.

Acknowledgements: Originally published as Working Paper 1 of the International Institute of Migration and Development, Kerala.

Notes

1 The terms "Global North and Global South" used in this chapter, do not necessarily denote the authors' agreement with what these terms stand for. However, in order to ensure consistency in exploring the arguments presented, both terms are used in this chapter as they are defined in the conventional literature.
2 There is a plethora of widely available literature critiquing the use and application of these two terms, particularly in the social sciences and development studies. This chapter does not delve into these critiques.
3 One attempt to produce an objective classification, uses the UNDP's Human Development Index to differentiate between North and South. In brief, the

Global North consists of those 64 countries which have a high HDI (most of which are located north of the 30th northern parallel), while the remaining 133 countries belong to the Global South with medium- to low HDI.

4 The term South–South migration was originally coined by international development agencies, including the World Bank and OECD to estimate

5 I say "discovered", because in terms of mobility, migration within the South began long before this. The 1970s and 1980s for instance, were some of the most prominent decades in terms of labour migration from South Asian countries to the Gulf and within African regions post-independence of many nations in the 1950s and 1960s onwards. This era has been relatively understudied in the literature as a historical basis for South–South migratory patterns. See, Mehdi Chowdhury and S. Irudaya Rajan, 2018, *South Asian Migration in the Gulf. Causes and Consequences*, Palgrave MacMillan.

6 I first referred to this term in an article written for *The Sociological Review* in June 2020; https://www.thesociologicalreview.com/research-by-the-developed -on-the-developing-view-from-the-researched/

7 There has been a great deal of discussion and literature on the divergences that these two terms create within both the social sciences, as well as in the international development sector. This chapter does not specifically build on those discussions.

8 In a disturbing turn of events, the website of the UN Agency for Migration claims that there is no universally accepted definition of migrant; https://www.iom.int/ who-is-a-migrant

9 See, https://www.coventry.ac.uk/research/research-directories/current-projects /2019/ukri-gcrf-south/

10 Critical race theory's founding members are usually identified as Derrick Bell, Richard Delgado, Charles Lawrence, Mari Matsuda and Patricia Williams.

11 This literature discusses the importance of economic contributions such as workers remittances to migrant-sending countries which could contribute to their economic growth, creating stability and security, therefore reducing financial dependence on the North. But in return, such growth could also create opportunities for the North for greater economic exploration in Southern countries.

12 See, https://www.mideq.org/en/blog/grappling-south-south-migration-and-ine qualities-development-studies-association-annual-conference/

13 Some argue that the theory and practice of decolonization actually originated from scholars in the Global South as a way to move beyond their post-colonial identity, such as Frantz Fanon, Paulo Freire and Eduardo Galeano. In contemporary and more recent literature, however, the discussion on decolonization has also been dominated by Northern scholarship and practice, who seek to investigate how they (the Global North) could shift perspective from the North to the South.

14 See, https://www.nytimes.com/interactive/2020/07/23/magazine/climate-migra tion.html?smid=tw-share

15 See commentary by Hien deHaas, http://heindehaas.blogspot.com/2020/01/cli mate-refugees-fabrication-of.html

16 See, https://www.dw.com/en/world-in-progress-italys-long-suffering-migrant -workers/av-47196190

17 See, https://www.weforum.org/agenda/2018/02/here-s-how-migration-can-ben efit-us-all/

18 See, https://thecorrespondent.com/235/europe-is-the-promised-land-and-noth ing-will-convince-these-migrants-otherwise/268987003780-79d885f6

19 Ameilie F. Constant (2014) "Do migrants take the job of native workers?" *IZA World of Labour*; 10.

20 See, https://www.oecd.org/dev/migration-development/south-south-migration.htm

21 This aspect has begun to receive greater traction in Northern literature when studying migration in these regions.
22 See arguments by Hien de Hass "Why development will not stop migration"; and Michael Clemens' research on the emigration life cycle.
23 Granted, many migrant-receiving countries of the South, particularly in the Gulf and South–East Asia, do not offer, or make it very difficult for migrants to achieve a pathway to citizenship or permanent residency, particularly low-skilled migrants.
24 See Google Scholar search; https://scholar.google.com/scholar?hl=en&as_sdt=0 %2C5&q=%22migrant+workers%22+AND+gulf+AND+abuse&btnG=
25 McKeown, Adam, 2004. "Global Migration 1846–1940." *Journal of World History* 15(2):155–189.
26 See for instance, https://www.berghahnjournals.com/view/journals/migration -and-society/3/1/migration-and-society.3.issue-1.xml
27 There are several emerging resources within the South, authored by the South on migration and development. See for instance, African migration, mobility and displacement at https://ammodi.com
28 In a Google scholar search of the term "North–North migration", only one response was returned; N Oishi, A Ono, "North–North migration of care workers: 'Disposable' au pairs in Australia", *Journal of Ethnic and Migration Studies*, 2019.

References

Awad, Ibrahim, and Usha Natarajan. 2020. "Migration Myths and the Global South." *The Cairo Review of Global Affairs*. 30: 46–56. (https://www .thecairoreview.com/essays/migration-myths-and-the-global-south/).

Bakewell, Oliver. 2009. *South-South Migration and Human Development: Reflections On African Experiences.* UNDP. (http://hdr.undp.org/sites/default/ files/hdrp_2009_07.pdf).

Bell, Derrick, A. 1995. "Who's Afraid of Critical Race Theory." University of Illinois Law Review. pp. 893–910. (https://heinonline.org/HOL/LandingPage ?handle=hein.journals/unilllr1995&div=40&id=&page=).

Black, Richard, Johnathan Crush, Sally Pederby, Savina Ammassari, Lindsay MsLean Hilker, S. Mouillesseaux, C. Pooley, and R. Rajkotia. 2006. "Migration and Development in Africa: An Overview." (https://scholars.wlu.ca/cgi/viewcon- tent.cgi?article=1014&context=samp).

Campillo-Carrete, Beatriz. 2013. "South South Migration - A Review of the Literature." International Institute of Social Studies (2). (https://pdfs .semanticscholar.org/f50d/6a23e881366eee4fe366fa8b2472ab897c7e.pdf).

De Lombaerde, Philippe, Fei Guo, and Helion Póvoa Neto. 2014. "Introduction to the Special Collection: South–South Migrations: What is (Still) on the Research Agenda?" *International Migration Review* 48(1): 103–112.

Deshingkar, Priya, and Benjamin Zeitlyn. 2015. "South-South Migration for Domestic Work and Poverty." *Geography Compass* 9(4): 169–179.

Fiddian-Qasmiyeh, Elena. 2020. "Introduction - Recentering the South in Studies of Migration." *Migration and Society* 3(1): 1–18. (https://www.berghahnjournals .com/view/journals/migration-and-society/3/1/arms030102.xml).

Golash-Boza, Tanya, Maria D. Duenas, and Chia Xiong. 2019. "White Supremacy, Patriarchy, and Global Capitalism in Migration Studies." *American Behavioral Scientist* 63(13): 1741–1759.

Hujo, Katja, and Nicola Piper. 2007. "South–South Migration: Challenges for Development and Social Policy." *Development* 50(4): 19–25.

Khattab, Nabil, and Hasan Mahmud. 2018. "Migration in a Turbulent Time: Perspectives from the Global South." *Migration and Development* 8(1): 1–6.

Mohapatra, Prabhu P. 2007. "Eurocentrism, Forced Labour, and Global Migration: A Critical Assessment." *International Review of Social History* 52(1): 110–115.

Ratha, Dilip, and William Shaw. 2007. *South-South Migration and Remittances.* Washington, DC: Development Prospects Group, World Bank.

Walzer, Michael. 1983. *Spheres of Justice.* New York, NY: Basic Books.

13 Non-payment of Wages Among Gulf returnees in the First Wave of COVID-19

S. Irudaya Rajan and C.S. Akhil

Wage Theft and Migrants

Wage theft occurs when an employer pays less than what is legally owed to the employee and is prevalent in almost every industry in the world. It consists of the total or partial non-payment of a worker's remuneration, earned through the provision of labour services, as stipulated in a written or non-written employment contract. It also includes the payment of salaries below the minimum wage, non-payment of overtime, non-payment of contractually owed benefits, the non-negotiated reduction of salaries as well as the retention of dues upon one's contract termination (MFA, 2021; Foley and Piper, 2021). International temporary labour migrants are known for their precarious working and poor living conditions, especially in major countries of destination including the GCC countries. Wage theft was poorly addressed across various migration corridors over the years due to the lack of access to justice mechanisms and labour-protection systems both at the country of origin and destination (Foley and Piper, 2021).

The COVID-19 pandemic has set this issue in a starker light. Many workers had their contracts abruptly terminated and most of them had been sent back home without the payment of their dues and wages. The GCC, well known for its stringent labour legislation and abject violation of labour rights and freedom of association, does not offer any method of recourse to this crippling issue. When it comes to the countries of origin, apart from registering complaints with the respective country missions and the various foreign affairs ministries of respective governments, grievances are often registered late and delayed responses do not help workers, which was especially true during the pandemic.

Academic literature approached the issue of wage theft during the pandemic from various angles such as the denial of access to justice, urgency and panic created to unplanned and massive repatriation of workers, absence of states when it comes to the protection of the rights of migrant workers and poor bilateral/multilateral co-operation between origin and destination countries (Foley and Piper, 2021; Piper and Foley, 2021; ILO, 2020; Ashwin and Akhil, 2021). Unlike the pre-pandemic period, the number of cases of

DOI: 10.4324/9781003315124-13

wage theft had multiplied due to the economic crisis and panic precipitated by the spread of the infectious disease among migrant communities. Among the workers who had lost their jobs, some were terminated and repatriated forcefully, some were given false promises about the payment of wages and dues and only a handful of the workers received all benefits and dues before repatriation (MFA, 2021). Some common forms of wage theft apart from a direct denial of wages during the pandemic are the following:[1]

- Wage deduction in the name of insurance, medical check-up and other services offered by the administration
- No timely payment of wages
- False promises on payment and dues in which worker cannot make claims after a particular period
- Malpractices in the calculation of leave entitlements
- Periodic payment of indemnity leading to the loss of money for the workers
- No mandatory payment of due and benefits during termination and deportation
- Lack of awareness of workers on the labour laws helped the employer escape from paying compensation for unjustified termination
- Establish false charges/cases against workers
- Extra hours of work

For a country like India, that received more than 2 million return-migrant workers during COVID-19, the impact of the wage theft is massive. The country carried out its largest repatriation process from 7 May 2020 to bring back the stranded migrants. Considering the persistent requests from the Indian diaspora and workers stranded overseas, the Indian government executed the repatriation of Indians using the national carrier and navy vessels and brought back the migrants in ten phases under a mission titled 'Vande Bharat Mission'.[2] From the point of view of the policymakers, they have addressed the immediate requirement of migrants (Rajan and Arokkiaraj, 2021). The rapid increase in the number of Indians affected in the gulf countries along with the loss of jobs and difficulty in identifying quarantine facilities for the workers in the labour camps made the Indian workers increasingly vulnerable (see Rajan and Batra, 2021; Rajan and Pattath, 2021). However, the state failed to understand and recognise their post-arrival grievances, especially the complaints of non-payment of wages and dues (Rajan and Sami, 2022). As per the Migrant Forum in Asia (MFA) data, the majority of the wage theft cases reported by Indians were group cases committed by medium to large firms involved in construction, hospitality, manufacturing, and transportation. It indicates that low-, medium-, and high-skilled migrants are uniformly affected by the non-payment of wages followed by loss of jobs. But, the class question is still relevant because the high-skilled and well-paid migrants had awareness of the issue and most of them had submitted the power of attorney to legal representatives in the destination countries to approach the legal mechanism. Since it put a huge financial burden on the migrants in terms of legal fees, only affluent migrants could afford such routes. The rest of the migrants require assistance from the stakeholders to access the justice mechanisms which is yet to happen in the Indian situation.

Among the Indian states, Kerala received the maximum number of temporary labour migrants during the pandemic period. According to the data gathered by Norka-Roots, until January 2021, 0.98 million Keralites have come back and 0.63 million among them reported that they came back due to loss of job. Considering this massive number of migrants who returned to Kerala, wage theft during the pandemic may account for millions of dollars. As a provincial state in India which has the most institutionalised migration management system that involves the government, migrant communities, diaspora groups and returnee associations, the response of stakeholders from Kerala towards the phenomenon of 'wage theft' would be an important question to analyse (Rajan, 2012; Rajan and Akhil, 2019).

In this context, the study aims to understand the extent of 'wage theft' in Kerala using a sample survey conducted among the returned migrants during the pandemic. The study also evaluates the responses of various stakeholders to the issue using qualitative narratives from the field.

Wage Theft Among Non-Resident Keralites (Nrks) During the Pandemic

With around 44% of the households having direct experience with international labour migration and 25% of the Gross Domestic Product being contributed by remittances, Kerala is a unique provincial state in India when it comes to international migration (Rajan and Zachariah, 2019). The widespread labour migration from the 1970s to various parts of the world had contributed immensely to the socio-economic development of Kerala state, which holds the highest position in almost every human development indicator (Zachariah et al., 2003; Zachariah and Rajan, 2012). So, every minor development in the international labour mobility regimes would have an impact on the state and on the migrants from the state. The socio-political and economic situations in the destination countries often lead to the massive return of Keralites. Kerala has had experiences of receiving large numbers of return migrants in the past due to political as well as financial reasons as in the case after the global financial crisis of 2008 hit economies all over the world severely. The current COVID-19 crisis appears to be another such catalyst for a large-scale return. What is different, however, is the sheer numbers of workers who have been affected all over the globe as well as the urgency in the repatriation, fuelled by the panic among the workers.

Unsurprisingly, among the returnees to Kerala during the pandemic, around 95% of the migrants returned from Gulf countries.[3] The data captures the reasons for return during the pandemic and portrays that 63.3% of the total returnees during the pandemic had come back after losing their jobs. The major destinations of Keralites – the six Gulf Cooperation Council (GCC) states of Saudi Arabia, the United Arab Emirates, Qatar, Bahrain, Oman and Kuwait had often reported cases of wage theft even before the pandemic. Most of the cases are not even fought legally if the workers are returned/repatriated to the home country. As per the Centre for Indian Migrant Studies,

> the massive cases of layoffs have been reported widely since 2014, especially from Gulf countries. The individual cases of non-payment of wages often go unnoticed. Only a few cases filed by domestic workers and low skilled workers are solved amicably with the intermediation from embassies and legal advocates.

Since many of the second-generation migrants from the state work in the service sector and industries that are covered under the domestic labour laws in the Gulf, the non-payment of wages often go to court. The poor success rate of the grievance mechanism of the Government of India (MADAD) and the absence of legal support do not help the migrants carry forward the legal fight and other negotiations upon return. The lawyers' panel established by the government of Kerala is not fully functional yet and the Indian lawyers in the destination countries, especially Gulf, are often interested in accident claims. In short, the non-payment of wages and dues experienced by the individual or small group of migrants from Kerala often go unnoticed and justice remained a distant dream in the pre-pandemic period.

Kerala has the largest and oldest institutional mechanism for the welfare of NRKs in the country. Non-Resident Keralites Affairs (Norka) and its field agency Norka-Roots had the automatic responsibility of addressing the crisis faced by migrants. Under the aegis of Norka-Roots, a self-documentation of returnees was established to capture the characteristics of returnees including the reason for return.[4] In this context, it is important to understand how the governments and other stakeholders responded to the question of wage theft faced by migrant workers. What are the actions taken by the government to address the problem and how big is the problem compared to the larger question of sustainable reintegration of the returnees during the pandemic? The major objectives of this chapter are as follows:

* To understand the extent and nature of wage theft during the pandemic among the Kerala returnee migrants from Gulf countries.
* To analyse the responses of various stakeholders to the question of 'wage theft' in the Kerala context.

Data and Methodology

A full-fledged scientific sample survey was impossible during the pandemic due to the mobility restrictions. In the case of returnees, the availability of reliable data was also limited. However, the study relied on the personal details of the returnees provided by the Kerala government and a stratified random sampling was conducted on this dataset. The survey was conducted among 1,559 migrant workers who had returned during the period from May 2020 to December 2020.

Sequential exploratory mixed method design is used for the study. The design involves an initial qualitative phase of data collection and analysis, followed by a phase of quantitative data collection and analysis, with a final phase of integration or linking of data from the two separate strands of data.[5] Apart from the simple quantitative tools such as ratios and cross-tabulation, the study relied on in-depth personal interviews conducted among the victims of wage theft identified from the survey. The respondents were identified from the sample survey and selected by ensuring country-wise, occupation-wise and gender-wise representation.

Observations From the Survey

This section discusses the evidence of wage theft from the survey and the field interviews. The narratives from interviews are used to substantiate the figures from the survey.

Profile of the Respondents

The survey was conducted among the returnees from Kerala who returned since the repatriation mission had been initiated by the Government of India. Since GCC countries account for the lion's share of temporary migrants from Kerala, the survey was conducted only among the migrants from GCC countries. As Table 13.1 indicates, among the total 1,559 respondents, UAE and Saudi contribute 54.3% of the total migrants which is equivalent to the proportion of the total population of Keralites in these two countries as per the KMS data (Rajan and Zachariah, 2019). Hence, these figures increase the reliability of the data.

Table 13.1 Return of Migrants to Kerala by Destination, 2021

Destination	Number	Per Cent
Bahrain	200	12.8
Kuwait	184	11.8
Oman (Muscat)	207	13.3
Qatar (Doha)	124	8.0
Saudi Arabia (Riyadh, Jeddah)	443	28.4
United Arab Emirates	401	25.7
Total	1559	100.0

Source: Author's own calculation from the survey conducted by the senior author.

Table 13.2 Occupation of Return Migrants Prior to Return, 2021

Occupation	Number	Percent
Business Owners	43	2.8
Construction Sector	242	15.5
Restaurant and Hospitality Industry	217	13.9
Medical Services	82	5.3
Domestic Workers Including Drivers	206	13.2
Government Employees	16	1.0
Industrial Employees	289	18.5
Banking and Financial Employees	52	3.3
Education related Employees	35	2.2
Other Services Including Human Resource Staffs	158	10.1
Others – not specified	219	14.0
Total	1559	100.0

Source: Same as Table 13.1.

Among the respondents, 18.5% of them were employed in the industrial sector, while workers from the construction and hospitality sectors constituted 15.5% and 13.9%, respectively. Considering the impact of COVID-19 on the economy of the Gulf region, this trend is predictable. As per the data, only 1% of the total returnees are government employees. The low share of government returnees indicates that the private and informal sectors in the Gulf suffered the most, a trend was seen in other regions of the world (Table 13.2).

About 47% of the workers reported that they returned due to job loss and 23.6% of the workers returned due to the fear/panic created by the pandemic. It reflects the sheer impact of COVID-19 among temporary labour migrants. If we take into account other reasons that indirectly led to job loss such as expiry of the contract and compulsory repatriation, the figure would be more than 55% of the total returnees. It is closer to the Norka data which says 60% of the returnees lost their jobs. However, compared to earlier return migrant surveys conducted as part of Kerala Migration Surveys, the present study indicate that the reasons for return are quite different (Table 13.3) (Zachariah et al., 2001, 2006; Zachariah and Rajan, 2010,; 2011).

Job Loss to Victims of Wage Theft

Among the 47% of the people who lost jobs and returned to Kerala in May 2020, 33.1% of the workers returned from Saudi Arabia. Even though UAE has the largest Kerala diaspora population, more workers from Saudi Arabia lost their jobs compared to UAE (21.5%). Qatar contributes 7.3% of the total workers who lost jobs. It could be due to the strong pro-labour policies of the country.

Table 13.3 Reason for Return Among Return Migrants in Kerala, 2021

Reason for Return	Number	Percent
To Retire	22	1.4
Missed Family	21	1.3
Care for Elderly	5	0.3
Accomplished Goals for Migration	11	0.7
Prefer to Work in Kerala	7	0.4
Lost Job/Laid Off	737	47.2
Illness/Accident	57	3.7
Expiry of Contract	82	5.3
Scared Due to COVID-19 and return by Own Choice	368	23.6
Compulsory Expatriation/Cancellation of Employment Visa	54	3.5
Low Wages	39	2.5
Poor Working Conditions	24	1.5
Nationalisation Issue	5	0.3
Visiting Visa Expired	18	1.1
Re-migrate to new Destination or Same Destination	14	1.0
Others – Not Provided	95	6.1
Total	1559	100.0

Source: Same as Table 13.1.

Table 13.4 Profile of Return Migrants Who Lost Job, 2021

	Number	Percent
Bahrain	88	11.9
Kuwait	97	13.1
Oman (Muscat)	95	12.9
Qatar (Doha)	54	7.3
Saudi Arabia (Riyadh, Jeddah)	245	33.1
United Arab Emirates	159	21.5
Total	738	100.0

Source: Same as Table 13.1.

Another surprising characteristic of the return migrants who lost jobs during the pandemic is their period of stay at the destination country. There is a general feeling among the public and policymakers that the freshers struggled to keep their jobs in the destination country. However, the survey shows that 67% of the respondents who lost jobs had spent more than two years in the Gulf countries. Among the returnees, 41% who lost their jobs had work experience of more than 10 years in the Gulf (Tables 13.4 13.5–13.6).

As indicated in the figures of return migrants, industrial workers (21%) followed by the workers in the construction (19%) and hospitality sector (17%) mainly lost their job during the pandemic. The government employees (0.8%) hardly lost their jobs. Among the workers, 15% of the domestic

Table 13.5 Duration of Stay Among Return Migrants
Who Lost Jobs, 2021

Years	Number	Percent
<1 year	67	9.1
1–2 year	72	9.8
2–5 years	146	19.8
5–10 years	151	20.5
10–20 years	194	26.3
Above 20 years	107	14.5
Total	737	100.0

Source: Same as Table 13.1.

Table 13.6 Occupation of the Return Migrants Who Lost Their Jobs, 2021

Occupation	Number	Percent
Business Owners	11	1.5
Construction Sector	140	19.0
Restaurant and Hospitality/Industry	126	17.1
Medical Services	17	2.3
Domestic Workers Including Drivers	116	15.7
Government Employees	6	.8
Industrial Employees	158	21.4
Banking and Financial Employees	23	3.1
Education Employees	10	1.4
Other Services Including Human Resource Staffs	57	7.7
Others – Not specified	73	9.9
Total	737	100.0

Source: Same as Table 13.1.

sector including drivers faced job loss. As the predictions indicate, the service sector is responsible for around 60% of the job loss during the pandemic, followed by the industrial sector.

It is important to understand the nature of job loss, how they lost their jobs and the responses of employers. Among the people who lost jobs, the majority of the workers (41%) were asked to resign by their employers. Notably, 11% of the workers were advised to travel back home without the payment of their salaries and a few workers (3%) were threatened with termination. Among these workers, only 14.8% of the workers received a favourable option of returning to Kerala with the wages and dues (Table 13.7).

As Table 13.8 indicates, 61% of the domestic workers were asked to resign from their job followed by 42% of the workers in the restaurant and hospitality industries. Even if the domestic jobs sector was the most vulnerable sector during the pandemic, the percentage of workers who were asked to resign is high due to the low protection for the employment of domestic

Table 13.7 Nature of Job Loss Among Return Migrants, 2021

	Number	Percent
Asked to Resign	302	41.0
Advised to Travel Back Home with Salary	109	14.8
Advised to Travel Back Home Without Salary	79	10.7
Threatened to Terminate	23	3.1
Offered Termination Option	114	15.5
No Extension of Work Visa	81	11.0
Others – Not Reported	41	5.6
Total	749	100.0

Source: Same as Table 13.1.

Table 13.8 Occupational of the Return Migrants Who Were Asked to Resign, 2021

Occupation	Number			Percent		
	No	Yes	Total	No	Yes	Total
Business Owners	10	1	11	2.3	0.3	1.5
Construction Sector	89	51	140	20.5	16.9	19.0
Restaurant and Hospitality/Industry	74	52	126	17.0	17.2	17.1
Medical Services	11	6	17	2.5	2.0	2.3
Domestic Workers Including Drivers	55	61	116	12.6	20.2	15.7
Government Employees	4	2	6	0.9	0.7	0.8
Industrial Employees	105	53	158	24.1	17.5	21.4
Banking and Financial Employees	13	10	23	3.0	3.3	3.1
Education Employees	6	4	10	1.4	1.3	1.4
Other Services Including HR Staffs	38	19	57	8.7	6.3	7.7
Others – Not Provided	30	43	73	6.9	14.2	9.9
Total	435	302	737	100.0	100.0	100.0

Source: Same as Table 13.1.

workers in the GCC countries. However, the workers in the industrial sector had a more cordial experience from the employers due to the labour protection system in the industrial sector in GCC. Among the industrial workers, 27% were offered a termination option and 22% were asked to travel back with salary. Only 2% of the industrial workers received threats or experienced forced termination from work. Apart from the medical and government sector workers, industrial workers are the only group of workers who experienced a dignified return from the destination country.

The data clearly reflect the loss of jobs in the sectors where Keralites dominate in the Gulf such as the service and hospitality sectors and industrial and domestic services. The profiling of returnees and a detailed narration of the characteristics of 'job losses indicate the need to explore the welfare and rights of the workers who lost their jobs during the pandemic. The next section analyses the phenomenon of wage theft among Keralites in the Gulf during the pandemic.

Evidence of Wage Theft During the Pandemic

Based on the literature and newspaper reports, it was evident that migrants in the Gulf state were the victims of large-scale job loss. A number of variables are analysed to establish the extent of wage theft among workers from Kerala in the sample survey.

As per the survey, among the 47% of the returnees who lost jobs, 39.1% of the workers have reported that they have faced non-payment of wages or dues and reduction in wages. Among the migrants who managed to work during the initial months of the pandemic also faced non-payment of wages. 8.8% of the workers who had lost jobs, worked during the pandemic without any wages and 18.2% of the workers had witnessed a reduction in their wages (Table 13.9).

Duration of the stay has a direct relationship with non-payment of wages and dues. More than 60% (61.1%) of the workers who did not receive their wages and benefits had work experience in the Gulf for more than five years. It indicates that workers who are eligible for higher amounts of dues and benefits were denied the payment. On the other hand, most of the newly joined or workers with fewer years of service received the benefits and wages before leaving the country of work.

Ramesh (not real name) was a foreman in an oil company, where he worked for the past 17 years. He returned home after having been terminated from his job. He stated that

> I did not take any leave with salary for the past six years since I thought I will get it once I leave this country forever. I considered it as savings for future. During the Covid-19 pandemic, company had to cut down its operation and asked to go on leave first and later on I was terminated. Now the employer owes me, leave salary of six years, gratuity and airfare for return flight ticket. They have terminated almost all workers with more than 10 years of work experience. Now we realise that it was an attempt by the company to steal our money

Table 13.9 Duration of Stay and Non-payment of Wages, 2021

Duration of Stay in Years	Yes
<1 year	8.6
1–2 year	10.5
2–5 years	19.8
5–10 years	20.4
10–20 years	26.7
Above 20 years	14.1
Total	100.0

Source: Same as Table 13.1

Table 13.10 Breakdown of Non-payment of Dues and Benefits
         Reported by Return Migrants, 2021

	Number	Percent
Air Ticket	41	5.6
Gratuity	47	6.4
Medical Benefits	12	1.6
COVID-19-Related Medical Benefits	5	.7
Family Visa	3	.4
Family Air Tickets	3	.4
HRA	6	.8
Incentives	26	3.5
Severance Pay	41	5.6
Others – Not Reported	44	6.0
No Dues Remaining	620	84.1

Source: Author's own calculation from Survey

The statement is a clear indication of the employer's attempt to terminate workers with more experience, especially during the time when the panic was created among the workers. Many of the elder and experienced workers rushed back home without even negotiating with the employers on the unpaid benefits since they were more prone to the virus.

A breakdown of dues and other benefits shows that 5% of the workers who lost jobs were denied all benefits such as gratuity, severance pay, air ticket and other benefits (see Table 13.10). Mary, a female domestic worker from Kuwait who returned home after the loss of job during the pandemic pointed out:

> I did receive hospital assistance and return ticket charges from the employer. However, I did not get incentives during termination because of the excuse that the employer paid my hospital bills. I requested them to provide some help during the two months lockdown period as I was physically unable to get anything done on my own. But they did not give me any help. I am planning to file a complaint with the help of Norka-roots to claim my unpaid wages.

Mary's experience reveals that during the pandemic, the employers tried to meet a cost which is the lowest to satisfy the workers. Hence, most of the respondents during the survey were reluctant to criticise the employers and supported them by citing the financial crisis. In this case, the workers were not aware of their labour rights and they made no attempts to claim their financial rights during the pandemic.

BOX 13.1: Narrative From a Returnee on Wage Theft

Rahul is one among the first returnees who boarded the first Vande Bharat Mission flight from Oman to Kochi on 9 May 2020. He is part of a Malayali football group and actively uses social media to document his life as a migrant. Rahul had an accident during a football match and which had seriously injured the ligaments of one of his legs. He was taken to the hospital and was referred for surgery. It was only then he realised that the insurance premium by his company covers only minor issues and will not cover any serious health issues. The employer was not ready to sponsor his journey from Oman to Kerala. However, he managed to return on one of the initial flights of Vande Bharat Mission and successfully underwent surgery.

Rahul will now have to arrange Rs.160,000 for the surgery under such difficult circumstances. He does not have any insurance in Kerala since he believes his medical expenses will be covered by the insurance provided by his company. He is very much dissatisfied with the high-ticket rate he had to pay to return after going through such a difficult phase.

Rahul experienced a 50-percentage reduction in March and April salaries after which he was sent on unpaid leave. They received this information over a phone call, after which there was no further enquiry from the employer to check the well-being of any worker. Rahul is currently on unpaid leave and has returned to Kerala but is still working for the company. He gets emails from his company and he is expected to respond no matter what time it is. As most of the emails are coming from different countries, he is expected to work day and night. While being asked about working for free he said that travel is his passion and he is happy to do any work related to it. However, he is not sure when the company is going to call him back after unpaid leave. He is also prepared to get a call informing his termination.

He did not claim leave salary for the past three years which is approximately equal to three months' salary (450 Riyal per month) before leaving. It was verbally notified that he would get it, but he is not very sure. The only assurance he has is a legal document which is valid till October 2021 and which says that he is eligible for pending incentives and salary in case of termination. But he has no idea what to do with it in case he will not be able to go back.

Occupation-wise Evidences Wage Theft

The previous analysis indicates that workers in occupations such as the hospitality sector, industry and domestic jobs were disproportionately affected during the pandemic and recorded a higher amount of job loss. As mentioned above, workers in the industry sector experienced relatively dignified returns. However, around 11% of the workers were advised to travel back without salary. They have not received any assurance from the employers about the payment of their wages at any stage of repatriation. The workers from construction (13.8%), hospitality sector (11.5%) and domestic workers (9.4%) suffered most because of the unwillingness from the employers to pay wages and dues. However, only 3% of the workers who lost their jobs were threatened with termination from the job. Apart from the 7% respondents in the construction sector, workers in all other sectors did not encounter any threat from the employer during the pandemic. The workers in the other service sectors such as medical services, banking and financial services and education did not face the issue of wage theft or forceful repatriation without paying their dues. The workers in the sectors that were affected severely during the pandemic were more prone to 'wage theft'.

Dinesh was the floor manager in a well-known restaurant chain in UAE. He was a victim of wage theft due to the closure of restaurants during the pandemic. Dinesh says:

> I was not receiving salary from the month of February as a result of the collapse of tourism industry. My employer provided free accommodation and food during this period but no other support. The owner could have paid if he wanted since they are financially sound, but I did not make any demand because I know that no business was happening now. I was asked to go on an unpaid leave by handing over a termination letter so that the firm won't be in trouble for not paying salary. Most of the restaurant and hotel owners in UAE did the same since there is not much protection of the hotel and restaurant staff.

The restaurant and hospitality industry consists of low-skilled and skilled workers. But their protection is often minimal since most of them, especially Keralites travel on visit visas and find employment after the job search. So, most of these workers are out of the protection system offered at least by the Indian government. There is a reproduction of vulnerabilities when they are thrown out of the job by the employer. There are hardly any means to claim the dues since most of them are terminated. If the reason is too harsh, a legal approach may harm the employee. Apart from the disproportionate economic impact by COVID-19, migrants in these sectors are identified to be more prone to wage theft due to less protection and lack of awareness about the grievance mechanisms.

Complaint Mechanisms and Grievance Redressal

Among the 737 respondents who lost jobs since March 2020, only 3.3% received advice about addressing the non-payment of wages. The advice was given by social workers or friends through lawyers and legal advocates and less than 1% of the workers received verbal advice regarding grievance redressal. Unsurprisingly, the respondents were reluctant to respond on the workplace concerns and on the behaviour of the employers. Even though there are grievance redressal and complaint mechanisms available in countries of origin and destination by Indian missions and Norka-Roots, the workers have shown hesitancy in accessing these services to share their grievances on wage theft.

Raju (not real name) spent 30 years as a foreman in Saudi Arabia. He was employed by a reputed firm in Saudi Arabia. He stated that:

> My relationship with the company was cordial throughout my tenure. I used to remit PF every month as an alternative to the pension. However, the company's financial situation was not promising during my retirement. Before leaving the country, the firm promised to pay the unpaid benefits within two months. I flew back to India, but never received the dues from the company. When I first inquired about it, the firm rejected my claim. I am not in a position to run the case in Saudi Arabia due to the lack of power of attorney and high legal charges. Unfortunately, I was not aware about the legal services offered by Norka-roots or the MADAD portal. Even if I was aware, I may not seek support from the government due to the fear of fighting a legal case against a big player in that country

The workers who faced non-payment of any type were in a confused state as to whether to file a complaint at the destination or give preference to the emergency repatriation. Most of them preferred the latter and travelled without any agreement or power of attorney submitted to the authorities or employer. Many of them were unaware of the services offered by the government and other stakeholders and the panic/lack of support to fight the case at the destination country also contributed to the poor access to grievance redressal mechanisms.

The respondents are afraid to ask for pending wages while some of them have already been mentally preparing themselves to meet any uncertain situation. It is almost as if everyone is expecting contact from their employer regarding salary cut, unpaid leave or termination. They are simply told about a decision in which they have no say. While some companies take the effort to call individual employees and tell the decision while some simply do it through a WhatsApp message. Unmarried and divorced women respondents are upset about losing financial independence and at the prospect of settling in Kerala as they think the society is not safe for single women. Married women with unemployed husbands, kids and parents as dependents find it hard to even think about future.

Large-Scale Wage Theft on NRKs – Evidences From the Field

The non-payment of wages and dues also are experienced due to large-scale layoffs and due to closure of businesses. One of the most notable cases during the pandemic had been reported from Saudi Arabia. A company named Nasser S. Al-Hajri Corporation (NSH) is accused of terminating workers without paying end of service benefits for up to 15 years. Out of 286 Indian workers who filed complaints in the wage theft portal by MFA, 188 were from Kerala.[6] One of the repatriated workers stated:

> I have been working in the Nasser S. Al Hajri (NSH) Corporation since 2007. I paid around one lakh Indian rupees as recruitment fee to join as a carpenter in the company. As time went by, I was assigned the job of a painter with 1200 Riyals as salary. Food and accommodation were provided however it was very difficult to make ends meet with the little salary I received. There are 150 other employees living in the same labour camp with me. I was working during COVID lockdown period as well with lesser working hours. The company terminated me without notice and they stopped the service benefits on 2nd July 2020. The manager asked me to write a letter asking for my 13 years' service benefits and I was asked to give an account number that is active in India. I gave my wife's account details and the manager said the company will be paying the money soon. I came back to India on July 12 on a chartered flight arranged by the company. It is September now and the manager keeps on saying excuses when asked for money. They will not be hiring me back for work even after pandemic since I'm 53 years old. My family is in a financial crisis and I need that money to survive.

The negotiations with the employer of the company have begun after Lawyers Beyond Borders (LBB), an international network of legal experts working for the rights of migrant workers filed a writ in the Kerala High Court requesting urgent interventions. The workers' representatives and civil society organisations are trying to provide justice for the workers through various ways. A number of group cases of wage theft other than the NSH, had been reported in the past five months. Six workers of a UAE-based company; Surface preparation Solutions & Technologies that operates in the UAE Free Zone complained about the non-payment of wages from March to July 2020. They were abandoned without a termination letter or end of service benefits including leave salary. They have come back to Kerala with the financial support of diaspora organisations. The owners of the company who are also Indians fled to India after dissolving the company. The workers are struggling to find a legal solution since the owners left the UAE.

Similar cases due to the closure of the business during the pandemic, had been widely reported across GCC countries.

> We are employees of a company functioning at UAE Free Zone. We used to live at the labour camp at Al Jazirah, UAE. All 6 of us joined this firm through a mutual friend who used to work here. We travelled to the UAE at different times on Visit visa and changed into work visa from there. We did not pay any kind of recruiting fee for this purpose. we used to get salary by hand and not always in full amount. We did not receive any salary after March 2020 and the management cheated us by dissolving the company in UAE and abandoning us without any notice. We have worked until the month of July without salary under the promise that they will pay us once their bills are settled. We received no protection during lockdown and were asked to work continuously. We came to know towards July end that the company owners, who are from Uttar Pradesh in India, left the country by abandoning us. We reached back India with the financial help provided by Radio Asia in UAE. We were not given any kind of termination notice or such because of which it became difficult for us to find new job as well

Another set of group that contains cases of wage theft that occurred even before the pandemic has also been registered.

Mushrif Trading and Contracting Co. in Kuwait has reportedly denied 8–15 months of salary and entire service benefits of 4–18 years of experience. Among the eight workers who have filed complaints, three have returned by the recent amnesty offered by the Kuwait government, two people have returned in 2019, one worker still remains in Kuwait and other returned with the support of diaspora philanthropists. Even though the workers have been facing the delay in payment since 2017 after the company suffered financially, the workers used the 'wage theft campaign' as an opportunity to fight for their rights. Similarly, many workers who worked in the destination countries even after facing non-payment of wages with a hope of receiving the wages at some point of time, found it extremely difficult to survive during the pandemic. The lack of access to food, proper housing and health facilities forced them to fly back to Kerala. However, some of them still stay back at the destination countries to fight for their wages. A group of 24 workers from Sagiya Contracting Company, a manpower-supply company in Bahrain had to stop working in June 2020 after being repeatedly denied wages. The workers decided to fight for justice by denying the tickets offered by the employer.

The victims of wage theft during the pandemic are predominantly semi-skilled workers, human resources professionals and construction workers. In the pre-pandemic period, apart from occasional cases of massive lay-offs, most of the cases of wage theft was reported among low-skilled workers and domestic workers in the destination countries. The major difference between the group cases and individual cases is that the collectiveness and possible sharing of information in the group cases increases the chances of claims. However, individual cases are often gone unnoticed and the victims of wage theft may not have the resources or information to claim the unpaid wages and dues. The two major aspects identified from the analysis is the lack of access to justice mechanisms in the destination countries before and after the repatriation. The absence of dynamic wage protection and labour rights protection systems in the Gulf countries prevents the uniform distribution of protection in all sectors of work. As Piper (2021) discusses, the role of non-state actors is crucial in this context to create further discussions on the transitional and multilateral justice mechanisms to address the issue of 'wage theft'. The final section of the chapter discusses the responses of both state and non-state stakeholders in Kerala.

Responses From Stakeholders and Recommendations

The issue of wage theft among returnees was widely discussed in the state after the initiation of the wage theft campaign by the Migrant Forum in Asia (MFA) and its partners. Migrant Forum in Asia (MFA) in association with a number of civil society and trade union collectives call upon countries of origin and destination to urgently put in place a transitional justice mechanism with the objectives of setting up an urgent justice mechanism to address grievances, claims and labour disputes of repatriated workers who have lost their jobs as a result of the pandemic; ensuring that cases are resolved as soon as possible, without delay, especially in cases involving labour disputes, safeguards must be put in place to ensure that migrants are able to pursue their case post-return.[7] The coalition released a total of five appeals that focus on actions to be taken by UN bodies, governments and businesses to take concerted action in engaging with existing cases of wage theft and lack of justice as well as the creation and maintenance of effective mechanisms. By establishing a website for the Justice for Wage Theft campaign, MFA documented the wage theft cases with the support from its partners.

A number of partners of MFA established helplines and online complaint fora in India to document and understand the extent of the problem. In Kerala, the Centre for Indian Migrant Studies (CIMS) led the campaign. Unlike the pre-pandemic period, the number of complaints about non-payment of wages and dues during the pandemic has increased multiple times. CIMS has already received around 700 cases of wage theft from the GCC region alone. The campaign unravelled the issues of wage theft even before the pandemic and a number of migrants described long-run cases of wage theft with the employers at the destination.

The Kerala government also began to respond to the requests for addressing the wage theft in the Gulf countries. As an initial step, the Norka department set up a toll-free number and complaint forms to report the cases of wage theft. They have received around 600 cases so far and have provided the information to the Indian missions in the Gulf countries. The poor responses made the Norka-Roots involve the lawyers' panel and handed over the cases to the Norka lawyers in the destination countries. However, these efforts did not make much successful results in the past one year. Norka-Roots and the Kerala government's reluctance to co-operate with the non-governmental organisations to fight the wage-theft campaign is a major hindrance. The limitation of collecting information from the destination countries can be solved by using the civil society and diaspora networks in the destination countries. But Norka's historic reluctance to associate with the non-government agents remains a key bottleneck. Moreover, Norka is yet to make use of its coveted Global Kerala Assembly Network to address the issue and to create awareness among migrants about the possible wage theft in the future.

An intervention at the global and regional platforms is the need of the hour. The stakeholders from the state should advocate for an effective intervention from the Government of India. Apart from the urgent justice mechanism, the stakeholders should push for comprehensive bilateral and multilateral agreements at the international level that ensures access to justice for the migrant workers. If the issue of wage theft is not addressed with due diligence, it will definitely have an impact on the economy of the state and the life of migrants as well.

Notes

1 Reported by migrant workers during Justice For Wage Theft Campaign by MFA. Accessed from http://mfasia.org/migrantforumasia/wp-content/uploads/2021/04/MFA_Crying-Out-for-Justice_04.12.pdf
2 https://www.thehindu.com/news/national/vande-bharat-becomes-one-of-top-civilian-evacuations/article34361996.ece\
3 https://www.thehindu.com/news/national/kerala/state-sees-largest-reverse-migration/article34163811.ece
4 http://202.88.244.146:8083/covidsupport/nrks/
5 https://escholarship.umassmed.edu/cgi/viewcontent.cgi?article=1104&context=jeslib#:~:text=The%20exploratory%20sequential%20mixed%20methods,two%20separate%20strands%20of%20data.
6 Reported by the Centre for Indian Migrant Studies.
7 https://justiceforwagetheft.org/en/page/c1cu5etiltr

References

Foley, L., & Piper, N. (2021). Returning home empty handed: Examining how COVID-19 exacerbates the non-payment of temporary migrant workers' wages. *Global Social Policy*, 21(3), 468–489.
International Labour Organisation (ILO). (2020). *Policy brief: Protecting migrant workers during the COVID-19 pandemic, recommendations for policy-makers and constituents*. Geneva: ILO.

Kumar, A., & Akhil, C. S. (2021). How migrants in the Gulf are fighting discrimination during the pandemic. Open democracy, 8 April. Available at: https://www.opendemocracy.net/en/openindia/how-migrants-gulf-are-fighting-discrimination-during-pandemic/

Migrant Forum in Asia (MFA). (2021). Crying out for justice: Wage theft against migrant workers during COVID-19. Migrant Forum in Asia, 7 April. Available at: http://mfasia.org/migrantforumasia/wp-content/uploads/2021/04/MFA_Crying-Out-for-Justice_04.12.pdf

Piper, N., & Foley, L. (2021). The other pandemic for migrant workers: Wage theft. Open democracy, 12 January. Available at: https://www.opendemocracy.net/en/pandemic-border/other-pandemic-migrant-workers-wage-theft/

Rajan, S. I. (2012). Assessment of NORKA-ROOTS (an implementing agency of the department of NORKA - Non-resident Keralites affairs of the government of Kerala) and the applicability of a similar organisation to other states in India. Migrant forum in Asia, Philippines.

Rajan, S. I., & Akhil, C. S. (2019). Reintegration of return migrants and state responses: A case study of Kerala. *Productivity*, 60(2), 126–135.

Rajan, S. I., & Arokkiaraj, H. (2021). Return migration from the Gulf region to India amidst COVID-19. Chapter 11. In A. Triandafyllidou (Ed.), *2021: Migration and pandemics: Spaces of solidarity and spaces of exception* (pp. 207–225). Singapore: Springer.

Rajan, S. I., & Batra, P. (2021). Return migrants and the first wave of COVID 19: Results from the Vande Bharat returnees. Chapter 6. In S. Irudaya Rajan (Ed.), *2021: India migration report 2021: Migrants and health* (pp. 57–76). New Delhi: Routledge.

Rajan, S. I., & Pattath, B. (2021). What next for the COVID-19 return emigrants? Findings from the Kerala return emigrant survey 2021. Chapter 14. In S. Irudaya Rajan (Ed.), *2021: India migration report 2021: Migrants and health* (pp. 181–195). New Delhi: Routledge.

Rajan, S. I., & Sami, B. D. (2022). Preliminary observations from Tamil Nadu return migrant survey 2021. Chapter 17. In S. Irudaya Rajan (Ed.), *2022: India migration report 2022: Health professionals migration.* New Delhi: Routledge.

Rajan, S. I., & Zachariah, K. C. (2019). *Emigration and remittances: New evidences from the Kerala migration survey 2018* (Working Paper No. 483). Thiruvananthapuram: Centre for Development Studies. Available at: http://cds.edu/wp-content/uploads/2019/01/WP483.pdf

Zachariah, K. C., & Rajan, S. I. (2012). *Kerala's Gulf connection, 1998–2011: Economic and social impact of migration.* Hyderabad: Orient Blackswan.

Zachariah, K. C., Mathew, E. T., & Rajan, S. I. (2003). *Dynamics of migration in Kerala: Dimensions: Differentials and consequences.* Hyderabad: Orient Blackswan.

Zachariah, K. C., Nair, P. R. G., & Rajan, S. I. (2001). Return emigrants in Kerala: Rehabilitation problems and development potential (Working Paper No. 319). Thiruvananthapuram: Centre for Development Studies.

Zachariah, K. C., Nair, P. R. G., & Rajan, S. I. (2006). *Return emigrants in Kerala: Welfare, rehabilitation, and development.* New Delhi: Manohar Publishers.

Zachariah, K. C., & Rajan, S. I. (2010). Impact of the global recession on migration and remittances in Kerala: New evidences from the return migration study (RMS) 2009 (Working Paper No. 432). Thiruvananthapuram: Centre for Development Studies.

Zachariah, K. C., & Rajan, S. I. (2011). From Kerala via Kerala via the Gulf: Emigration experiences of return emigrants (Working Paper No. 443). Thiruvananthapuram: Centre for Development Studies.

14 Do Remittances Affect Labour Supply Decisions at a Household Level in India?

Amaani Bashir

Introduction

Remittances have had a key role to play in developing India's financial flows during the past 40 years. Remittances have been a key financial flow in South Asian countries as well; indeed, India is currently the highest remittance-earning state in the world, with the Indian diaspora sending home $80 billion in 2018 (KNOMAD, 2019). The fact that there are nearly 30 million Indians overseas, only further contributes to the profound effects of migration on the country. The Reserve Bank of India stipulates that nearly 60% of remittance funds are used for sustenance purposes (Reserve Bank of India, 2018). Remittances can serve as an important source of household credit and can instate several welfare and economic benefits for household members. The IMF defines remittances as transfers sent by migrants to relatives who live away from the household (Asiedu and Chimbar, 2019); this means that there are significant implications on the labour decisions of the household due to the missingness of certain 'labour'. Labour Force Participation (LFP) is an important consideration in this regard (Acosta et al., 2007; Adaku, 2013; Alpa and Harriss-White, 2011; Adams, 1998).

LFP is defined as the population of the labour force divided by the total working-age population. While India's remittance receipts have increased 180% since 1975, India's tryst with premature de-industrialisation has raised concerns with LFP rates in India. Literature citing a Dutch Disease type phenomenon state that remittances can cause an exchange range appreciation, leading to uncompetitive trading sectors for the country (Acosta et al., 2009). Interpolating this on a micro-level implies that remittances can be used as a cushion against falling labour income, withdrawing from the labour force in tradable industries. Along these lines, this study aims to look at how household decisions are impacted by remittances, specifically the decision to partake in the labour force (Amuedo-Dorantes and Pozo, 2006; Azizi, 2018; De la Brière et al., 2002; Eromenko, 2016).

Using large representative data from the National Sample Survey of India (NSS), we find that remittances have negatively impacted the average

DOI: 10.4324/9781003315124-14

marketable work intensity of the household. After correcting for endogeneity issues, this study finds that the remittance impact is deepened, more so in the rural sector which displays a higher elasticity to remittances. Using a Multinomial Logistic Regression, we also find that remittances cause a slight substitution effect in changing work activity statuses of individuals into more household enterprises or domestic tasks from being salaried employees; this effect is once again deeper in the rural sector. Missingness of labour in a household can be compensated by the effect of remittances. We also find that remittances have some unobservable effect on the decision-making of the household, after factoring out the various uses of remittances (Hanson, 2007; Puhani, 2000).

Theoretical Motivations

Neoclassical Theory of Labour-Leisure

According to the neoclassical theory of labour, individuals make decisions about how to allocate their time between work (labour) and rest (leisure). This decision is made based on a constraint determined by (i) individual market wage w, (ii) a time budget (hours a day) and (iii) the individuals non-labour income N. Readers are recommended to read Koutsoyiannis (1975) for an in-depth reading of this theory.

In our study, while the conceptual basis follows the neoclassical theory, leisure can be replaced by the concept of non-market activity such as domestic work or informal work. This implies that the time allocation is a trade-off between marketable (labour) and non-marketable (defined as unpaid) activities, which will serve as the base to understand substitution effects in the study.

In the neoclassical theory, a person's consumption of goods and leisure is constrained by time and income (earned by wages w and by non-labour income N); we amend this to argue that a person's engagement in market activities (hence consumption) and non-market activities are constrained by time and income in the same way. Assuming non-market activities are a normal good, an increase in consumption must be compensated by a decrease in non-market activities. The elasticity of this tradeoff is determined by w. Given that some part of an individual's income is independent of the hours of work, this implies that consumption can be increased independently of hours worked or the wage rate.

$$C = (w * Y) + N \qquad (1)$$

Using this and assuming that time can only be split between market and non-market activities, to keep consumption constant, an increase in N can indicate a preference in allocating more hours from market to non-market activities, known as a 'Substitution Effect'. However, an increase in N

shifts also allows the individual to increase consumption, which is known as 'Income Effect'. The combination of the Income and Substitution effect sees the individual increase their consumption, while decreasing their market activities as a result of an increase in non-labour income.

Lucas and Stark's (1985) Theory of Remittances

While the most common assumption under which Econometric studies of the effects/determinants of remittances are those pertaining to altruistic or self-interest purposes (Lueth and Ruiz-Arranz, 2008; Adams and Cuecuecha, 2010), Lucas theorised the model of tempered altruism such as:

$$U_m = U\left[c_m(w-r), \sum_{h=1}^{n} A_h u(CHH)\right] \tag{2}$$

where C_m is their consumption and A_h are 'altruism weights' attached to various household members and consumption per capita is expected to increase with income per capita of the household and r is the amount remitted. The main premise is that the migrant's utility function (Um) depends on utility of their remaining family members UHH which is a function of consumption (CHH).

Then, maximising the optimal amount of remittances sent becomes a function of the income per capita (y), the migrants wage wand the number of household members *n*, like so:

$$C_h = C\left(y + \frac{r}{r}, n\right) \tag{3}$$

However, altruism and self-interest are not binary but rather a ratio of preferences for remitting which manifest themselves in the volume of remittances. Lucas reconciles self-interest and altruism under a 'tempered altruism' framework while offering separate hypotheses, taking into account level of education, sector of living, and household income among others. Lucas also stated that remittance volumes are usually seen as an implicit contractual agreement between a migrant and the remaining family, which is only adhered to until it is in the migrants benefit to do so, for a multitude of reasons such as those expressed above. Interestingly, this theoretical analysis assumes complete and voluntary contracting which are self-imposing, hence making it challenging to understand the true motives for remittances and their effects on labour supply decisions. To specify its effect on work intensity, the hypothesis must be extended to involve the assumed income effect of non- labour income. The monotonicity of remittances as non-labour income implies that remittances will decrease the household's work requirement, hence reducing the time spent in market activities.

Empirical Motivations

Macroeconomics of Remittances

Lueth and Ruiz-Arranz (2006) find a positive relationship between remittance receipts and the dependency ratio in the home country of a sample of 11 countries in Europe and Asia, affirming an altruistic motive. Tempered altruism has a more ambiguous result in their story as they find a positive relationship between volumes of remittances and countries with high inflation rates (to compensate for lower purchasing power), which shows a protection against price uncertainty. Chami et al. (2018) argue that remittances can have macroeconomic supply and demand implications. On the demand side, remittances reduce unemployment but tend to benefit lower wage, low-productivity nontradable industries whereas on the supply-side, remittances do reduce labour force participation and interestingly, increase the informality of the labour market. Citing a Dutch Disease type phenomenon, Acosta et al. (2009) study El Salvador to state that remittances decline labour supply and increase consumption that is biased towards non-tradables. Higher non-tradable prices incentivise expansion of that sector away from the tradable sector. They argue that smoothing income flows makes remittance receiving households increase consumption and leisure levels. Using a DSGE model, Guha (2013) shows that an increase in the non-wage income results in a fall in the labour supply in the tradable sector and a decline in the output of the traded sector, signalling a Dutch Disease effect of foreign remittances.

Labour Supply and Remittances

While much of the literature has focused on the determinants of remittances, their inter linkedness to the labour supply decision implies that it is important to look at both as key household decisions. Adam and Cuecuecha (2010) point to three views on how remittances could affect household decisions:

i. Remittances are firstly used like additional income from any source and have similar uses to other sources of income, depending on the household's utility maximisation function.
ii. Remittance can induce `behavioural changes' at the household level, spending more on consumption, rather than investment goods.
iii. If remittances are regarded as a transitory type of income, households are less dependent on them for consumption and use them for one on investment purposes.

Ramos and Jadotte (2016), looking at this relationship in Haiti, find that there is a decline in labour supply as well as hours worked with the presence of remittances, where the response of female-headed households is less sensitive than male-headed households. Their study indicates the existence of an income effects dominating the substitution effect with additional income.

Cox-Edwards and Rodriguez-Oreggia (2009) look at the labour force participation decisions as one dependent on the reservation wage and that remittance has the effect of increasing the reservation wage. They also argue that migration and remittances are endogenous; if the migrant's decision on how much to remit depends on whether the family members are looking for a job or not, reverse causality exists. Omitted variable bias may exist if remittances are related to the remittance-recipient family members' wealth or ambition, which may be correlated to the labour supply by the recipient. However, by using Propensity Score Matching, they find limited evidence of labour force participation effects of persistent remittances. This is consistent with the 'neutral' view of remittance as a method to generate in-household income as opposed to additional income augmenting effects. However, care must be taken to apply the neoclassical concept of the reservation wage to the coercive nature of labour markets in developing countries, implying that workers may not respond to reservation wages.

Descriptive Statistics

Using the NSS 64th Round – the Employment, Unemployment, and Migration survey, we find a sample of 125,578 households. There are 53,855 migrant households, of which 3,961 have international migrants and 49,905 households have domestic migrants. International migrants tend to be from urban areas more than rural areas. About 42.97% of the households have reported at least one member migrating out; this number increases to 46.36% in the rural sample. 0.48% of the households reported migrating internationally, and this percentage drops to 0.45% in the rural sample, indicating the prevalence of rural to urban migration. The majority of migration takes place within the same district, nearly 45.72%.

The average remittances of the sample are ₹6287. Consequently, the rural sector is ₹5370, contrasted with ₹8022 in the urban sector. There is a general monotonically increasing relationship for the remittance returns to education. An illiterate migrant receives an average of ₹4,764 which then increases to ₹14,546 at the post graduate level or above. While there is a slightly monotonically increasing relationship with land size classes, there is a significant increase in the amount of remittances sent for individuals who own more than 8 hectares of land. While all other land classes show remittances under ₹10,000, households that own more than 8 hectares of land see an average remittance transfer of ₹22,878. There is also an increasing number of migrants for increasing land size, which implies that there may be wealth effects that come into play when making the decision to migrate and hence remit. This is very important as the predominant motive for remittances are often assumed to be poverty as a push factor, but this rarely considers the costs of migration and transaction costs of remittances as well.

Unsurprisingly there is a positive relationship by monthly expenditure quintiles and the amount remitted to the household suggesting the need for remittances to ease consumption constraints. Using remittances on food items is by far the most popular first use of remittances (65%), followed by education as a popular second use (35%), implying that human capital development may be an important goal of remittance-recipient households and thirdly healthcare and other household items as popular third uses (20% and 37%, respectively). However in terms of absolute volume, the highest average remittance usage is for saving/investment (₹64,404) purposes, followed by housing improvements (₹ 40,000) and debt repayment (₹36,012). Since a large percentage of household's report remittance use on basic necessities, it shows that standards of living at the household are a popular channel through which remittances alleviate household constraints; these considerations will serve as an important determinant in the choosing of explanatory variables.

General Model

Ordinary Least Squares

An Ordinary Least Squares regression is used to specify the labour supply decision will be used. Since there is truncation in remittances and an endogeneity of remittances, this may be a somewhat imperfect methodology for estimating this relationship. However, it provides an appropriate functional form to continue further analysis. The regression will look at the effects of remittance volumes on the average work intensity of a household per week, which was constructed by looking at the household's marketable activities.[1] In running a naive regression on *work intensity$_i$* socioeconomic controls to determine the true effect of remittances on the decision to work are used, the choice of which are elaborated in Appendix A.

$$workintensity_i = \pm + \beta_1 lremit_i + \beta_2 HHtype_i + \beta_3 lconsumption_i + \beta_4 HHsize_i$$

$$+ \beta_5 landpossessed_i + \beta_6 firstuse_i + \beta_7 averageperiodout^2$$

$$+ \beta_8 teched_{ia} + \beta_9 State_i + \beta_{10} totalmigrants_i + \beta_{11} gened_i + s_i$$

Looking at the log of remittances *lremit$_i$*, we find a negative relationship; for a 1% increase in the volume of remittances, the average work intensity reduces by 0.172 days, with a statistically significant result. This is the expected sign of the relationship, if you assume remittances act as additional income that would induce members of the remittance-recipient households to withdraw from labour force participation (Table 14.1). Once remittances are accounted for show that a 1% increase in *lconsumption$_i$* induces the household to increase work intensity by 0.114 days. This could be because if remittances are not used to absolve consumption constraints, then consuming goods becomes a strong determinant to work as remittances are instead supporting investment

Table 14.1 General Ordinary Least Squares Regression

Table X: General OLS Regression

Variables	Coefficients	Standard Errors
lremit$_i$	−0.172***	(0.00367)
lconsumption$_i$	0.114***	(0.00961)
landpossesssion$_i$		
0.005–0.01	0.0333***	(0.0124)
0.002–0.20	0.0270**	(0.0129)
0.21–0.40	0.116***	(0.0151)
0.40–1.00	0.305***	(0.0156)
1.01–2.01	0.353***	(0.0170)
2.01–3.00	0.398***	(0.0221)
3.01–4.00	0.431***	(0.0297)
4.01–6.00	0.433***	(0.0360)
6.01–8.00	0.639***	(0.0462)
Greater than 8.00	0.571***	(0.03656)
Averageperiodout^2	−0.000377***	(2.42e-0.5)
Totalmigrants$_i$	0.0123***	(0.00234)
Constant	3.281***	(0.0790)
Observations		128,642
R-squared		0.313

type purchases. This seems especially plausible since the consumption variable consists of sustenance purchases of the household in the past 30 days and also durable purchases like healthcare and education. *lconsumption$_i$* takes a negative and significant coefficient when remittances are removed, implying that remittances are not being used for consumption, but are rather freeing up households to increase labour force participation to satisfy consumption by satisfying long-term credit constraints (Bucheli et al., 2018).

The use of remittances by recipient household was used as a control to isolate the use of remittances from the decision-making effects of remittances. This variable is different from the remittance volume because it identifies whether it is consumption, investment, or financial uses of remittances that frees up the household to make labour force decisions. All remittance uses have positive relationships with work intensity suggesting that these consumption, investment, or financial satisficers of remittances are not how remittances reduce household work intensity. Since these coefficients are measured against a base category (food items in this case) that is consumption based, it can be said that consumption motives lower work intensity compared to other credit uses. However, the coefficient on education as a use of remittance is negative indeed an increase in remittance used for education reduces the average work intensity of the household by 0.255 days. This implies that education payment in these households is a significant good that imposes constraints on leisure.

The *averageperiodout$_i$* of migrants in the house was squared to capture non-linearities of inheritance motives over time. Here *averageperiodout^2* shows a significant (albeit, not very substantive) negative relationship; as total time away from the household increases, the work intensity increases and consequently decreases as time increases even more (Table 14.2). This can serve as a rudimentary analysis in disproving the inheritance motive as the work intensity does not decline with migrants spending time out initially, only to decrease later. However, this could be explained by the increasing age of remittance recipients, hence a natural withdrawal from labour force participation under the lifecycle hypothesis. This implies that remittance acts as an additional income to the household and may not induce any unusual behavioural changes. *Land possession$_i$* has a positive effect on work intensity with the amount of land; increasing land possession increases work intensity of 0.03 to 0.571 days by increasing land possession (Table 14.1). This implies that land possession is largely being used for marketable agricultural practices such as cash crops. It also implies that in isolation it doesn't possess any independent wealth effects. Parida (2015) equates this to being

Table 14.2 Structural Equation (Heckman Correction)

Variables	Heckman Correction
lremit$_i$	−0.274***
	(0.00357)
firstuse$_i$	0.0488***
	(0.00130)
landpossesssion$_i$	0.123***
	(0.00195)
Averageperiodout^2	−0.000794***
	(2.69e-05)
Averageperiodout$_i$	−
lconsumption$_i$	(0.0634***)
	(0.312***)
Technicaleducationi	
Technicaldegree:	0.796***
Graduatei	(0.0729)
Technicaldegree:	1.108***
Postgraduatei	(0.124)
Diploma:	0.578***
BelowGraduate$_i$	(0.0474)
Diploma:	0.831*** (0.0984)
Graduate$_i$	
Diploma:	1.232*** (0.176)
Postgraduate$_i$	
Lambda	0.157***
Constant	3.371***
Rho	−0.11285
Observations	567,929

consistent with Engels Law, where families having more land (typically better off families in the rural sector) are spending generally less portion on sustenance and moreover on physical and human capital investments.

Selection Bias Correction

There are several migrants that do not remit back as well, perhaps due to some 'reservation remittance' or transaction costs of sending money back (Freund and Sapatora, 2008). It would be incorrect to group migrant non-remitters and non-migrants (hence having no remittances) in the same group as there are surely characteristic differences between migrant and non-migrant groups in addition to a remitting/non-remitting household which cause a selection bias in the analysis.

While this problem can be absolved by running a double-hurdle model or a 3-stage least squares model, the lack of socioeconomic variables in the dataset means that valid exclusion-restrictions cannot be attained between multiple simultaneous equations. With a valid exclusion-restriction, the Inverse Mills Ratio, and the regressor vector in the substantive equation will be less correlated, reducing multicollinearity among predictors as well as between the error terms.[2] However, since we are studying the effects of remittances and not migration, the second selection bias problem will be focused on and the former will be controlled for using variables to capture migration effects. Moreover, due to non-linearities in Probit models, the correction term will not be perfectly correlated with the regressors, even in the absence of exclusion-restrictions (shown by a low rho value). This means that the Heckman procedure can technically be carried out without exclusion-restrictions.

Selection Equation

$$\alpha + \beta_1 Religion_i + \beta_2 HHsize_i + \beta_3 Marital_i + \beta_4 Gened_i$$

$$+\beta_5 Sector_{i(rural,urban)} + \beta_6 State_i + \beta_7 lconsumption_i + s_i$$

Structural Equation

$$workintensity_i = \alpha + \beta_1 lremit_i + \beta_2 firstuse_i + \beta_3 averageperiodout^2_i$$

$$+\beta_4 totalmigrants_i + \beta_5 landpossession_i$$

$$+\beta_6 lconsumption_i + s_i$$

The theoretical motivations for the Selection Equation are that demographic characteristics have often been anecdotal push factors in migrations (Selection Equation). For example, the movement of the Indian Muslim community to the Middle East has been characteristically documented in migration literature. Marital status and household size indicate pressures for higher incomes that arise from migrating and remitting. Certain states also have a higher propensity to migrate than others i.e., Kerala internationally and Bihar domestically. Factors determining the volume of remittances (Structural Equation) such as *averagetimeout,*[2] *totalmigrant*$_p$ *firstuse*$_i$ which closely models altruism, insurance, and intergenerational loan motives isolate remittance effects on the household's work intensity. For example, increasing migrants from the same household will have an ambiguous effect on labour force participation through (a) migration effects manifesting themselves in lower household labour supply and (b) remittance effects which may cause the household to withdraw from the labour force with increasing migrants.

The correction deepens the remittance effect on decreasing work intensity, implying that the truncation was leading to a downward bias in estfimating the remittance impact on labour supply.[3] Following Funkhouser's theories, consumption can be both in the Selection and Structural Equations, the Lambda correction is significant at the 1% level. A 1% increase in remittances leads to a decrease in work intensity of 0.274 days a week (Table 14.2). Indeed, the literature above has pointed to how consumption is an important determinant in volume of remittances. Yet, wanting to ease credit streams is a push factor for the decision to remit. The positive and significant coefficients of *lconsumption*$_i$ in both equations imply that consumption of the household is a channel through which hours worked are affected more so in the presence of remittances (Bettin and Zazzaro, 2009). Consumption affects the decision to remit which then in turn affects the hours worked in the household due to the income effects of remittances; Remittances are positing an income effect which dampen the requirement for labour force participation in households (even if consumption expenditure that is independent of remittances displays a positive relationship with work intensity). However, *lconsumption*$_i$ has a larger positive effect in determining the volume of remittances as opposed to the decision to remit, implying that consumption may not be a strong push factor but does affect household labour-time allocations once the decision is made.

The effect of *averageperiodout*[2] has become marginally stronger than the OLS model. Even if they have migrated with the precedent of sending remittances (Positive Selection), the missingness of labour in the house is seen to induce an increased work intensity (Table 14.3).

Instrumental Variables

McKenzie and Sasin (2007) argue that endogeneity issues can arise from trying to discern motivations to remit and motivations to migrate. While motives are often overlapping, the significant number of non-remitting migrants in this dataset would suggest otherwise. Though migration effects have been controlled to avoid corner solutions this does not completely rectify the problem as it is impossible to take non-monetary transfer costs, or the ease

Table 14.3 OLS vs. Heckman Correction

Variables	OLS	Heckman Correction
$lremit_i$	−0.172***	−0.274***
	(0.00367)	(0.00357)
$firstuse_i$	−	0.0513***
		(0.00129)
$landpossesssion_i$	0.1213***	0.123***
	(0.00197)	(0.00195)
$averageperiodout^2$	−0.000377***	−0.000794***
	(2.42e-05)	(2.69e-05)
$lconsumption_i$	0.114***	(0.0634***)
	(0.00961)	(0.312***)
$technicaleducation_i$		
$technicaldegree:$	0.2640***	0.7960***
$Graduate_i$	(0.0724)	(0.0729)
$technicaldegree:$	0.2290	1.1080***
$Postgraduate_i$	(0.140)	(0.124)
$Diploma:$	0.07820	0.5780***
$BelowGraduate_i$	(0.0623)	(0.0474)
$Diploma:$	0.2150**	0.8310***
$Graduate_i$	(0.103)	(0.0984)
$Diploma:$	0.4180*	1.2320***
$Postgraduate_i$	(0.217)	(0.176)
Lambda		0.157***
Constant		3.371***
Observations		567,929

of remitting into quantitative account, hence some endogeneity problems continue to exist. The endogeneity issues arising from the activity status of a household; i.e. family enterprises would induce more remittances being sent but the reverse causality would argue that the labour force decision (i.e. the decision to start a family enterprise) is determined by remittances instead. Lianos (1997) argues that the improper treatment of endogeneity might explain why income elasticities in micro-econometric data are smaller than 1, which suggests that remittances are a basic good, whereas remittances often show a cyclical elasticity of more than 1 in macro-econometric data. The instruments chosen for this are number of times a household has received remittances in the past 365 days ($timesremitted_i$) and the reason for migration ($migrationreason_i$) can serve as instruments for the volume of remittances for the following reasons:

i. The times remitted can be assumed to have a monotonically increasing relationship with the log of remittances due to a positive correlation coefficient (0.4931), but also a low correlation with the outcome variable $workintensity_i$ (−0.07).

ii. The number of times remitted is a good proxy for the migrants income and consumption abroad as it implies that transaction costs of remittances can be borne by a migrant with higher incomes. Furthermore, the reason for migration can serve as an effective categorisation of remittance motivations which in turn can explain volumes of remittances, yet does not pre-empt work intensity decisions of the household.

iii. Certain transactions like big investments or large asset purchases often require a one-time transfer, but multiple remittances can imply consumption motives. Hence, the number of times remitted can be revealing of the reason for remittances yet have similar effects to volumes of remittances on labour force decisions in a household, absolving reverse causality concerns.

iv. Additionally, correcting the selectivity problem using the appropriate Inverse Mills Ratio is important as it helps to discern the actual effect of remittances on labour supply decisions as opposed to the characteristic effects of a migrant household.

Running an IV equation with the variables in the naive equation as opposed to the Structural equation posited in the Heckman correction absolves the problem of trying to separate Structural and Selection equations via exclusion-restrictions by including the chosen Inverse Mills Ratio. This allows for the determinants of labour supply to be determined with more detail using a full range of controls to isolate the effect of remittances. The Heckman-corrected IV regression is modelled as:

$$Work\ intensity_i = \alpha + \beta_1 lremit_i + \beta_2 HHtype_i + \beta_3 lconsumption_i$$

$$\beta_4 HHsize_i + \beta_5 landpossessed_i + \beta_6 firstuse_i$$

$$+ \beta_7 averageperiodout^2 + \beta_8 teched_i + \beta_9 State_i$$

$$+ \beta_{10} totalmigrants_i + \beta_{11} gened_i + s_i,$$

where

$$lremit_i = timesremitted_i\ and\ migration\ reason_i$$

In running *timesremittedi* and *migrationreasoni* as instruments to *lremiti*, we find that there are indeed exogenising instruments, since they do not reject the null hypothesis of exogeneity in the Durbin-Wu-Hausman test ($p = 0.7269$). Interestingly, while the test for over-identifying restrictions is significant at the 1% level ($p = 0.0108$), using each instrument separately fails the Durbin-Wu-Hausman tests, implying that the instruments have joint significance in exogenising the remittance effect on labour supply.

Table 14.4 Heckman-Corrected IV

Variables	Coefficients	Standard errors
lremit$_i$	−0.293***	(0.0492)
lconsumption$_i$	0.197***	(0.0778)
landpossesssion$_i$		
0.005–0.01	0.0681	(0.102)
0.002–0.20	−0.358**	(0.0912)
0.21–0.40	0.0835	(0.0110)
0.40–1.00	0.490***	(0.112)
1.01–2.01	0.542***	(0.114)
2.01–3.00	0.189	(0.130)
3.01–4.00	0.735***	(0.163)
4.01–6.00	−0.535*	(0.147)
6.01–8.00	0.356***	(0.205)
Greater than 8.00	1.527***	(0.141)
Averageperiodout^2_i	−0.00465*	(0.000225)
Totalmigrants$_i$	−0.00465	(0.0256)
Constant	4.262***	(0.548)
Observations		2,357
R-squared		0.445

Instrumenting the log of remittances increases the strength of its effect on work intensity: A 1% increase in remittance now reduces work intensity by 0.293. The R-squared has increased to 0.445 which implies that instrumenting out *lremiti*; indicating that remittances were capturing other effects in determining labour supply decisions of the households. The coefficient of consumption has become stronger on work intensity. Additionally, lower levels of land possession now display a negative coefficient. Shah and Harris-White (2011) argue that dependency on migrant wage labour, rural livelihoods are combining both micro-agricultural work on small plots of land and petty commodity production to reproduce households, implying that land possession at low levels is more dependent and volatile to remittances in determining household labour supply decisions. *averageperiodout²* displays a deeper coefficient, implying that the missingness of labour has a deeper effect on work intensity (Table 14.4). This points to the confounding effects of migration and remittances on the labour supply decisions, showing that the volatility in labour supply comes from remittances as a function of migration, and isn't necessarily exhibiting a purely remittance-based income effect.

Cross Validation

While the true elasticity of remittances is challenging to discern due to the limitations of data, the aforementioned analysis has given rise to 3 models:

Table 14.5 Average Model Cross Validation

OLS	Heckman-corrected OLS	Heckman-Corrected IV
1.234209955	1.397106506	1.396475217

OLS, Heckman-corrected OLS, and IV. To make meaningful comparisons between these models, one can conduct across validation analysis. To do this, we run k-fold iterations of testing, and take the average Root Mean Square Error (RMSE). These averages can then be compared across models; the lower the RMSE, the lesser the average deviation of the testing data from the training data.

Table 14.5 shows that while OLS has the lowest RMSE, this is because it has minimised the squared residual to obtain its fit. The Heckman correction and IV are both trying to treat issues of endogeneity which means that often there are large standard errors in these estimators caused by instruments that aren't highly correlated with the endogenous regressor, hence higher RMSE's. The analysis above suggests that the Heckman-corrected OLS with the Inverse Mills Ratio is a better fit than the Heckman-corrected IV equation in estimating the impact of labour supply on remittances. In the study, as both the OLS and Heckman model's RMSE's are lower as k-fold iterations increase and are converging, the IV equation has an increasing RMSE with higher k-fold iterations, implying that there may be a problem of over fitting which is consistent with the IV over-identifying test taken above.

Rural Model

Rural migration in the past was seen predominantly as a marital phenomenon which was incentivised by spatial income differential; in 1981 the net outflow from rural to urban areas represented 2.2% of the total rural population and the gross outflow of migrants for employment reasons only represented 1.6% of the Indian population. Now, rural migration and remittances are characterised by the engagement with places of origin through socioeconomic activities. Parida (2015) state out-migration that has taken place in rural areas is highest in agricultural dependent and poorer states like Odisha, Bihar, UP, MP, AP, Chhattisgarh, and Jharkhand, remittances have had a larger role to play in poverty reduction and changing consumption patterns.

Banerjee (1984) argues that remittances sent to rural areas are sent mainly for 'house-hold expenses' and 'aiding agriculture' in contrast to the Kenyan rural context, where remittances are used for the 'consumption needs' of individual rural dependents. More recently however, Rempel and Lobdell (1978) argue remittances in their study was seen as a means of maintaining their families which they cannot afford to move into town whereas others use remittances to represent a payment of social debt for the household that has provided past assistance received in the past, such as an intergenerational loan repayment. They state that consumption, education, and housing are significant reasons but only if strengthened by the social capital considerations.

Remittances to urban areas have a much different effect to those in rural areas because of their differences in purchasing parity, social group, gender, and class dynamics, meaning that remittances can ease credit constraints for some groups much more than others in the rural sector. For example, Singh and Oberoi (1980) find that remittances were more likely to be received by richer rural households, hence increasing the gap between the rich and poor in the rural sector. This means that the general model above should be focused on the rural sector to understand how remittances can affect labour supply decisions.

Ordinary Least Squares – Rural Model

$$work\ intensity_i = \alpha + \beta_1 lremit_i + \beta_2 HHtype_i + \beta_3 lconsumption_i + \beta_4 HHsize_i$$

$$+\beta_5 landpossessed_i + \beta_6 firstuse_i + \beta_7 averageperiodout^2$$

$$+\beta_8 teched_i + \beta_9 State_i + \beta_{10} totalmigrants_i + \beta_{11} gened_i$$

$$+\beta_{12} socialgroup_i + \beta_{13} HHHeadgender_i \left(male, female \right) + s_i$$

In running an OLS for specifically the rural sector on the average work intensity of the household, we find that the effect of the log of remittances on work intensity is stronger; an increase of the remittances sent to a household by 1% will lead to a reduction in the average work intensity of the household by 0.186 in the rural sector, whereas it is reduced by 0.095 in the urban sector and 0.172 in the general model (Table 14.6). This confirms the theory that the remittance effects are often stronger in the rural sector.

Social dynamics of the rural sector often tend to be more pronounced in which case, the variable $socialgroup_i$ to account for the individual being a part of Scheduled caste, Scheduled Tribes or Other Backward Classes are included. The [socialgroup]_i exhibits a dampening effect as well after controlling for remittances, albeit very little. Interestingly, the coefficients in being part of a Scheduled caste/class or Other Backward Class has a negative impact on average work intensity, perhaps due to the systematic exclusion of such social groups from formal marketable employment as well as their lack of affluence in having non-labour income (Annapuranam and Inbanathan, 2017) (Table 14.6).

Table 14.6 Rural Ordinary Least Squares

Variables	Naive Rural	Augmented Rural
lremit$_i$	−0.186***	−0.138***
	(0.00457)	(0.0117)
lconsumption$_i$	0.197***	0.188***
	(0.0129)	(0.0297)
landpossesssion$_i$		
0.005–0.01	0.0336*	0.0376
	(0.0193)	(0.0412)
0.002–0.20	0.0988**	0.117***
	(0.0190)	(0.0415)
0.21–0.40	0.203***	0.218***
	(0.0206)	(0.0459)
0.40–1.00	0.377***	0.372***
	(0.0210)	(0.0479)
1.01–2.01	0.418***	0.456***
	(0.0227)	(0.0531)
2.01–3.00	0.444***	0.445***
	(0.0271)	(0.0665)
3.01–4.00	0.451***	0.534
	(0.0349)	(0.0906)
4.01–6.00	0.424***	0.594***
	(0.0405)	(0.108)
6.01–8.00	0.729***	0.599***
	(0.0515)	(0.143)
Greater than 8.00	0.554***	0.617***
	(0.0422)	(0.125)
Averageperiodout^2_i	−0.000480***	−0.000344***
	(2.94e-05)	(7.15e-05)
Totalmigrants$_i$	0.0198***	0.000997
	(0.00279)	(0.00710)
HH Head Gender [Female]		−0.603***
		(0.0277)
Social Group		
SC		−0.101**
		(0.00443)
OBC		−0.115***
		(0.0401)
Other		−0.162***
		(0.0420)
Constant	2.711***	3.222***
	(0.107)	(0.241)
Observations	89,477	19,793
R-squared	0.282	0.336

The elasticity of work intensity in a female-headed household is stronger than a male-headed household after controlling for remittances in the rural sector: After accounting for remittances, the elasticity of work intensity in a female-headed household falls to–0.603, which implies that remittances dampen the dependency on work intensity for female-headed households more than male-headed households in the rural sector which falls in line with the literature discussed above. Female-headed households would use remittance money for household expenditures and hence be less dependent on market-based activity, withdrawing labour force participation as a result (Bui and Kugler, 2011). An increase of remittances to a household by 1% leads to a reduction in work intensity by 0.138; the stronger effects of gender and social dynamics in the rural sector are more pronounced hence affecting economic determinants like remittances in the process (Table 14.6). *land-possession* exhibits a positive relationship to *workintensity*, with increasing semi- elasticity as land size increases to *workintensity* when, implying that ownership of land in rural areas is intrinsically tied to employment due to the predominance of agricultural jobs in the market-based sector, regardless of non-labour income (Table 14.6).

Selection Bias Correction

Selection Equation

$$\alpha + \beta_1 Religion_i + \beta_2 HHsize_i + \beta_3 Marital_i + \beta_4 Gened_i$$

$$+\beta_5 Sector_{i(rural,urban)} + \beta_6 State_i + \beta_7 lconsumption_i$$

$$+\beta_8 HHHeadgender_i + s_i$$

Structural Equation

$$workintensity_i = \alpha + \beta_1 lremit_i + \beta_2 firstuse_i$$

$$+\beta_3 averageperiodout^2 + \beta_4 totalmigrants_i$$

$$+\beta_5 landpossession_i + \beta_6 lconsumption_i + \beta_7 socialgroup + s_i$$

The Heckman selected above was applied to the rural sector with the addition of *Socialgroup_i* in the Selection Equation because it tends to the literature which implies that demographic characteristics serve as push factors for remittance behaviour. The gender of the head of household, as stated above often determines the uses of remittances, but shouldn't affect the decision to remit, unless a female-headed household faces structurally different credit constraints than a male-headed household (Kugler and Bui, 2011).

Table 14.7 Heckman Correction – Rural

Variables	Structural	Variables	Selection
$lremit_i$	-0.238***	$HHsize_i$	-0.0560***
$firstuse_i$	0.0365***	$lconsumption_i$	-0.180***
$totalmigrants_i$	-0.00399	$Socialgroup_i$	
$landpossesssion_i$		SC	-0.0727***
0.005–0.01	-0.042	OBC	0.000691
0.002–0.20	0.0365	Others	-0.0147
0.21–0.40	0.360***	$Gened_i$	
0.40–1.00	0.634***	Literate-NFEC	0.0578
1.01–2.01	0.746***	Literate-TLC	0.218
2.01–3.00	0.800***	Others	0.168***
3.01–4.00	0.866***	Below Primary	0.0366***
4.01–6.00	0.997***	Primary	-0.00565***
6.01–8.00	0.958***	Upper primary	-0.0871***
Greater than 8.00	–	Secondary	-0.135***
$HHHeadGender_i$	-0.888	Higher Secondary	-0.240
$averageperiodout^2_i$	-0.000562***	Diploma	-0.296***
		Graduate	-0.396***
		Postgraduate and above	-0.553***
Lambda	-0.448		

The remittance effect after correcting for Selection Bias, increases significantly; an increase in remittances by 1% lowers the average *workintensity* of the household by 0.238 days as opposed to 0.138 in the naive model (Table 14.7). An increase this significant gives some indication of the severity of the selectivity problem in unearthing the true effect of remittances on the decision to work. Contrary to the general model, the *totalmigrant-sout_i*'s effect on the *workintensity* is insignificant perhaps due to remittance accounting for the economic impact of missing labour in the household. Being in a female-headed household displays a negative and significant effect on workhours, further reconciling the stronger elasticity of female-headed households to remittances as opposed to male-headed households. The size of the family has a stronger effect in the rural sector on the selection decision to remit (–0.0560), displaying a preference on retaining members at home rural sector as opposed to the urban sector.

Instrument Variable

$$workintensity_i = \alpha + \beta_1 lremit_i + \beta_2 HHsize_i + \beta_3 landpossessed_i$$

$$+ \beta_4 firstuse_i + \beta_5 teched_i + \beta_6 State_i + \beta_7 averageperiodout^2$$

$$+ \beta_8 totalmigrants_i + \beta_9 gened_i + \beta_{10} socialgroup_i + s_i,$$

$whererlremit_i = timesremitted_iandmigrationreason_i$

The correction for Selection Bias shown above can indicate that endogeneity problems pervade the rural analysis as well. In running an IV regression using the same instruments times remitted and migration reasons. This increases the effect of remittances more than the IV of the general model: A 1% increase in remittances decreases the average work intensity of the household by 0.470. The R-squared has increased to 0.516, indicating the highest fit of all the models so far (Table 14.8). The effect of consumption has a massive increase showing nearly half a day more of work. The effect of a female-headed household is now insignificant, where remittances are instrumented by the $timesremitted_i$ and $migrationreason_i$. The latter of these instruments, when excluded, make the gender of the head of a household significant and have a negative effect on the average work intensity of the household (Table 14.8). This runs in conjunction with the theoretical claim that female- and male-headed households have different motivations to migrate or remit, which is being accounted for with the migration reason instrument.

In the rural sector, both these instruments serve to exogenise the $lremit_i$, since they do not reject the null hypothesis of exogeneity in the Durbin-Wu-Hausman test (p=0.1737). The test for over-identifying restriction are also rejected (p = 0.3710), implying that the instruments used are exogenous and appropriately.

Similar to the general model, we see that the OLS has the lowest RMSE from the 3 models. The Heckman-corrected OLS model has an RMSE that is decreasing as k-fold cross validation iterations are increasing, but more importantly it is converging to the OLS model, implying that the Inverse Mills Ratio is not adding issues of over fitting to the OLS model. However, the Heckman-corrected IV equation has a significantly higher RMSE average than the other 2 models, which calls into question the validity of the instruments and/or the inflated standard errors (Table 14.10). Between the OLS and Heckman model, the Heckman model's RMSE falls below the OLS models implying that the Heckman model attests a better t due to its correction of the Selection Bias, absolving this endogeneity issue.

Table 14.8 Heckman Correction

$lremit_i$	Lambda Z	Rho
–0.238***	–0.4484895***	–0.30069

Table 14.9 Heckman-Corrected Rural IV

Variable	Coefficient	Standard Error
lremit$_i$	–0.470***	(0.215)
lconsumption$_i$	0.724**	(0.282)
landpossesssion$_i$		
0.005–0.01	–0.481	(0.362)
0.002–0.20	–0.651**	(0.375)
0.21–0.40	0.0823	(0.394)
0.40–1.00	0.809***	(0.396)
1.01–2.01	0.649*	(0.388)
2.01–3.00	0.115	(0.470)
3.01–4.00	0.475	(0.617)
4.01–6.00	–1.347***	(1.059)
6.01–8.00	0.684*	(1.010)
Greater than 8.00$_i$		
Averageperiodouti2	–0.000558*	(0.000833)
Totalmigrants$_i$	–0.0167	(0.0794)
HHSize$_i$	–0.0357	(0.0615)
Constant	1.598	(2.100)
Observations		2,357
R-squared		0.516

Table 14.10 Average Rural Model Cross Validation

OLS	Heckman-Corrected OLS	Heckman-Corrected IV
1.4004171417	*1.4033493*	*1.899388441*

Multinomial Logistic Regression

The analysis above is consistent with the literature that remittances ease credit constraint of consumption constraints which then leaves income for investments, further transitory expenditure or savings. However, the hypotheses above also suggested than remittances can cause a substitution effect, one where individuals in a household can substitute market-based activities, such as salaried employment with other types of work, such as increased domestic work, or household enterprises with the introduction of remittances (Jadotte and Ramos, 2016). The neoclassical theory of labour and leisure says that a substitution effect can cause withdrawal from the labour force to spend more time on leisure when there is an increase in the wage rate or if on-labour income increases (Imbens et al., 2001). This substitution effect can also be induced by changing the activity status of a household as seen in Table 14.11.

Table 14.11 Multinomial Logistic Regression

Activity Status	Multinomial Logistic Coefficient	Marginal Propensity of Iremit$_i$	Rural-Multinomial Logistic Coefficient	Rural-Marginal Propensity of Iremit$_i$
HH Enterprise-Own account worker	0.1779	0.0017564	0.0339924	0.003831**
HH Enterprise – Employer	0.3176	0.0004331**	0.1715902	0.001116***
HH Enterprise – Unpaid worker	0.0925	0.0056933***	-0.0764016	-0.0112959***
Salaried Employee	Base	-0.004545***	Base	-0.0029666***
Public Worker – Casual wagelabour	-0.0036	-0.0001497**	0.0678728	-0.0003236**
Public Worker – NREGA Worker	0.2723	0.0000495	0.2621288	-0.0000717
Public Worker – Others	-0.04	0.0069711***	0.0423127	-0.0080719***
Did not work – Sickness	-0.232	0.004486***	-0.2449475	-000006495***
Did not work – Other reasons	0.047	-0.000807***	0.1408586	-0.0008667**
Salaried but didn't work – Sickness	-0.334	-0.0000594**	-0.5279769	-0.000458
Salaried but didn't work – Other	-0.214	-0.0001743***	-0.2429696	-0.0000793
Salaried but didn't work – Seeking employment	0.052	0.0033****	0.0988869	-0.0026939*
Salaried but didn't work – Available but not seeking employment	0.1437	0.0001962	0.2112419	-9.76e-06
Education	-0.0016894	-0.0016894	0.2072667	-0.0017421
Domestic duties	0.011223	0.011223***	0.2484834	0.007305***
Domestic duties and external household duties	0.0085133	0.0085133***	0.2790697	0.0073909***
Rentiers and Pensioners	0.0065803	0.0065803***	0.4281011	0.0028926***
Disability	-0.0006619	-0.0006619**	0.0778905	-0.0012726***

The rural context displays some interesting trends of its own. While remittances have a similar effect on household enterprises in terms of own account worker and employer, remittance tends to incite a negative effect on being an unpaid worker in a household enterprise. Furthermore, while in the general model casual wage labour had a negative remittance coefficient, in the rural sector specification it displays a positive coefficient implying that remittance induces a withdrawal from the formal sector as compared to salaried employment. It displays stronger positive coefficient in salaried workers who seeked/don't seek employment, implying an enhanced cushioning effect of remittances. Both activities regarding domestic duties are significantly larger than those in the general model. This arms the literature that posits that remittances induce a strong elasticity in the rural sector due to increased dependence on non-labour income as the wage rate in the rural sector is low (Table 14.11). There is also a much stronger propensity to be in education in the rural sector as opposed to the general model, which displays a negative coefficient of remittances for education. As seen here there is a significant, albeit not significant substitution effect of remittances.

Conclusion

Regardless of the treatment that remittances have been subject to throughout the chapter, the direction and significance of its effect on work intensity is unchanging (albeit the intensities vary based on the concern of endogeneity). This chapter finds that the Heckman-corrected OLS suggest the least biased estimate of the effect of remittances on work intensity on a household level. This chapter is consistent with literature from not only India, but around the world with regard to the dependency of a rural household on a migrant member supporting their spending habits, which leads on to the knock on effect of 'Declining' Labour force participation or 'Dropping-out' of the Labour Force entirely. However, conducting a multinomial analysis also entails that there are small, albeit significant substitution effects of remittances as well. This is consistent with neoclassical literature positing that non-labour income will induce an income effect. Considering Leisure (or non-market activity) as a normal good will also induce a substitution effect shown here by an increasing propensity to partake in domestic duties, or to start household enterprises which implies withdrawing from the 'salaried' industry. However, there are several considerations that need to be taken into account when interpreting results.

As mentioned in the section, Selection Bias Correction, the changing signs of the Heckman Correction in different Heckit iteration implies that there is an ambiguity in understanding the true g nature of selection bias, and this ambiguity may be exploited leading to confirmation bias, which is why this study conducted a cross validation and RMSE analysis. A better method of tackling Selection Bias would be to undertake a Propensity Score Matching Multiple Imputation method. This has the added benefit of using nearest neighbour matching to impute synthetic remittance values to assess the true severity of selection bias. However, limitations of computation power mean that this chapter could not adopt this technique to assess the complete effect of remittances on labour force decisions. Furthermore, as mentioned above, the double selection bias of the study means that migration controls would at most control for some confounding effects of migration from remittances. However using a double-hurdle or 3 SLS model was not possible due to data limitations but is an interesting avenue to explore for further research.

Conclusively, this study has found that, while there are a multitude of reasons that affect work decisions of household, remittances pose a significant weight in the decision-making process. This chapter proves the micro-foundations of the literature surrounding remittances inducing a Dutch Disease effect by positing that remittances have a persistently negative and significant impact on the decision to work in Indian households. This has significant impacts for the growth of the country, where premature de-industrialisation and precarious labour markets are posing tremendous challenges in sustainable self-sufficient economic development and will hopefully serve as a reminder to be wary of the vagaries of financial flows nature of financial flows such as these.

Notes

1 Only marketable activities were included in creating the dependent variable. The intensity of the activity is marked by whether household members worked less or more than 4 hours, in which he will be considered to have worked at 'full intensity'. It is also possible to have worked multiple jobs or partake in non-market activities and this is classified as 'full intensity'.
2 In running the Heckman 2-step procedure, Qin (2019) notes that the variables that are used to construct the Selection Equation cannot be used to estimate the Structural Equation. Failure to satisfy exclusion-restrictions yield inconsistent estimates and inflated standard errors in the second stage equation.
3 While other Heckman corrections exhibited lower RMSE against the OLS model, this Heckman correction has best Probit model in determining selection into a remitting group (highest Lambda value). Moreover, this Heckman model's lower RMSE also takes into consideration a better Structural equation than the others and hence serves as an appropriate correction for the Selection Bias problem between remitters and non-remitters.

References

Acosta, P., Fajnzylber, P., and Humberto, L. J. 2007. *The impact of remittances on poverty and human capital: Evidence from Latin American household surveys* (English). Policy Research Working Paper no. WPS 4247. Washington, DC: World Bank. http://documents.worldbank.org/curated/en/446091468046772511 /of-remittances-on-poverty-and-human-capital-evidence-from-Latin-American -household-surveys

Acosta, P., Lartey, E., and Mandelman, F. 2009. Remittances and the Dutch Disease. SSRN Electronic Journal.

Adaku, A. 2013. The effect of rural-urban migration on agricultural production in the northern region of Ghana. *Journal of Agricultural Science and Applications*, 2(4), pp. 193–201.

Adams, Jr., R. 1998. Remittances, investment, and rural asset accumulation in Pakistan. *Economic Development and Cultural Change*, 47(1), pp. 155–173.

Adams, R., and Cuecuecha, A. 2010. Remittances, household expenditure and investment in Guatemala. *World Development*, 38(11), pp. 1626–1641.

Alpa, S., and Harriss-White, B. 2011. Resurrecting scholarship on Agrarian transformations. *Economic and Political Weekly*, 46, pp. 13–18.

Amuedo-Dorantes, C., and Pozo, S. 2006. Remittances as insurance: Evidence from Mexican immigrants. *Journal of Population Economics*, 19(2), pp. 227–254.

Annapuranam, K., and Inbanathan, A. 2017. What really causes for exclusion? An analysis with special reference to scheduled castes. *Contemporary Voice of Dalit*, 9(2), pp. 123–135.

Asiedu, E., and Chimbar, N. 2019. *Does remittance to Africa really reduce labor force participation and increase reservation wage? A Quasi-experimental evidence from Ghana*. Accra, Ghana: University of Ghana & University of Passau.

Azizi, S. 2018. The impacts of workers' remittances on human capital and labor supply in developing countries. *Economic Modelling*, 75, pp. 377–396.

Banerjee, B. 1984. The probability, size and uses of remittances from urban to rural areas in India. *Journal of Development Economics*, 16(3), pp. 293–311.

Bettin, G., Lucchetti, R., and Zazzaro, A. 2009. Income, consumption and remittances: Evidence from immigrants to Australia, Mo.Fi.R. Working Papers 34, Money and FinanceResearch group (Mo.Fi.R.) - Univ. Politecnica Marche - Dept. Economic and Social Sciences.

Binci, M., and Giannelli, G. 2018. Internal versus international migration. *International Migration Review*, 52(1), pp. 43–65.

Bucheli, J., Bohara, A., and Fontenla, M. 2018. Mixed effects of remittances on child education. *IZA Journal of Development and Migration*, 8(1). https://izajodm.springeropen.com/track/pdf/10.1186/s40176-017-0118-y.pdf.

Chami, R., Ernst, E., Fullenkamp, C., and Oeking, A. 2018. Are remittances good for labor markets in LICs, MICs and Fragile States? IMF Working Papers, 18 (102), p. 1.

Cox-Edwards, A., and Rodríguez-Oreggia, E. 2009. Remittances and labor force participation in Mexico: An analysis using propensity score matching. *World Development*, 37(5), pp. 1004–1014.

De la Brière, B., Sadoulet, E., de Janvry, A., and Lambert, S. 2002. The roles of destination, gender, and household composition in explaining remittances: An analysis for the Dominican Sierra. *Journal of Development Economics*, 68(2), pp. 309–328.

Eromenko, I. 2016. Do remittances cause Dutch disease in resource poor countries of Central Asia?, MPRA Paper 74965, University Library of Munich, Germany.

Freund, C., and Spatafora, N. 2008. Remittances, transaction costs, and informality. *Journal of Development Economics*, 86(2), pp. 356–366.

Funkhouser, E. 1992. Mass emigration, remittances, and economic adjustment: The case of El Salvador in the 1980s, NBER chapters, in: Immigration and the work force: Economic consequences for the United States and source areas, pp. 135–176. National Bureau of Economic Research, Inc.

Guha, P. 2013. Macroeconomic effects of international remittances: The case of developing economies. *Economic Modelling*, 33, pp. 292–305.

Hanson, G. H. 2007. Emigration, remittances and labor force participation in Mexico, IDB Publications (Working Papers) 2637, Inter-American Development Bank.

Imbens, G. W., Rubin, D. B., and Sacerdote, B. I. 2001. Estimating the effect of unearned income on labor earnings, savings, and consumption: Evidence from a survey of lottery players. *American Economic Review*, 91(4), pp. 778–794.

Jadotte, E., and Ramos, X. 2016. The effect of remittances on labour supply in the Republic of Haiti. *The Journal of Development Studies*, 52(12), pp. 1810–1825.

KNOMAD. 2019. Migration and development brief 31. Migration and development brief [online]. Washington, DC: World Bank Group. Available at: https://www .knomad.org/sites/default/files/2019-04/Migrationanddevelopmentbrief31.pdf [Accessed 2 Sep. 2019].

Koutsoyiannis, A. 1975. *Modern microeconomics* (2nd ed.). London, UK: The Macmillan Press Ltd, pp. 35–36.

Kugler, A., and Bui, S. 2011. Are remittances in the hands of women more elective? Evidence from Vietnam, 4th AFD-WB International Migration and Development Conference, 10–11 June.

Lianos, T. P. 1997. Factors determining migrant remittances: The case of Greece. *International Migration Review*, 31, pp. 72–87.

Lueth, E., and Ruiz-Arranz, M. 2006. A gravity model of workers' remittances. IMF Working Papers, 06 (290), p. 1.

Lueth, E., and Ruiz-Arranz, M. 2008. Determinants of bilateral remittance flows. *The B.E. Journal of Macroeconomics, De Gruyter*, 8(1), pp. 1–23.

McKenzie, D., and Sasin, M. J. 2007. Migration, remittances, poverty, and human capital: Conceptual and empirical challenges. Policy Research Working Paper no. 4272. Washington, DC: World Bank. #c World Bank. https://openknowledge .worldbank.org/handle/10986/7453 License:CC BY 3.0 IGO

Oberoi, A. S., and Singh, H. K. 1980. Migration, remittances and rural development: Finding of a case study in Indian Punjab. *International Labour Review*, 199(2), pp. 229–241.

Parida, J. 2015. Remittances, household expenditure and investment in rural India: Evidence from NSS data. *Indian Economic Review*, 50, pp. 79–104.

Puhani, P. 2000. The Heckman correction for sample selection and its critique. *Journal of Economic Surveys*, 14(1), pp. 53–68.

Qin, D., van Huellen, S., Elshafie, R., Liu, Y., and Moraitis, T. 2019. A principled approach to assessing missing-wage induced selection bias, SOAS Department of Economics.

Rempel, H., and Richard, A. L. 1978. The role of urban-to-rural remittances in rural development. *The Journal of Development Studies*, 14(3), pp. 324–341.

Reserve Bank of India. 2018. Annual Report 2017–2017. Reserve Bank of India. Mumbai.

15 COVID-19 and International Migrants

Results from Post-Flood Migrant Survey in Kerala

S. Irudaya Rajan and Roshan R. Menon

Introduction

Floods are considered to be among the most frequently occurring and deadly forms of natural disasters (WHO, 2009). Floods are caused by a combination of factors which could be natural or man-made, and the unpredictability of the event makes it all the more destructive in nature especially in the case of flash floods. Such flood-related disasters though cannot be stopped, steps can be taken towards mitigating the impact of the flood through proper monitoring mechanisms.

In 2015, a study by the World Resources Institute (WRI), positioned India as the most flood-prone county in the world compared to 164 countries considered in the study. Floods in India mostly occur as a consequence of multiple extreme precipitation episodes, which occur during the monsoon period (Mishra, 2021). The country though witnesses regular episodes of floods, over the past decade, there has been an increase in the occurrence of catastrophic floods with states like Uttarakhand (2013), Kashmir (2014), Tamil Nadu (2015), Kerala (2018 and 2019), Maharashtra (2019) and Karnataka (2019) having been affected in the recent years (Chopra, 2014; Malik and Hashmi, 2021; Patnaik et al., 2019; Lal et al., 2020; Patil et al., 2020; IFRC, 2020; Rajan et al., 2022).

Kerala is a narrow strip of land lying between the Western Ghats in the east and the Arabian Sea in the west. The state has been undergoing a rapid socio-economic transformation over the years, which changed Kerala from being an agrarian state to a highly urbanised and consumerist state. The state of Kerala is vulnerable to natural disasters and is categorized as a multi-hazard zone state (KSDMA, 2018, 2019). Floods are the most common natural hazards in the state with close to 14.5 per cent of the state's land area being prone to floods. The steep gradient slopes of the Western Ghats also make it prone to landslides, with the districts of Wayanad, Kozhikode, Idukki and Kottayam being extremely susceptible to landslides (KSDMA, 2018).

The state of Kerala witnessed two devastating floods in 2018 and 2019. The 2018 flood, caused due to incessant rains in the month of August, was one of the largest floods to have affected the state after the floods of 1924.

DOI: 10.4324/9781003315124-15

The torrential rains which lashed its territories forced the state to release excess water from dams across the state, while landslides also aggravated the impact of the floods. The state was ravaged by floods in the year 2019 as well, with a majority of the northern districts being affected this time. While the state was better equipped to fight the floods in 2019, the 2019 floods not only caused huge economic impacts but also claimed many lives.

Impact of Floods – An Overview

Several studies undertaken on the impact of floods indicated that the economic impact of the natural disaster shows a marked upward trend over the past several decades (Najibi and Devineni, 2017;Tripathi, 2015). Developing countries are more prone to be hit by natural disasters which increase their vulnerability and thus hampers their social and economic growth. Theron (2007), in his study, has found that social impacts of floods include changes in people's way of life, culture, community, political systems, environment, health and wellbeing, their personal and property rights and their fears and aspirations.

The frequency of natural disasters is seen to have been increasing over the years, resulting in loss of life, damage to property and destruction of the environment (United Nations, 2002). Flooding has also had a major role in the displacement of people worldwide and the number of those displaced by natural disasters has been on the rise, as the adverse effect of climate change continues to mount (Holmes, 2008). Floods reduce the assets of households, communities and societies through the destruction of agricultural crops, home dwellings, public infrastructure, machinery and buildings, apart from the tragic loss of life. In some cases, the effect of extreme flooding is dramatic, not only at the individual household level but also in the country as a whole (Integrated Flood Management Concept Paper, 2009).

Impact of the 2018 Floods

The 2018 floods, one of the deadliest floods of the century in Kerala, was a result of the torrential rains that lashed the state in the month of August 2018. The state witnessed an excess of 42 per cent rainfall than the normal average during the monsoon period, but it was the period between August 1 and 20 that the state witnessed the heaviest of the spells. All the districts in the state barring Kasaragod received excess rainfall during the month of August, with the districts of Pathanamthitta, Idukki, Kollam, Thiruvananthapuram, Malappuram and Palakkad receiving more than twice the rainfall that they normally receive. The incessant rains also led to several landslides across the state with over 341 landslides having been reported from 10 districts, and the district of Idukki alone having witnessed 143 landslides (Table 15.1).[1]

Table 15.1 District-wise Rainfall During the Period from 1 August to 30 August 2018

Districts	2018		
	Normal Rainfall (mm)	Actual Rainfall(mm)	Excess Rainfall (Per cent)
Kasaragod	636.3	636.9	0
Kannur	540.9	665.3	23.0
Kozhikode	500.9	836.0	67.0
Wayanad	592.9	1053.5	78.0
Malappuram	395.3	913.7	131.0
Palakkad	333.8	848.8	154.0
Thrissur	440.1	734.7	67.0
Ernakulam	401.3	648.3	62.0
Alappuzha	343.1	608.2	77.0
Kottayam	386.0	619.2	60.0
Idukki	527.3	1478.9	180.0
Pathanamthitta	352.7	764.9	117.0
Kollam	258.7	644.1	149.0
Thiruvananthapuram	142.0	373.8	163.0

Source: Indian Meteorological Department (IMD)

The devastating flood and landslides had in all affected 5.4 million people in the state, with over 1.4 million being displaced and having caused a death toll of 433. Relief camps were set up across the state to accommodate the affected, and people also took shelter at their friends' and relatives' houses. The report also suggests that access to piped water was disrupted for 20 per cent of the state's population and over 1.75 lakh buildings were fully or partially damaged across the state as a result of the floods. The floods also affected the educational sector across the state with over 1,600 schools being turned into relief camps, and the closure of schools for long periods as a result of being affected or damaged by the floods. The low turnout was also witnessed in schools with students owing to trauma and stress caused due to the loss of family/friends or large-scale damages to their homes or the neighbourhood.

The impact of the floods of 2018 is said to have affected 2.6 per cent of the state's GDP. The damage to the agricultural sector was immense, with thousands of hectares of agricultural land being washed away. Along with farming, numerous types of allied livelihoods were affected due to the floods and there has been an estimated loss of Rs.26,850 crores to the primary sector alone in the state.

The total damage caused by the floods as estimated by the Post Disaster Need Assessment (PDNA) was Rs.10,557 crores and total losses were around Rs.16,163 crores amounting to a total disaster effect of around Rs.26,720 crores (USD3.8 billion). The figure does not include damages caused to private properties and buildings that include shops, showrooms, business units, private hospitals/educational institutions and private vehicles and also does not take into account the losses incurred by private traders and business units.

Impact of the 2019 Floods

The state of Kerala witnessed a deluge for the second year in a row, in 2019, during the month of August, as witnessed in the year 2018. Unlike the 2018 floods, the 2019 floods largely affected the northern districts of the states, many of which weren't much affected by the 2018 floods. Similar to the 2018 floods, the state witnessed heavy rainfall during the month of August and received 123 per cent excess rainfall than the normal during the period. Most affected districts were Kozhikode (176 per cent), Wayanad (110 per cent), Malappuram (176 per cent), Palakkad (217 per cent), Thrissur (127 per cent) and Ernakulam (140 per cent), all of which received more than 100 per cent excess rainfall during the period (Table 15.2).

The peak of the rainfall which eventually led to devastating floods and landslides happened from 6 August to 14 August 2019. During this period, Kerala received 602.2 mm of rainfall which is 394 per cent excess of the normal rainfall (122.0 mm) expected. All districts received more than 300 per cent excess rainfall during the peak period. In all, 1,038 villages from

Table 15.2 District-wise Rainfall During the Period from 1 August to 30 August 2019

Districts	2019		
	Normal Rainfall (mm)	*Actual Rainfall (mm)*	*Excess Rainfall (Per cent)*
Kasaragod	658.9	1194.5	81.0
Kannur	554.0	1107.2	100.0
Kozhikode	510.8	1,407.8	176.0
Wayanad	568.3	1,190.8	110.0
Malappuram	392.7	1,084.2	176.0
Palakkad	324.8	1,030.6	217.0
Thrissur	467.9	1,062.0	127.0
Ernakulam	398.5	957.7	140.0
Alappuzha	339.1	676.1	99.0
Kottayam	375.7	763.0	103.0
Idukki	590.5	979.4	66.0
Pathanamthitta	333.6	717.7	115.0
Kollam	258.2	549.3	113.0
Thiruvananthapuram	144.0	325.0	126.0

Source: Indian Meteorological Department (IMD)

13 districts were affected by floods and landslides during the 2019 monsoon period. The resulting death toll was 125 and 42 were injured as a result of the floods and landslides. An estimated 1,967 houses have been reported fully damaged and 19,297 houses severely damaged (>75%) (KSDMA, 2019).

Scope of the Study

The floods of 2018 and 2019 are seen to have had a major impact on the state of Kerala. The floods have resulted in widespread destruction of public as well as private infrastructure and are also seen to have affected the lives and livelihoods of the people.

The current study is in continuation to two earlier studies conducted by the Centre for Development of Studies in 2018, one of which was conducted across 20 first sampling units (FSUs) and the second, in 40 FSUs across the state. The studies conducted in 2018, immediately looked at the aftermath of the 2018 floods in Kerala and studied how the floods affected the livelihood of the people in the state by employing the Sustainable Livelihoods Approach Framework of DFID to understand the effect of the 2018 Kerala floods on the livelihoods, including both physical and financial; the effect on human capabilities, by looking at the health indicators in the post-flood period; and the effect the floods had on plans of migration, among both individuals and households, and whether migration acted as a strategy for rehabilitation or as a coping strategy for the households in Kerala (Rajan et al., 2020).

Following the results of the two earlier studies, which clearly showed the severe impact of the floods in terms of affecting the livelihood of the people in the state, it becomes pertinent that we look at how the individuals and households in other parts of the state are affected by the floods of 2018 and 2019. Thus, the current study looks at localities that weren't a part of the earlier attempts to understand the impacts the 2018 and the 2019 floods have had on individuals and households across the state of Kerala.

Methodology

This survey follows the methodology of the KMS 2018 Survey. A subset of the total sample from KMS 2018 is selected (Rajan and Zachariah, 2019).

The total sample taken for the KMS 2018 Survey was 15,000 households using a stratified multistage random sampling method. The 14 districts of Kerala are divided into 28 strata with one rural and urban stratum in each district. The households are distributed between the district's rural stratum and urban stratum proportional to the district's rural-urban households in the 2011 Census. The villages and the wards given by the census are taken for each rural and urban stratum respectively selected by a proportional sampling method. Systematic random sampling methods were used to select samples from each ward from the available list of households at the time of the survey.

The proposed study is following the same sample of households because the majority of the households were affected by the devastating disaster in Kerala.

Sampling

The Survey was conducted amidst the COVID-19 pandemic, from August 2020 to December 2020. Before the start of the survey, the district coordinators collected and verified the household details of the selected wards from the selected localities. District coordinators also made surprise field visits to evaluate the integrity of the survey. The sampling was thus done across 9 districts in a total of 67 FSUs, each containing 30 households. Samples were, thus, taken from 2010 households. Post-survey scrutiny of questionnaires as well as data cleaning and entry was done by the research staff at the Centre for Development Studies (CDS) with which the first author was earlier associated.

The current report focuses on 1,785 households that were surveyed in the year 2020, to understand the impact of the 2019 and 2018 floods on the households across the state (Table 15.3).

Findings and Analysis

The findings from the study are grouped under three heads, focusing on the impact on the land and assets, the impact on agriculture and lastly the impact on the economic activities of the people of the households. Given below is a summary of such findings based on the data collected from 1,785 households across 9 districts in Kerala.

Impact on Land and Assets

The section focuses on how the floods of 2018 and 2019 had an impact on the land and assets of the households across Kerala. We also look at how the basic necessities were impacted by the floods and also into the compensation received from the government towards the damage to such assets.

Table 15.3 Breakdown of Sampling Units

Districts	Number of FSUs	Sample HH	Traced HH	Untraced HH
Alappuzha	3	90	83	7
Kannur	10	300	261	39
Kollam	10	300	269	31
Kozhikode	7	210	196	14
Malappuram	8	240	207	33
Palakkad	5	150	124	26
Pathanamthitta	7	210	189	21
Thrissur	10	300	268	32
Wayanad	7	210	188	22
Total	67	2010	1,785	225

Table 15.4 Households Affected by the Floods

Effect on House	2018		2019	
	Frequency	Per cent	Frequency	Per cent
Affected by the flood	210	11.8	159	8.9
Not Affected by the flood	1,575	88.2	1,626	91.1
Total	1,785	100.0	1,785	100.0

Table 15.5 Houses Damaged by the Floods

Effect on House	2018		2019	
	Frequency	Per cent	Frequency	Per cent
Damaged by the flood	82	39.0	46	28.9
Not damaged by the flood	118	56.2	109	68.6
Non-Response	10	4.8	4	2.5
Total	210	100.0	159	100.0

Table 15.4 shows the number of households that were affected by the flood. We see that while the 2018 floods had an impact on 11.8 per cent of the total households in the sample, the impact of the 2019 floods in the surveyed area was comparatively lower with only 8.9 per cent of the households being affected by the floods.

Among the households that had reported being affected by the floods in 2018, 39 per cent had suffered damages to their houses during the floods. In the case of the 2019 floods, we see that the number is relatively lower with 28.9 per cent of the households having reported to have suffered damages to their houses (Table 15.5).

While insurance does act as a cushion to reduce the impact of the floods on the assets being damaged due to the floods, we see that in 2018 as well as in 2019, very few houses among the households affected by floods have been insured (Table 15.6). While this number is 1.4 per cent during the 2018 floods, the same for the 2019 floods is 1.9 per cent.

Among the households that were affected by the floods, only about 22.4 per cent of the households have reported to have received any form of compensation from the government for the losses suffered (Table 15.7). The 2019 figures are seen to be even lower, with only 10.7 per cent of the households having reported to have received compensation towards the damages caused by the floods.

From the households that possess non-agricultural land, it was observed that the floods haven't had a major impact on the non-agricultural lands during both the floods. While only 4.2 per cent of the households have

Table 15.6 Insurance Status of Houses

Insurance Status	2018		2019	
	Frequency	Per cent	Frequency	Per cent
House insured	3	1.4	3	1.9
House not insured	193	91.9	145	93.6
Non-response	14	6.7	7	4.5
Total	210	100.0	159	100.0

Table 15.7 Compensation Received from the Government Towards the Damage Caused

Compensation Status	2018		2019	
	Frequency	Per cent	Frequency	Per cent
Compensation received from government	47	22.4	17	10.7
Compensation not yet received	108	51.4	95	59.7
Non-response	55	26.2	47	29.6
Total	210	100.0	159	100.0

Table 15.8 Damage Caused to Non-agricultural Land Due to Floods

Effect on Agricultural Land	2018		2019	
	Frequency	Per cent	Frequency	Percent
Land damaged due to floods	63	4.2	46	3.1
Land not damaged/not applicable	1,266	85.0	1,173	78.8
Non-response	160	10.8	270	18.1
Total	1,489	100.0	1,489	100.0

reported to have suffered damage to their non-agricultural land during the 2018 floods, the 2019 figures show that a relatively lower share of only 3.1 per cent of the households have reported to have suffered damages to their non-agricultural lands (Table 15.8).

Among the households that have reported to have suffered damage to their non-agricultural land as a result of the 2018 and 2019 floods, 30 per cent of the households have reported to have received compensation from the government towards the same in 2018, while in 2019, only 15 per cent of the households have reported to have received this compensation (Table 15.9).

A major impact of the floods was on the availability of electricity and freshwater, with power lines and freshwater pipelines and wells being

Table 15.9 Compensation Received From the Government Towards the Damage Caused to Non-agricultural Lands

Compensation Status	2018		2019	
	Frequency	Per cent	Frequency	Per cent
Compensation received from government	19	30.2	7	15.2
Compensation not yet received	28	44.4	31	67.4
Non-response	16	25.4	8	17.4
Total	63	100.0	46	100.0

Table 15.10 Number of Days without Electricity after Floods

Days Without Electricity	2018		2019	
	Frequency	Per cent	Frequency	Per cent
0	852	47.7	941	52.7
1–5	574	32.2	518	29.0
6–10	286	16.0	239	13.4
11–15	49	2.7	65	3.7
16–20	14	0.8	15	0.8
21 or more days	10	0.6	7	0.4

damaged as a result of the floods. On looking at the impact of the 2018 floods, we see that, while 47.7 per cent of the households haven't had to face disruption of the power supply as a result of the floods that year, 32.2 per cent of the households did not have power for 1–5 days (Table 15.10). Restoration of power can be longer challenged depending on the extent of damage caused to the power lines, and as a result, what we see that 16 per cent of the households did not have power for 6–10 days and at the very extreme, just around 0.6 per cent of the total households have reported of not having power in their household for over three weeks.

As far as the 2019 floods are concerned, we see that 52.7 per cent of the households did not face any disruption in the power supply as a result of the floods, while 29 per cent of the households reported to have not had power for 1–5 days. 13.4 per cent of the households reported to have not had power for 5–10 days. At the very extreme, just about 0.4 per cent of the households had a disruption in their power supply for over three weeks.

On looking at the disruption of the availability of freshwater to the households, we see that in the case of both the 2018 floods and the 2019 floods, there hasn't been much impact during both the floods. Over 90 per cent of the households had not faced such issues during both the floods and around 6 per cent of the households had faced short-term disruptions in terms of availability of water (Table 15.11).

Table 15.11 Number of Days without Water after Floods

Days without Water	2018		2019	
	Frequency	Percent	Frequency	Percent
0	1,611	90.2	1,631	91.4
1–5	117	6.6	105	5.9
6–10	33	1.9	27	1.5
11–15	13	0.7	10	0.5
16–20	3	0.2	7	0.4
21 or more days	8	0.4	5	0.3

Impact on Agriculture

The impact of the floods on agricultural land and agricultural crops would impact the very livelihood of the people depending on it. Thus, it is pertinent to understand the impact the floods have had on the agricultural holdings (see Tables 15.12 and 15.13).

Among the households having agricultural lands, 11.2 per cent reported to have had damage to their agricultural land as a result of the 2018 floods. The number for the same as a result of the 2019 floods, stands at 10 per cent.

In terms of the compensation received from the government for the damage to their agricultural lands, only 10.7 per cent of the households have reported to have received such compensation after the 2018 floods and 18 per cent after the 2019 floods.

Floods as mentioned earlier, have a direct impact on the agricultural produce being grown. While 18.9 per cent of the households have reported to have suffered crop damage as a result of the 2018 flood, 18.5 per cent of the households have reported to have suffered damage to their agricultural crops following the 2019 floods (Table 15.14).

Impact on the Economic Activities of the People

A major impact of the floods is seen in the form of disruption of work, which could be in the form of reduced work in the days during and succeeding the floods or leaving them with no work during the period. The following section looks at the impact the floods have had on the economic activities of the people in 2018 and 2019 (Tables 15.15 and 15.16).

Among the working-age population in the sample, we see that over 28 per cent of the individuals have experienced some disruption to their work as a result of the 2018 floods and over 26 per cent of the individuals as a result of the 2019 floods.

Table 15.16 shows the nature of disruption caused to the work as a result of the 2018 and 2019 floods. Among the different economic activities

Table 15.12 Damage Caused to Agricultural Land Due to Floods

Damage to Agricultural Land	2018		2019	
	Frequency	*Percent*	*Frequency*	*Percent*
Land damaged due to floods	56	11.2	50	10.0
Land not damaged/not applicable	356	71.5	448	56.6
Non-response	86	17.3	166	33.4
Total	498	100.0	498	100.0

Table 15.13 Compensation Received from the Government Towards the Damage Caused to Agricultural Land

Compensation Status	2018		2019	
	Frequency	*Percent*	*Frequency*	*Percent*
Compensation received from government	6	10.7	9	18.0
Compensation not yet received	35	62.5	31	62.0
Non-response	15	26.8	10	20.0
Total	56	100.0	50	100.0

Table 15.14 Effect on Agricultural Crops Due to Floods

Effect on Agricultural Crops	2018		2019	
	Frequency	*Per cent*	*Frequency*	*Per cent*
Agricultural crops damaged	94	18.9	92	18.5
Agricultural crops not damaged	355	71.3	301	60.4
Didn't grow crops	38	7.6	30	6.0
Non-response	11	2.2	75	15.1
Total	498	100.0	498	100.0

Table 15.15 Impact of the Floods on Usual Economic Activities

Economic Activity Status	2018		2019	
	Frequency	*Per cent*	*Frequency*	*Per cent*
Economic activity affected due to floods	603	28.1	562	26.2
Economic activity not affected	1,537	71.8	1,578	73.7
Non-response	2	0.1	2	0.1
Total	2142	100.0	2,142	100.0

Table 15.16 Economic Activities Affected Due to the Floods and Reasons for Disruption

Economic Activity	2018			2019		
	No. of Working Days Reduced	Wage Reduced	Lost Job	No. of working days reduced	Wage reduced	Lost job
Employed in state/central government	11	1	0	13	0	0
Employed in semi government aided school/ college, co-operative / local admin bodies	18	1	0	13	1	0
Employed in private sector	64	1	0	65	2	2
Self-employment	149	2	5	139	3	3
Unpaid family work	6	0	0	5	0	0
Agricultural labour	59	4	3	47	5	4
Labourers in non-agricultural sector	197	4	5	186	2	3
NREGA	26	0	0	29	0	0
Total	530	13	13	497	13	12

Table 15.17 Impact of Floods on Businesses

Status	2018		2019	
	Frequency	Per cent	Frequency	Per cent
Business Affected	49	38.9	52	42.6
Business Not Affected	75	59.5	62	50.8
Non-Response	2	1.6	8	6.6
Total	126	100.0	122	100.0

considered, we see that in the 2018 floods, the major impact has been on the self-employed and on the labourers in the non-agricultural sector and the disruption caused was mainly in terms of reduced workdays for the affected. In the 2019 floods as well, the major impact was experienced in the form of reduced workdays for the people, again mostly felt by non-agricultural labourers and the self-employed.

Among the households with members involved in various businesses, 38.9 per cent have been reported having been affected by the 2018 floods. The figures for the same after the 2019 floods stood at 42.6 per cent (Tables 15.17 and 15.18).

On examining the extent of loss to businesses as a result of the two floods, we see that close to 45 per cent of the households have reported to

Table 15.18 Extent of Loss to Businesses Due to Floods

Loss	2018		2019	
	Frequency	Percent	Frequency	Percent
No loss	0	0.0	2	3.9
Minimal loss	14	28.6	18	34.6
Average loss	22	44.9	28	53.8
Total loss	2	4.1	4	7.7
Non-response	11	22.4	0	0.0
Total	49	100.0	52	100.0

have suffered an average loss to their business while 28.6 per cent of the households have reported to have suffered a minimal loss. After the 2019 floods, over 53 per cent of the households have reported to have suffered an average loss in their respective businesses as a result of the floods, while 34.6 per cent of the business have been reported to have suffered minimal losses during the period.

Conclusion

The Kerala floods of 2018 and 2019 have had a devastating impact at both micro- and the macro levels. The current study looked at a total of 1,785 households, spread across 9 districts of Kerala, focusing on a variety of aspects involving the impact on the livelihoods of its people. The study thus provides us an insight into how the lives of the people in Kerala were affected as a result of the two floods that lashed the state in 2018 and in 2019.

In the current study, we have focused on aspects ranging from the impact of the floods on the assets of the households to its impact on agriculture as well as other economic activities undertaken by members of the households considered in the study. The floods are seen to have a major impact on the households in varied forms, with the impact being in the form of damages to the house in general and to their landholdings. Along with that, we also come across the fact there is a lower tendency among the households to get their homes insured against such natural disasters. Coming to the aspect of the compensation received from the government towards such damages to physical assets, we also see that the general receipt of compensations is on the lower side. The absence of insurance mechanisms and lower receipt of compensation from the government cause a devastating financial impact on the households during natural calamities, whereby, they are left to bear by themselves the complete expenses in terms of restoration of the houses or rehabilitation in some cases.

Coming to the aspect of the impact on agriculture across the two floods, there has been evident damage to agricultural produce caused by both the floods. While damage to the agricultural land is seen to be on the lower side compared to the non-agricultural land, the receipt of compensation for the damage caused to agricultural land is also seen to be relatively on the lower side.

When it comes to the impact on the work of the individuals, what has been observed is that the most affected sections of the population are the non-agricultural labourers and the self-employed. The impact among them is seen to be mainly in the form of reduced working days, with people reporting lower wages and loss of jobs being negligible across the two floods. Businesses across Kerala are seen to have been significantly affected by the floods with a good proportion of the respondents having reported to have suffered average losses owing to both the floods.

The results of the current study are in line with the findings from the earlier studies conducted across 60 FSUs across the state. In the earlier study, it was seen that the floods of 2018 had caused a considerable effect on the assets of the households across the state, especially the physical assets and access to livelihoods, which in turn impacted the financial assets of the households. The floods were seen to have severely impacted the economic activities of the individuals in terms of disruption of work and reduced working, especially among the people employed as labourers in the non-agricultural sector, those employed in the private sector and the self-employed. Along with this, as seen in the earlier study, the current study also observes that a considerable number of households have suffered immense losses to land and property, particularly the agricultural land, thus severely impacting the households directly dependent on agriculture as a form of livelihood. Apart from these, people engaged in various businesses were also severely impacted by the floods with many of them reporting an average to total loss in their business (Rajan et al., 2020).

Thus, it is clearly visible that the 2018 and 2019 floods have had a significant impact on the households across Kerala. With the threat of climate change looming and the state being subjected to regular floods over the past few years, there is a need to adopt measures both at the government and at the individual levels to be resilient towards any future floods or other forms of natural disasters that may affect the state. There needs to be an increased awareness among the general population on how to be prepared for and equipped against such adversities and also strong policies directed towards minimizing the impact of any future natural disasters along with effective compensatory measures should be adopted in the event of any such natural disaster in the future.

Note

1 For the entire UNDP report on the Post Disaster Needs Assessment report, please see: https://www.undp.org/content/dam/undp/library/Climate%20and %20Disaster%20Resilience/PDNA/PDNA_Kerala_India.pdf

References

Chopra, R. (2014). *Uttarakhand: Development and Ecological Sustainability*. New Delhi: OXFAM India.

Department of Environment Affairs and Tourism. 2007. Impacts, Vulnerability and Adaptation in Key South African Sections: An Input into the Long-term Mitigation Scenario Process. Energy Research Centre. University of Cape Town. Cape Town.

Holmes, J. (2008). At Home but Homeless. *Zambia Sunday Post*, 26 October.

IFRC. (2020). *India: Monsoon Rains and Floods*. Geneva: The International Federation of Red Cross and Red Crescent Societies.

KSDMA. (2018). *Kerala Floods – 2018 1st August to 30th August 2018*. Thiruvananthapuram: Kerala State Disaster Management Authority, Govt. of Kerala.

KSDMA. (2019). *Floods & Landslides 2019*. Thiruvananthapuram: Kerala State Disaster Management Authority, Govt. of Kerala.

Lal, P., Prakash, A., and Kumar, A. (2020).Google Earth Engine for Concurrent Flood Monitoring in the Lower Basin of Indo-Gangetic-Brahmaputra plains. *Nat Hazards*, 104, 1947–1952.

Malik, I. H., and Hashmi, S. N. I. (2021). The Great Flood and its Aftermath in Kashmir Valley: Impact, Consequences and Vulnerability Assessment. *Journal of the Geological Society of India*, 97, 661–669.

Mishra, A. (2021). Observing a Severe Flooding Over Southern Part of India in Monsoon Season of 2019. *Journal of Earth System Science*, 130. https://doi.org /10.1007/s12040-020-01509-7.

Najibi, N., and Devineni, N. (2017). Recent Trends in Frequency and Duration of Global Floods. *Earth System Dynamics Discussions*, 1–40. https://doi.org/10 .5194/esd-2017-59.

Nott, J. (2006). *Extreme Events: A Physical Reconstruction and Risk Assessment*. New York: Cambridge University Press.

Patil, J., Shinde, M., and Kanthe, R. (2020). Flood Disasters 2019 in Maharashtra (India), Aftermath and Revival for Natives and Tourists. *Ecology, Environment and Conservation*, 26, 693–698.

Patnaik, I., Sane, R., and Shah, A. (2019). Chennai 2015: A Novel Approach to Measuring the Impact of a Natural Disaster. Working Paper: (19/285). Delhi: National Institute of Public Finance and Policy.

Rajan, S. I., Suresh, A., and Rohit, I. (2022). Footloose Workers in Times of Calamities: A Case Study of the 2018 Kerala Floods. *Insight Turkey*, 24(1), 11–22.

Rajan, S. I., Taylor, S., Shajan, A., and Hardisty, L. (2020). Climate Change, Migration and Development: The Aftermath of the 2018 Floods in Kerala. Chapter 21. In S. Irudaya Rajan (Ed.), *India Migration Report 2020: Kerala Model of Migration Surveys* (pp. 385–406). Oxon: Routledge.

Rajan, S. I., and Zachariah, K. C.. (2019). Emigration and Remittances: New Evidences from the Kerala Migration Survey, 2018. Centre for Development Studies Working Paper No. 483. Thiruvananthapuram, Kerala.

Tripathi, P. (2015). Flood Disaster in India: An Analysis of Trend and Preparedness. *Interdisciplinary Journal of Contemporary Research*, 2(4), 91–98.

United Nations. (2002). *Living with Risk a Global Review of Disaster Reduction Initiatives Preliminary Version (INIS-XU–010)*. New York: United Nations.

WHO. (2009). *Protecting Health from Climate Change, Connecting Science, Policy and People*. Geneva: World Health Organization.

World Resource Institute. (2015). Aqueduct Global Flood Risk Country Rankings. World Resource Instiute, Washington.

16 Internal Migrant Enumeration and Service Provision

A Municipal Governance Approach

Ananta Kukreja and Asmeeta Das Sharma

Introduction

Internal Migration in India

The macroeconomic drive towards fiscal austerity, combined with the concentrated focus on urban development, has led to an economic decline in the rural areas of India. Uneven urban development has further led to regional disparity pushing people out of the declining agricultural sector to the margins of the city in search of livelihoods (Action Aid, 2019). India particularly faces strong migration flows both inter-state and inter-district, with the latter being the more prominent trend (Census, 2017). While there have been repeated attempts by the Centre to highlight and define internal migration through the Inter-State Migrant Workmen Act (1979) and the Building and Other Construction Workers Act (1996), on-ground implementation and actual transfer of envisioned benefits has been very poor. Neoliberal policies, pro-market reforms and increased competitiveness have compounded the struggle of the migrant workers, leaving them devoid of basic social security. While India moved up from rank 139 to 52 in the Ease of Doing Business in 2018, its ITUC's Employment Protection Index ranking fell by 7 percentage points (International Trade Union Confederation (ITUC), 2020).

Over 455.8 million Indians were found to be migrants for various reasons during the enumeration exercises of Census 2011 (NCERT, 2020). Out of the total migrant population 146.1 million (32%) were males and 309.6 million (68%) were females. Internal migration figures for India show that migration is dominated by female migration, mainly due to the prevalent social custom of exogamous marriages. For males, economic reasons have been cited as the most important reason for migration. Further, the rate of inter-state migration in India doubled between 2001 and 2011, growing 4.5% annually with an average of five to six million migrants a year (World Economic Forum, Price Waterhouse Coopers, 2017). Internal migration flows in India are driven by regional economic inequalities. Uttar Pradesh and Bihar are responsible for the greatest number of migrants, with 20.9 million people residing outside the states. This is 37% of the total number of inter-state migrants as per the Census enumeration. Maharashtra has the

DOI: 10.4324/9781003315124-16

highest share of in-migrant population with around 57.4 million (Census, 2017). Between 2011 and 2016, 9 million people migrated annually between states in India, contributing roughly 10% to the GDP (Deshingkar, 2020). Despite their contribution to development, migrants remain outside the purview of governance in the city. Lack of political will and policy gaps in the existing ecosystem deprive the migrants of even the basic services, including housing, food, healthcare, sanitation amongst others making them heavily dependent on their contractors ('Thekedaars' or 'Dalals').

However, the COVID-19 pandemic has brought a change in the long history of exclusionary urban policies and the image of the migrant in the city. The early lockdown caused one of the largest exodus from the city despite the multitude of relief efforts by various agencies. The migrant workers emerged as one of the most vulnerable groups, who stopped receiving their daily wages due to the lockdown. Further, the precariousness of their employment, lack of security of housing tenure, the fear of the virus and the belief that the city is not their home led to the deliberate decision of returning to their homes. City administration, who were at the forefront of the situation, were taken aback by the large number of workers trying to exit the city, highlighting the lack of data, acknowledgement and policy gaps in the existing governance system.

This chapter investigates the condition of the migrant worker in the city and the practical gaps in municipal governance to address their issues through the case of Surat. It presents these gaps from the migrant's and government's perspective, advocating the need for data enumeration for adequate service delivery. It proposes a strategic approach to implementing this at the municipal level as a way to circumvent the challenge of centralisation of power and have a direct impact on the migrant population.

This chapter is an outcome of a year of research and on-ground investigation under the Ministry of Housing and Urban Affairs, India Smart Cities Fellowship Program, 2020. The project team consisted of four members – the aforementioned authors, Ms Yogada Sandeep Joshi and Mr Thomas Krishna Pegu and was mentored by Dr Irudaya Rajan (Professor, Center for Development Studies, Thiruvananthapuram) and Dr Debolina Kundu (Professor, National Institute of Urban Affairs, New Delhi). The programme required the authors to deductively investigate the prevalent issues in the internal migration sector and design a tool in response. The methods used in this phenomenological research were a combination of desk research and empirical investigations. The proposed tool was then piloted in the city of Surat together with the Surat Smart City Development Limited and the Surat Municipal Corporation.

Prevalent Issues

Migrants are perceived as a burden and threat to the host cities and communities, overlooking the developmental benefits of their movement. One of the greatest challenges faced is to reverse this hostility towards migrants and build a narrative based on the positive reality of migration. Ten out of the seventeen Sustainable Development Goals have targets addressing migrants. SDG 10 for reducing inequalities, particularly advocates that migrant mobility must be properly managed for it to benefit all (IOM GMDAC, 2020).

As a consequence of this negative image and the lack of inclusive governance, migrants face multiple challenges in the city. Poor access to housing and basic amenities, no entitlements, exploitative working conditions and labour market discrimination being a few. These issues mostly arise due to lack of identity in the destination cities; absence of ration/voter card; violating their basic right to the city. The right to freedom of movement is constitutionally protected [clauses (d) and (e) of Article 19(1)], but it does not guarantee access to entitlements, voting rights in local, state and national elections or even access to government schemes. While the responses from the state and market have failed in promoting the welfare of migrant workers, Civil Society Organisations (CSOs) have been able to come up with solutions that have helped migrants access their basic rights. The efforts by CSOs and NGOs, however, remain scattered and the organisations work in silos, with a focus on their respective geographies and industries.

Ongoing Efforts by the Centre, States and Urban Local Bodies for Social Security of Migrants

The Centre and the states governments had initiated a few efforts towards the protection of migrants even before the COVID-19 crisis hit. One of the first interventions for the migrants was the Inter-State Migrant Workmen (Regulation of Employment and Conditions of Service) Act, 1979 enacted by the Central Government aimed to regularize movement of migrants and protect them against exploitation by providing them with social security benefits (ActionAid, 2019). However, despite the mandates and amendments, it has seen very poor implementation and failed in fulfilling its purpose. The Central Government also announced three social security schemes in the 2015–16 budget focusing on financial inclusion of all including Pradhan Mantri Suraksha Bima Yojana: Accident risk insurance, Pradhan Mantri Jeevan Jyoti Bima Yojana: Life insurance, and Atal Pension Yojana which provides pension to workers in the unorganized sector. The outreach and implementation of these schemes along with the evaluation of their successes is still underway (ActionAid, 2019).

Some host states in India are more responsive and proactive towards the protection of their migrants. The states of Odisha and Andhra Pradesh signed an MoU in 2012 (Odisha Labour Directorate, 2012) to implement a project under International Labour Organisation (ILO) aiming to improve the living and working conditions of migrant workers from Odisha at brick kilns in Andhra Pradesh. Its objective was to facilitate the strengthening of the inter-state coordination mechanism with a focus on improving education, housing and Public Distribution System benefits. Also, Kerala introduced the 'Interstate Migrant Welfare Scheme' back in 2010, 'Awas', an insurance scheme and the 'Apna Ghar' accommodation network (Peter, Sanghvi and Narendran 2020). The state provided healthcare including consultation and medication is free for migrants and locals in Kerala. In the same vein, the Gujarat government aimed to provide education to children of migrant workers especially in the city of Surat which sees over seven lakh migrants from Odisha working in the textile sector. While the States of Gujarat and Kerala were pioneers in according significance to the plight of migrant workers, there was still a need to deliver a concrete policy change encompassing all migrants in these states. The labourers in Gujarat continue to live in housing that lacks basic necessities and persistent insecurity due to threat of eviction and harassment by the police. ('Unlocking The Urban', 2021).

There has been a paradigm shift in how the Centre, states, Urban Local Bodies and CSOs approach the issues of migrants in the country to fight the COVID-19 pandemic. As vulnerabilities exacerbated due to the pandemic, the migrant workers were most susceptible to economic, social and financial losses. Dealing with a pandemic of such intensity required support at all levels of governance and the assistance of all stakeholders. While the Central Government arranged Shramik trains to transport back migrants to their home states, the state governments undertook multiple efforts to ensure that the migrants had access to ration, shelter and healthcare. Some of the notable steps taken up by various institutions in support of migrants include:

- National Migrant Information System (NMIS): National Disaster Management Authority (NDMA) developed an online dashboard to capture a central repository of migrant workers. The NMIS aims to help in speedy inter-state coordination to facilitate smooth return migration and contact tracing.
- Atal BeemaVyakti Kalyan Yojana: This scheme provides unemployment insurance to workers who have subscribed to the Employees' State Insurance (ESI) scheme, and will cover such workers during the pandemic. The Ministry of Labour and Employment (MoLE) is looking to extend the scheme and allow workers to avail this insurance if they are impacted by the virus.
- Pradhan Mantri Gareeb Kalyan Yojana: Announced ₹1.70 lakh crore package 'Pradhan Mantri Gareeb Kalyan Yojana', targetting 80 crore people affected by lockdown. Under this scheme, free ration is being distributed for next three months under this scheme.
- PM CARES Fund Trust: Out of ₹3,100 crore allocated for the fight against COVID-19, a sum of approximately ₹1,000 crores will be used for the care of migrant labourers. (NDTV.com, 2020).

- Seva Sindhu App (Karnataka government): The Seva Sindhu Portal allows people to register themselves before travelling or returning to the state. Focused on aiding migrant labourers, the app also allows one-time financial assistance meant for daily wage workers and labourers.

One of the most distinguishable aspects of governance at the advent of the COVID-19 crisis was the role that municipal bodies and civil societies played in curbing the spread of the virus. While the Centre and the State directed policies and strategies, it was the municipal bodies which ensured their implementation. For instance, the proactive steps undertaken by the Brihanmumbai Municipal Corporation in Dharavi, the largest slum area in India, reduced the growth rate of COVID-19 cases from 4.3% in May 2020 to 1.02% in June 2020 (Sohini Sarkar, Hindustan Times, 2020). The interventions included barrication of exit and entry, disinfection of public toilets, door-to-door screening and partnerships with local NGOs. Similarly, the municipal workers in Delhi sanitized containment zones of Delhi while the staff of municipal corporations in Chennai assumed the role of survey-ors for identifying people with COVID-19 symptoms. Non-governmental Organizations also sprung into action immediately after the lockdown was announced.

Municipal governance was given constitutional power by the 74th Amendment Act, 1992. Eighteen functions were devolved to the local bodies including urban planning and town planning, water supply and fire services, public health, slum redevelopment and (under the 12th Schedule) along with preparation of economic plans and ensuring social justice (Statement of object and purpose of the 74th Amendment Act of Constitution India, Article 3, Section (g)). Bearing this in mind, the role played by the municipal bodies during the COVID-19 crisis and the exponential increase in urbanisation in the country, it is increasingly important to strengthen urban local bodies. It becomes imperative that the ULBs guarantee fundamental rights for all its citizens to create instruments for the independence of its migrants.

The following section analyses the relationship between the urban local body and the migrant in the city of Surat.

The Case of Surat

The state of Gujarat receives 4.20 per cent of the total inter-state migrants in India, standing third to Delhi and Maharashtra. Surat, Vadodara, Rajkot and Ahmedabad are the main destinations in Gujarat with Surat district absorbing the highest share of 38.93% (Sughande, 2017), and 58% of Surat city's population being migrants (UNESCO, 2013, p 6). A major manufac-turing hub, the district is home to textile, diamond, construction, chemi-cal, petrochemical and small production industries. The workers undertake long-term and short-term migration from Odisha, Uttar Pradesh, Rajasthan,

Bihar, Jharkhand and West Bengal among others. The semi-skilled and skilled workforce in the diamond sector majorly comes from the larger Saurashtra region.

Globally the fourth fastest growing city in the world, Surat produces 40% of the nation's man-made fabric and 28% of the fibre. Further, 9/10 of the world's diamonds are cut and polished here (Surat Smart City Development Limited, 2017). The exponential growth in population is because of the unpredictable surges of in-migration. Migrants come to the city seeking employment with a majority aiming to stay for a long time. Coming from long distances, this migration is undertaken through known kin or next of kin with the assurance of a job in the city. One of the major migrant groups hail from the distressed district of Ganjam in Odisha. With a 35-hour train journey, a majority of the Odia migrants come to work in the textile sector, majorly in the power looms industry. The general issues of the migrant population in the city can be highlighted through the plight of this group of migrants. (Refer to Surat city resilience strategy, The Rockefeller Foundation (Asia), April 2011, p. 14 for a detailed overview of the Surat economy.)

In pre-COVID times, there were approximately 650,000 power looms, 150–200 wholesale textile markets, 20,000 manufacturers – including 10,000 weavers, 75,000 traders, 450 processing units – and 50,000–60,000 embroidery machines in the Rs 500-billion synthetic textile hub of Surat. According to the Federation of Gujarat Weaver's Association, the industry has an annual turnover of 50,000 crore rupees (Umarji, 2019). It is safe to draw the parallel that this can be attributed to a contribution of the inter-state migrants as Gujaratis constitute only one-fifth of the total workforce. This is due to the economic benefits of cheap labour, lack of unionisation and lesser demands or expectations that the inter-state migrants bring with them. The Odia migrants particularly come across as one of the most exploited groups, as per previous research. Migration is typically undertaken by individual male migrants who visit their family back home once or twice a year or in the event of an emergency. In the city, they often reside in dormitories or slums within their own cultural communities. An 8 × 8 m room typically houses ten people who rotate as per their day or night shifts. All of them share one bathroom or the community toilet facilities. This quality of life is a product of their detachment from the city and priority to maximize their savings and remit them home.

The workers are typically paid on a bi-monthly basis, calculated on the number of metres of cloth or yarn they produce. This is recorded informally in handwritten registers or marked on the cloth itself. The industrial units also register the names of the workers; however, these are often the short informal names used in their social circles. This system has however improved after the extensive penetration of the Aadhar card and some employers have started capturing the Aadhaar details of their workers. The remuneration received is remitted home mostly through third-party local shops who charge proportionate amounts (like Rs. 20 for a transfer of Rs.

1,000) as commission. A study reported that a migrant in Surat typically remits 35.3% of their income, which amounts to about 52.9 per cent to 61.7 per cent of the migrants' household's income in the source state (Das, Sahu, 2020).

Further, the migrant dense settlements facilitate a parallel economy which revolves around the daily routine of a migrant. Local messes provide Odia food to the workers twice a day on a subscription basis. They record the names and Aadhaar numbers of the subscribers and typically charge between 1,500 and 2,000 rupees a month – to be paid on a bi-monthly basis. Lunch is provided in tiffins while dinners are served in the dining area of the mess. Additionally, markets pop up and shop timings are determined by the incoming and outgoing times of the migrant workers. Near the residential areas and labour nakas, (areas where labourers congregate for daily wage employment) groceries, food and other essentials are sold formally and informally between 6 and 8 am in the morning and 7 pm onwards in the evening catering to the workers returning home from work at these times. The area is bustling with workers on cycles or on foot and a variety of middlemen looking to contract them for the day.

Preliminary surveys also revealed that most workers preferred going to private clinics or local chemists for healthcare rather than availing the public healthcare facilities. This is due to the lack of trust in the system and the unwillingness to lose out on daily wages by spending half a day or a full day at the civil hospital due to a long waiting time. Hence, schemes like the ESIC are redundant as they can only be available predominantly at public healthcare facilities. Considering that the workers' life revolves around his or her workplace and long working hours, it is almost impossible to interact with them for primary surveys other than the time when they are in transit between work and home. This, combined with the fear of losing their source state identity and benefits is the reason why workers hesitate to change their addresses on their Aadhaar cards. This highlights that any efforts that are made for the betterment of the migrant need to be made keeping his or her daily routine and user mindset at the core of the strategy.

While this picture may not be representative of all the migrants in the city, some who have been following the same lifestyle for more than 15–20 years, it highlights the key issues faced across the spectrum. A workshop with the city government officials and non-governmental organisations working in the migrant space in Surat also revealed that identity, housing and legal aid were the top three priority areas of work. The primary issue being of identity. Migrant workers lack a sense of ownership and identity in the city. A visual proof of this is the mass exodus during the lockdown imposed in India to contain the spread of COVID-19. The lack of job security, uncertain housing tenure, fear of losing family and the worker's belief that the city governments are not responsible for them, led to people undertaking arduous journeys purely based on hearsay. The crisis is a pivotal moment in India's migration narrative as it was a visual display of the worker's distrust in the system, the system's paralysis due to the lack of migrant data and the realisation that the city's industry is run by migrants. The temporary shortage of workforce during the initial unlock phases saw desperate measures by employers to bring back workers by offering them flight tickets, raised wages and other compensations.

Migrants and Local Governance

Accessing the local administration has always been a challenge and moreover, daunting for the migrant workers. While it must be acknowledged that there is a behavioural aspect that needs attention, this chapter focuses on how local governance can address this gap.

Most Indian states pose the problem of a compulsory domicile to access city or state benefits. For example, the Maa Card, a state healthcare card in Gujarat or a direct water connection or university education. Residing in informal rental accommodations, the workers usually don't have a proof of address and hence don't possess a domicile in the city, at times, despite fulfilling the minimum domicile requirements. This also excludes them from most citizen schemes floated by the city and state administration. Further, the lack of awareness and fluency in Gujarati excludes them from accessing citizen services like visiting the local police station or any other grievance redressal system. Despite Surat being a relatively multilingual city, the language and cultural barriers have led to the creation of ethnic pockets in the city with Odia, UP and Bihar, Maharashtrian and Bengali settlements spread across the city's landscape. These migrants move to the city through their next of kin, who are their only support systems in the city. The fear of losing their cultural identity, for the comfort of language and limited interaction with the host population leads to ghettoism in the city.

A study by the Centre for Development Alternatives, Ahmedabad, on migrant workers in Ahmedabad and Surat highlighted that a small proportion of workers have access to social security. The provident fund facility was availed by 1.85 per cent of workers in construction and 10.78 per cent in textile (Hirway, Singh, Sharma, 2014). However, interactions with community organisations revealed that most workers don't have the knowledge or awareness to retrieve these funds. Health and life insurance were also highlighted as a major concern. Frequent accidents on-site or in factories often leave workers and families without adequate compensation, rendering them helpless and vulnerable to debts. Employers do not provide social security benefits to all employees and often under-report their workforce strength.

Efforts by the Local Government

In order to overcome these gaps, the Surat Municipal Corporation has been taking some steps to ensure benefits are delivered to the migrants. SMC has been focusing on providing state and central schemes to the masses through 'Lok Kalyan Melas' in the city every six months, even before the pandemic.

These *melas* brought together various departments of the government at a given place where the public applied for eligible schemes and gained welfare benefits. These *melas* were attended by citizens of the city as well as the migrants with necessary documents for the applications.

With the plight of the workers compounding during the COVID-19 crisis, the SMC took numerous steps to warrant the safety and security of its migrants. As discussed earlier, the actual burden of execution of policy and guidelines lies in the hands of the urban local body.

Following the nationwide lockdown in March 2020, the SMC not only curbed the spread of COVID-19 but also initiated one of the biggest food distribution tasks in the state of Gujarat, feeding more than 5.5 lakh people twice a day (VijaySinh Parmar *Times of India*, 2020). The city officials took up a multitude of well-coordinated efforts including conversion of schools and shelter homes into food distribution centres, synchronising their activities with the prevalent NGOs and 'community samaj' belonging to various states. The SMC also funded the Akshaya Patra Foundation to feed over one lakh migrants in the city.

Once the lockdown was lifted, the stranded workers commenced their travel back to their home states. Despite the efforts adopted by the SMC to keep migrants in the city and well-fed, there was resistance because of the insecurity experienced by the migrants. The SMC accompanied by other authorities organized the movement of over 18 lakh migrants through road and rail transport. Municipal Corporation also undertook the task of collecting migrant information including name, Aadhaar card number and contact number. A group of city officials were deployed for the smooth movement of the migrant workers.

Dearth of employment opportunities in the home state, diminishing levels of savings and the exhaustion of sitting idle propelled the movement of the migrants back to the city. The industry as well as the urban local bodies realized the importance of migrants in the city and made arrangements for their return. The Federation of Gujarat Weavers Association and the SMC officials devised a plan to bring back migrants through special Shramik trains especially from the Ganjam district of Odisha. The SMC laid down the following processes to enable smooth returns: (a) Gathering information on migrant name, phone numbers, place of stay in Surat, the industry address and COVID-19-related information from the entry points in the city including bus addas and railway stations. (b) Setting up of a tracking body at SuratiiLab- a start-up innovation centre by the Surat Smart City Development Limited. This body analysed and managed the collected data, calling up the migrants to check their symptoms and finally creating zonewise reports on the number of migrants present in each zone. (c) Mandating industry employers to follow quarantine and testing guidelines laid out by the state health department.

Affordable Rental Housing Complexes Scheme (ARHC) as a subset of Pradhan Mantri Awas Yojana was announced to provide housing on rent to migrants/urban poor. In November 2020, the SMC became the first city to finalize an ARHC with 393 bedrooms (The Hindu, 2020).

Why Are the Migrants Still Suffering?

In 2019, Oxford Economics projected an average growth rate of 9.2% p.a. in the 2019–2035 period for Surat city (Richard Holt Oxford Economics, 2019). The driving force behind such a growth rate is the internal migrant who travels far and wide for work to Surat. The local governments always realized the significant role played by the migrants which became further noticeable during the lockdown. With return migration in full swing, the industrial units shut down while the profits plummeted leaving the economy vulnerable. Despite the importance of migrants, their conditions are not actively supported by the city government for three reasons. (a) 'Labour' is a subject under the State as well as Centre belonging to the Concurrent List of Subjects under the Constitution of India. It does not show prevalence in the 12th Schedule of the 74th Amendment Act notwithstanding the effects it has on the city and its people. The jurisdiction of the city for the purpose of migrants is not defined. (b) As per a discussion with the SMC, 'the city cannot work for a particular user group i.e. the migrants. The city could work for the upliftment of all labour and the entire group of urban poor but not particularly the migrant'. (c) Finally, the city government lacks power and funding to single-handedly drive a narrative in support of the migrants.

The presence of Inter-state Migrant Workmen Compensation Act 1979 put prime focus on registration of inter-state labourers to protect them against exploitation by the industry and middlemen. According to a practicing labour lawyer in Surat, the industry deems it more feasible to pay penalties rather than actively registering its employees and providing them benefits under provident fund and ESIC benefits. The non-compliance to the existing legal frameworks for assistance of migrants is also because of the tedious nature of compliance procedures for the employers.

While the migrant workers suffer numerous hardships in the city, including police brutality, long working hours, lack of social security and legal help; they accept their fate in the city. The earnings of the migrants is one of the biggest incentives and a behavioural challenge which prevents the migrant from aiming for a better life. Also, a migrant worker is not a vote bank for either the state or the local governments rendering him/her powerless and completely at the mercy of the employer.

One of the crucial aspects of security in the city is the sense of belongingness that a migrant perceives. These migrants move to the city through their next of kins and kin who are their only support systems in the city. Losing out on a cultural identity after moving to Surat and their exclusion in social gatherings leads to ghettoism in the city.

It is the CSOs who took up the mettle of aiding the migrants through the COVID-19 crisis. In the face of it all, these organizations work on similar causes in the space of migration not limited to healthcare, housing, legal aid and registrations. They are funded by donor organizations aiming at a particular community of migrants without reconciliation amongst each other on the kind of work undertaken by them. This siloed approach of the CSOs does not allow the ecosystem to flourish. The fight for migrant rights and necessities continue to remain individualistic in nature.

Our Approach

This chapter proposes a strategic approach to address the gap between local governance and the migrant population. It presents that the first step to improving the migrant's quality of life is to impart an identity to him or her in the city. This identity can only be provided to the migrant by enumerating data on migrant population, mobilizing resources and using the data to plan an effective delivery system.

Registration and Service Delivery

The strategy presents a registration and service delivery mechanism to be undertaken by the urban local body. Registration can initially be undertaken by third parties to spread awareness and knowledge of the process, with the ultimate aim of encouraging self-registration by the migrants. A digital tool, like a mobile application or website can be used for efficient data capture with user-friendly interfaces that can be easily navigated by the migrant. In order to process this data and ensure delivery of services, a Migrant Cell could be instituted within the urban local body to overlook all the migrant-related activities. The Migrant Cell could link the registered migrant with benefits ensuring social security, financial inclusion, identity and/or food security by checking their eligibility and processing their applications for the relevant schemes. This will require collaboration with various government departments and third-party agencies to ensure effective delivery. An accountability system must be set in place by the urban local body to ensure that transparency is maintained in the system.

Various funding models can be instituted to raise funds for the Cell and its activities, based on the existing migrant welfare funds collected like the BOCW Cess. Further, CSR funding or other market-driven sources of funding can also be devised.

Collaborative Action

Further, the migrant welfare space sees a host of stakeholders working in silos, trying to achieve their individual agendas. While this agenda might not be the same for all the end goal of migrant welfare remains a common point of interest. Since the sector has a dominant presence of NGOs and academic institutions, government collaboration with these actors will ensure effective resource use and collective action. This partnership can further be used to onboard the employer industries as well as other market forces to work towards it. Market-driven solutions can be devised for migrant issues like affordable housing, rental housing, financial support – remittances or loans and access to job markets.

The Migrant Cell can also play the role of a knowledge bank where data collected by all the stakeholders can be shared and collectively analyzed for targeted interventions. It is essential to bring all the stakeholders on board and propagate the benefits of collective action.

Data-Driven Decision-Making

Data is the key to ensure desired impact for this system. From carefully designed data variables to be captured at the time of registration to using the input data, anonymizing and analyzing it, data can be a powerful tool for decision-making and ensuring that benefits are delivered transparently. The COVID-19 crisis highlighted the gross lack of data on the floating population present in the city, catching the city administrations off guard at the time of the exodus. The most recent datasets available on the migrant profile are Census 2011, many details of which are yet to be published, NSSO 2014–15 and Economic Survey of India 2016–17. All these datasets consider different definitions of migrants and capture scattered data variables. The registration drive will ensure dynamic data is collected and processed to define the migrant demographic profile, skill profile, migrant patterns, access to amenities and its usage. The data can also be used to spatially map the population, the population density and the housing conditions to enable urban local bodies to initiate targeted housing interventions. Spatial mapping can also help in identifying wards which have higher densities of migrants and their quality of life to route adequate funding for the ward's development. Further, grievance redressal systems can be put in place and speedy responses can be planned through geotagging and referring the issues to the nearest NGOs or CSOs.

However, it is important to mention that data privacy issues must be addressed throughout the process to protect the migrant's personal details and ensure that it is not used for further discrimination, exploitation or exclusion.

Discussions

The model proposed above is currently being piloted in Surat. However, on-ground experience and a keen understanding of the basics of the processes, proves that it is essential to understand the context or existing situation. The model and approach need to be altered as per the needs of every city, its migrants and the presence of various stakeholders in the sector. This will require a detailed analysis of the migrant population of the city to gain an understanding of why they have migrated, what is the nature of migration and profile of the migrant workers.

Further, the model emphasizes the need for encouraging and empowering municipal bodies to undertake the responsibility of the migrant population. The top-down approach of centralized databases and schemes is ineffective as the local implementation reality is starkly different, given the country's cultural diversity. The data and initiatives need to be managed at the city level to ensure effective service delivery. Considering the scale of the population in question, the municipal boundary is a more effective size to administer and ensure benefit transfer to the workers within its limits.

Outcomes and Conclusions

This chapter highlights the key issues faced by inter-state migrants through the case of Surat. It further presents the core governance gaps, which if addressed, can be instrumental in improving migrant welfare. The approach proposed is an instrument to help the various stakeholders understand the gravity of the situation in a city. The mammoth challenge of data collection, ensuring it remains dynamic, while addressing the issues of privacy and exclusion, can be overcome by ULBs if adequate support is provided by the state and central agencies. Apart from financial assistance, resources and procedural guidance, they will need adequate technical assistance to effectively implement the model. The ULB needs to be financially, administratively and technically empowered and motivated to address the migrant issues, imparting a city-specific identity, good quality housing and adequate legal aid for grievance redressal.

Further Recommendations

a. **Breaking silos:** Bringing together all departments responsible for providing services and schemes to the migrants. There is a need to raise awareness amongst them and facilitate knowledge sharing and streamlining of processes for better service delivery.
b. **Using quadruple helix for social innovation:** Synchronizing the activities of all four actors of the quadruple helix framework – academia, civil societies, government and industry to ameliorate the lives of migrants.
c. **Empowering the migrants:** Improving access to markets and civic services by streamlining grievance redressal systems and spread of legal knowledge. There is also a need to disseminate information and enable outreach in local languages about the welfare schemes and rights of the migrants. Outreach and knowledge dissemination is the most challenging facet. There is a need to factor in the behavioural differences and priorities of the migrant population to enable optimal results.
d. **Building a collaboration network:** Building a knowledge portal for collaboration between the existing network of non-profits in the city and further the country to share resources and best practices.

Bibliography

Action Aid. 2019. "Workers on the Move, Exploring Issues Related to Circular Migration and Labour Market Dynamics in India". 2019. In *Improving Conditions of Work and Living for Circular Migrants in India*, p. 125. New Delhi.

Bihari Sahu, Gagan, and Biswaroop Das. 2020. "Lockdown Effect: Surat's 10 Lakh Migrant Workers 'Lose' Rs 9,000 Per Month Each". *Counterview.Net*. https://www.counterview.net/2020/04/lockdown-effect-surats-10-lakh-migrant.html.

"Census of India: Migration". 2017. *Censusindia.Gov.In.*

Deshingkar, Priya. 2020. "Why India's Migrants Deserve a Better Deal". *Live Mint*, May 2020.

Hirway, Indira, UdaiBhan Singh, and Rajeev Sharma. 2014. *Migration and Development: Study of Rural to Urban Temporary Migration to Gujarat*, pp. 8–10. Ahmedabad: Centre for Development Alternatives.

"How are the Children in India Receiving their Mid-Day Meals Amid the COVID-19 Pandemic? | Nutrition". 2021. *NDTV-Dettol Banega Swasth Swachh India*. https://swachhindia.ndtv.com/how-are-the-children-in-india-receiving-their-mid-day-meals-amid-the-covid-19-pandemic-47940/.

"In Sharp Turnaround, Covid-19 Growth Rate Dips to 1.02% in Mumbai'S Dharavi in June". 2020. *Hindustan Times*. https://www.hindustantimes.com/india-news/in-sharp-turnaround-covid-19-growth-rate-dips-to-1-02-in-mumbai-s-dharavi-in-june/story-LJfJSJsZu7XISfAe0gQWaO.html.

International Trade Union Confederation (ITUC). 2020. "2020 IUTC Global Rights Index - The world's worst countries for workers". Brussels, Belgium: ITUC. https://www.ituc-csi.org/IMG/pdf/ituc_globalrightsindex_2020_en.pdf.

Labour Directorate. 2012. "Signing of MoU with Andhra Pradesh". https://labdirodisha.gov.in/?q=node/87.

Migration and Sustainable Development. 2020. "Migration, Sustainable development and the 2030 Agenda". Geneva, Switzerland: International Organisation for Migration.

Peter, Benoy, Shachi Sanghvi, and Vishnu Narendran. 2020. "Inclusion of Interstate Migrant Workers in Kerala and Lessons for India". *The Indian Journal of Labour Economics*. https://link.springer.com/article/10.1007/s41027-020-00292-9

Rockerfeller Foundation. 2011. *Surat Resilience Strategy*. Surat: Rockerfeller Foundation.

"Rs 1000 Crore from PM Cares Fund Used for Migrant Labourers". 2020. *Ndtv .com.* https://www.ndtv.com/india-news/rs-3-100-crores-from-pm-cares-fund-for-fight-against-coronavirus-says-pms-office-2228336.

""SDG's", Migration Data Portal - The Bigger Picture". 2020. https://migrationdataportal.org/sdgs?node=0

Sarkar, S.. 2020. "Covid-19 Count in Mumbai's Dharavi Rises to 2,218, Eight New Cases Emerge". Hindustan Times, New Delhi.

Sugandhe, Anand. 2017. "Gujarat Becoming New Destination for Inter-State Migrants". *Journal of Economic & Social Development*, XIII (40–51).

"Surat Initiates Biggest Food Distribution Task in State". 2020. *Times of India*. https://timesofindia.indiatimes.com/city/surat/surat-initiates-biggest-food-distribution-task-in-state/articleshow/75130757.cms.

"Surat Smart City - About Surat". 2017. *Suratsmartcity.Com*. https://www.suratsmartcity.com/Surat/AboutSurat.

"The Constitution (Seventy-Fourth Amendment) Act, 1992 | National Portal of India". 2021. *India.Gov.In*. https://www.india.gov.in/my-government/constitution-india/amendments/constitution-india-seventy-fourth-amendment-act-1992.

Umarji, Vinay. 2019. "Surat Textile Industry Still Under Subdued Capacity Utilisation". *Business Standard*, 2019. https://www.business-standard.com/article/economy-policy/surat-textile-industry-still-under-subdued-capacity-utilisation-118010100692_1.html.

"Unlocking the Urban". 2021. *Aajeevika Bureau*. https://www.aajeevika.org/assets/pdfs/Unlocking%20the%20Urban.pdf.

United Nations Educational, Scientific and Cultural Organization [UNESCO]. 2013. *Social Inclusion of Internal Migrants in India*. New Delhi: UNESCO.

"Unit 1; Chapter 2, Migration: Types Causes and Consequences". 2020. *India: People and Economy* (NCERT), p. 16.

World Economic Forum, Price Waterhouse Coopers. 2017. *Migration and its Impact on Cities*. World Economic Forum, Geneva.

17 Shutdown Workers and Role of Agents in Tamil Nadu

S. Irudaya Rajan and Bernard D'Sami

Introduction

Human mobility has taken a huge dip like never before in recent history. Social distancing and staying home have been the imposed norm all around the globe in this war against the microscopic parasite. The pandemic which had its origin in the Hubei province of China has witnessed a rapid spread all over the world claiming more than 6 million lives globally as of March 2022. The curtailment of all kinds of cross-border movements has dampened the labour migration and has forced the migrants to return to their home countries (lee *et al*, 2020). The disruptions caused by the pandemic have blurred the boundaries of labour markets. These disruptions along with the economic downturn and high levels of unemployment have aggravated the already worse situation of low-skilled migrants.

According to International Labour Organization, migrant workers constitute 4.7 per cent of the global labour pool, comprising 164 million workers. Nearly half of the migrant population are women.[1] The oil boom in the 1970s led the Gulf region to be one of largest recipients of labour migration flows. India is one of the foremost countries of origin for migrant labourers, whose number is pegged at 17.5 million. It is also one of the topmost recipients of remittances from migrant labourers, which plays a crucial role in the national development (World Bank, 2020; Khanna, 2020). The arbitrary and uncoordinated closure of international borders to curb the spread of COVID-19 infection has caused an anomalous wave of return migrants to India. (Boillat and Zähringer, 2020; International Organization for Migration (IOM), 2020; Migration Data, 2021).

The state of Tamil Nadu has a long and continuing history of considerable overseas migration with distinct dynamics, destinations and implications. Based on a survey conducted by the International Institute of Migration and Development (IIMAD), Kerala and Loyola Institute of Social Science Training and Research (LISSTAR), Chennai, this chapter will examine the state of shutdown workers in Tamil Nadu and the ramifications of COVID-19 among them.

DOI: 10.4324/9781003315124-17

Tamil Nadu and International Migration

Tamil Nadu, like the other southern states of India, could be classified as a middle-income state. It shares a maritime border with Sri Lanka. Tamil Nadu is the tenth largest state in terms of area and is also the sixth most populous state. Tamil Nadu fares better than the all-India average in terms of human development, as measured by the Human Development Index. Its performance is better than the neighbouring states of Andhra Pradesh and Karnataka, but not as well as that of Kerala.

Tamil antecedents can be traced to the Caribbean islands (West Indies) and to the Asian countries such as Sri Lanka, Myanmar, Mauritius, Malaysia and Singapore, and South Africa in the African continent. In the 1830s, the system of indentured labour provided a cheap workforce from India. Tamils constituted a major chunk of the indentured labourers in the colonial plantation economies of the Caribbean, islands in the Indian Ocean, South and Southeast Asia, Africa and some islands in the Pacific. During the first stage, convicted labourers were forcefully sent to far-off countries as indentured labourers in the sugar plantations and the second stage witnessed the assimilation and acclimatization of the indentured labourers in the destination communities. The third stage followed the change in pattern from the colonial periphery to the centre of the decolonization process which left some Tamils 'stateless' and the consequences haunt them even today. In the fourth stage, the character of Indian migration increasingly changed and a new diaspora began to emerge (Judith & Rosemary, 1994: Robinson, 1986). The latter decades of the 20th century saw the return of demand for contract labour in oil-rich states of the Gulf and the 'tiger' economies of Southeast and East Asia. It is estimated that around 9 million Indians live and work in the Gulf alone (Rajan, 2012; 2017; 2018a; 2019; 2018b).[2] These labourers became part and parcel of India because of the dependency of the country on their remittances. These new contingents of labourers withstood the oppressive conditions of their indentured forefathers in the 19th century but unlike them they were generally not allowed to settle in their host societies.

The Tamil Nadu Migration Survey 2015 estimates that there are around 2.2 million emigrants from Tamil Nadu around the world, with Singapore constituting the largest number of emigrants (4.1 lakh). With the critical changes in the world economy and the increased integration of the economies of Southeast Asia into the global capitalist system propelled the migration. The Gulf Cooperation Council (GCC) countries of Saudi Arabia, Oman, Kuwait, Bahrain, Qatar and United Arab Emirates (UAE) on the other hand account for 11 lakh Tamil emigrants, which is half of total emigrants from Tamil Nadu. The United States, the home to one of the largest Indian populations in the world, constitute 3 lakh emigrants and Malaysia with 1.9 lakh.

The Research Process

Drawing upon the survey data, this chapter examines the extent of the COVID-19 pandemic in the return migration phenomenon of shutdown workers from Tamil Nadu. The chapter also suggests certain measures for the reintegration and recruitment process of these shutdown workers.

COVID-19 brought new imperatives for the movement around the world which forced the governments in several countries to impose lockdown within their boundaries (IMF,2020). Restriction of movement became an obligation as the pandemic exerted pressure on the governments around the globe to implement stricter containment measures (Hadzic,2020; Marchant,2021). The repatriation measure adopted by several governments for the panic-ridden population was beneficial for the trapped emigrant workforce. India also adopted the same strategy to bring back the stranded migrants who were caught up with the socio-economic vulnerabilities associated with the lockdowns.[3] In this spirit, a return migrant survey was conducted and return emigrants who came to Tamil Nadu were interviewed. Along with this, we looked specifically into the shutdown workers and their recruitment process, socio-economic political vulnerabilities.

The survey was carried out from December 2020 to May 2021 with a sample size of 386 shutdown workers using Computer Assisted Telephonic Interview (CATI) method. The sample was randomly drawn from expatriates who returned to Tamil Nadu from international destinations from April 2020 to November 2020. The sample is not weighted by the population of the districts, and which in turn lacks representativeness in terms of district and is broadly a non-probability sample. The questionnaire is categorized regarding the emigration history of the shutdown worker, the demographic and family characteristics, return experience, future plans, remittances and household assets. The study relied heavily on the personal details provided by the respondents during the survey. Each interview lasted around 30 minutes to one hour.

Shutdown Workers

By the late 1990s, the migration sector got major attention and scholars started to look into the processes which propel migration (Xiang and Lindquist, 2014). Many earn their livelihood by organizing migratory movements as travel agents, brokers, interpreters and housing agents (Castles and Miller 1998, 97). This chapter takes its place alongside those studies that focus specifically on shutdown workers and recruiters. An emigrant worker who is working for one or less than a year for preventive maintenance or the shutdown of a company can be called a shutdown worker.

There has been a change in the trend and patterns of emigration workers for some time now. While some workers are directly hired by employers who eschew agencies or agents, there is an overwhelming majority who are still dependent on recruiters.

These people work in origin countries, taking up the role to make sure labour is available for the interested clients. Shutdown workers are in high demand across GCC. Shutdown work is also known as preventive maintenance. Based on the company policies and for their ease, a vendor company would take up the responsibility of shutdown work usually. They facilitate the process of striking up a relationship with the manpower and consultancy groups in various countries. Prior to the arrival in the destination country, the employment agencies spread information through advertisements and mediate interviews that are conducted over the phone or internet. These workers who are recruited are taken to the destination countries under tourist or visiting visa category. Generally, shutdown work is undertaken in the winter season (October to April). It is because companies prefer winters as most of the workers are compelled to do overtime in winter compared to summer. Although most of the workers stay in their destination countries illegally, both the employer as well as the government turns a blind eye towards them. The workers' medical insurance and rules and regulations are flouted most of the time, which leave the shutdown emigrant workforce in a precarious position, especially in terms of health and labour standards

The above pictures depict a typical advertisement in an Indian English daily. Our research has brought to light that some of them are also engineers who are taking up the shutdown work. Shutdown workers are mostly employed in oil and gas companies; offshore and onshore, power stations and manufacturing units which are undertaken from one month to a year, depending on the size of the company. Maintenance work such as cleaning, refill, replacement of machine parts, leakage issues are rectified during the shutdown period. Shutdown work involves skilled, semi-skilled and low-skilled and even unskilled work. Also, the existing shutdown through their network paves way for their friends and members from their own community/village to migrate.

The workers who are interested in shutdown work view it as an escape from their liabilities because it is for limited time. The average cost of migration incurred by an emigrant from Tamil Nadu is ₹1,08,112 compared to ₹ 76,243 for a Kerala emigrant. On an average, emigrants from Tamil Nadu pay ₹32, 000 higher than their counterparts in Kerala (Rajan et.al, 2021). The recruitment companies do their interviews directly through their recognized (by the PGE and PoE) agents/consultancy in their own native language like Tamil, Malayalam, Hindi etc. Thus it is easy for the workers to appear for such interviews and take up the job. Prior to workers' arrival, the agent or the company ensure accommodation for the emigrant worker in dormitory, food and overtime allowances. As there is less exploitation compared to normal low-skilled migration, most of the workers prefer to do short-term shutdown work.

This section delves into the issue of shutdown workers and the narratives drawn out from the interviews.

Profile of the Respondents

The survey was conducted among the shutdown workers from Tamil Nadu and respondents were those who came through Vande Bharat mission or chartered flights. Among the total 332 respondents, United Arab Emirates and Saudi Arabia constitute the highest number of return shutdown workers (Table 17.1).

Characteristics of the Return Emigrants

Majority of the return emigrants were between the age of 21 and 30 years with 59.1 per cent and only 1.2 per cent was between 51 and 58 years of age. More than half of the return emigrants were Hindus with 81.1 per cent, whereas Christians constituted 13.8 per cent and Muslims only 5.1 per cent. Most of the return emigrants belonged to the rural area with 68.3 per cent and urban population was only 31.7 per cent (Table 17.2).

Occupation of the Return Emigrants

About 42.8 per cent of the respondents said that they worked as pipe fitters, quality engineers, general fitters, inspection supervisors, helpers, oil refiners and masons while 14.5 per cent worked as the engineers (mechanic, electric and civil) and welders and Mechanics constitutes (23.1 per cent). Any advertisement (enclosed in the article) for shutdown work required a team of workers who range from engineers (qualified as well as experienced) to that of unskilled helpers (Table 17.3).

Total Period of Stay

Duration of stay in the last location, the majority (68.9 per cent) of the respondents stayed for less than six months and 31.1 per cent stayed for 7 months to 12 months duration in the last location for the job. This is clearly indicating the nature and duration of the shutdown work. It is usually three to six months and, in some cases one year (Table 17.4).

Return Flight Expenses

Most of the emigrants' return flight expenses were taken by their employers (85.9 per cent). Few of them managed to take their expenses from their own savings (7.2 per cent) whereas others received half of the expenses from their employers (Table 17.5) and the other half they had to borrow from friends (3 per cent), while some got sponsored by the Tamil Nadu government embassy (1.8 per cent).

Table 17.1 Destination of Returned Shutdown Workers, 2021

Destination	UAE (United Arab Emirates)	Saudi Arabia	Qatar	Kuwait	Bahrain	Oman	Maldives	Singapore	Myanmar	Nigeria	Others	Total
Number	105	96	39	21	11	8	7	3		2	33	332
Percentage	31.6	28.9	11.7	6.3	3.3	2.4	2.1	2.1	0.9	0.9	9.9	

Source: Tabulation from the Tamil Nadu Return Migration Survey 2021 conducted by the authors.

Table 17.2 Characteristics of the Return Shutdown Workers, 2021

Characteristics	Number	Percentage	Characteristics	Number	Percentage	Characteristics	Number	Percentage
Age Group			Religion			Type of Locality		
21–30	196	59.1	Hindu	269	81.0	Rural	227	68.3
31–40	94	28.3	Christian	46	13.9	Urban	105	31.7
41–50	38	11.4	Muslim	17	5.1			
51–58	4	1.2						

Source: Same as Table 17.1.

Table 17.3 Occupation of the Return Shutdown Workers, 2021

Occupation	Number	Percentage
Cable layer related work	4	1.2
Construction worker/labourer	12	3.6
Crane/lift operator, safety officer	10	3.1
Electrician	11	3.3
Engineers	48	14.5
Fabrication worker	11	3.3
Welder	38	11.4
Mechanic	39	11.7
Painter	4	1.2
Welder	38	11.4
Plumber	3	0.9
Site Supervisor	10	3.0
Others*	142	42.8

Source: Same as Table 17.1; *Others include (Pipe fitter, Quality Engineer, General Fitter, Inspection Supervisor, Helper, Oil Refiner and Mason)

Table 17.4 Duration of Stay at the Countries of Destination by Return Shutdown migrants, 2021

Duration of Stay	Number of Return Emigrants	Percentage
1 to 6 months	229	68.9
7 to 12 months	103	31.1

Source: Same as Table 17.1.

Table 17.5 Sponsorship of Return Flights as Reported by Return Shutdown Workers, 2021

Return Expenses Sponsored by	Number	Percentage
Employer	285	85.9
Own savings	24	7.2
Family back home	1	0.3
Borrowed from Friends/Employer	2	0.6
Tamil Nadu Government Support	7	2.1
Received half of the expenses from the Employer and borrowed the other half from friends	10	3.0
From own savings and borrowed money	1	0.3
Others (donation from Indians in Romania, Indian Embassy)	2	0.3

Source: Same as Table 17.1.

Reason for Return of Emigrants

As for the primary reasons for leaving the last location, 45.7 per cent of them said that they lost the job/laid off and 28.6 per cent of them were scared due to COVID and decided to return (Table 17.6). Shutdown workers were badly caught because shutdown work was undertaken in the Gulf countries between October and April (supposed to be winter months). As the COVID-19 pandemic hit the countries from February onwards some of them were on the verge of completing the work but could not complete and take up the salary. Some of them completed the work but could not return. Many of them were caught when they were halfway through. They were already given accommodation but were provided only with food and the employer arranged for their return and so no salary was given. Wage loss was a major problem faced by the workers.

Salary Drawn in the Last Location

Less than half (48.9 per cent) of the respondents reported that their salary range is between ₹ 21,000 to ₹ 50,000, but most of them preferred not to disclose their salary details. On an average ₹ 36,800 is the salary drawn from shutdown emigrants (Table 17.7). Skilled workers such as qualified engineers with experience receive a decent salary between ₹ 70,000 and ₹ 80,000, while most of the diploma holders and workers with experience only receive a salary of ₹ 40,000 to ₹ 50,000. Only 1.9 per cent of the returned emigrants received a salary above ₹ 1,00,000. A general decline in the salary package was observed, due to prevailing competition in the labour market.

Future Plans of the Return Emigrant

Most of the return emigrants plan to re-emigrate to do the same job as before (33.1 per cent) and whereas some seek a new job (32.8 per cent). Only 2.1 per cent of them wish to start a new business in Tamil Nadu after

Table 17.6 Reason for Return Shutdown Migrants

Reason	Number	Percentage
Lost job/laid off	152	45.7
Scared of COVID-19 and returned on their own choice	95	28.6
Expiry of contract	74	22.3
Illness/accident	2	0.6
Missed family	2	0.6
Others	7	2.1

Source: Same as Table 17.1.

Table 17.7 Salaries Received by the Return Shutdown
Migrants in the Destination, 2021

Salary received	Number	Percentage
₹ 11,000 to ₹ 20,000	25	7.5
₹ 21,000 to ₹ 30,000	55	16.5
₹ 31,000 to ₹ 40,000	53	15.9
₹ 41,000 to ₹ 50,000	55	16.5
₹ 51,000 to ₹ 60,000	20	6.1
₹ 61,000 to ₹ 70,000	13	3.9
₹ 71,000 to ₹ 80,000	10	3
₹ 81,000 to ₹ 90,000	2	0.6
₹ 91,000 to ₹ 1,00,000	3	0.9
Above ₹ 1,00,000	6	1.9
Not willing to say	90	27.1

Source: Same as Table 17.1.

Table 17.8 Future Plans of the Return Shutdown Migrants, 2021

Future Plans	Number	Percentage
Re-emigrate to the same job as before	110	33.1
Re-emigrate to get a new job	109	32.8
Seek new job in Tamil Nadu	78	23.5
Others (Planning to start agricultural works, seek job abroad, Not planned anything, going to work in Tamil Nadu)	28	8.5
Start a new business in Tamil Nadu	7	2.1
Start-up in Tamil Nadu		
No	320	96.4
Yes (Agricultural work, Driver, Milk shop, Petty shop etc.)	12	3.6

Source: Same as Table 17.1.

their return while more than half of the return emigrants (96.4 per cent) are not interested in investing in any start-ups. Few others (8.5 per cent) are not sure about their future plans whereas others plan to start agricultural works and start working in Tamil Nadu. Though the pandemic situation has made them return to their native land, the majority of the emigrants wish to go back abroad for work. Over the years they have become comfortable in doing the same job that they had been trained to do and even the wages that they earn abroad were higher (Table 17.8).

Shutdown Workers: New Evidences from Case Studies

The large-scale layoffs and forced leave, with no wages and social security benefits have put their life in disarray. The pandemic pushed the state of shutdown workers to much severity. When the pandemic started, the shut-down workers were asked to stay in their own rooms and they were given a meagre amount of ₹ 2,500 per month for the food. One of the respondents said:

> Lockdown was implemented in the month of March, 2020. They asked us to stay in the room and they provided ₹ 2500 per month for food. This is not sufficient for us. We all have stayed for three months, these three months did not go for a job and at the same time the company has not provided the salary.
>
> (Respondent 1, Dubai)

The respondents were asked to register with any Indian Government portal. Most (66.9 per cent) of the respondents said that they were not able to register and later the company took the initiative to pack them to India. While 24.7 per cent of the respondents reported that they have registered in the MEA (Ministry of External Affairs) and 2.7 per cent of them registered in Non-Resident Tamil (NRT) portal. About 32.7 per cent of the respondents said that there is no communication from the Indian government following the registration in MEA, whereas 78.6 per cent of the respondents said that there is no communication from NRT. Most (62.9 per cent) of the respondents reported that they came to India through chartered flights. Most (85.6 per cent) of the respondents stated that the employer purchased the flight ticket. Even though the employer purchased the flight ticket, one of the shutdown workers said

> We have not worked for three months because of the lockdown. In these three months the company did not pay us a salary. I am currently withdrawing ₹ 40000. If you calculate this for three months it comes around ₹ 1,20,000. If you calculate the flight ticket and other expenses to return to India it will hardly come around ₹ 30,000. This is the profit for the company.
>
> (Respondent 2, Qatar)

Majority (66.9 per cent) of the respondents said that they have not paid any money from their pocket to return to India. There are few cases reported where they spent half of their money from their pocket and the company spent half of their money to return to India.

There is extensive literature on the importance of income transfers and the impact of remittances on growth and development in the origin countries but also the remit motivations (Boccagni and Decimo, 2013). Most of the migrants, during their time abroad, were constantly in touch with their family members back home through telephone and e-mails. Remittances play a crucial role in the socio-economic development of these shutdown workers and as most of them are laid off during the pandemic, financial distress is going to creep in along with a shrink in living standard. Drawing from the narratives, it is understood that the migrant workers who were stranded and quarantined in shabby places suffered from financial and psychological stress due to concerns about their jobs and families. Along with global inequalities migrant workers are exposed to extreme financial, physical and psychological risk in return for modest wages (Wise and Covarrubias, 2009) and COVID-19 exacerbated it. Some of the hometowns of shutdown workers whom we interviewed during the time of survey were deemed epicentres of the COVID-19 outbreak, which made them worried about their families. However, with the loss of these remittances, the shutdown workers and their dependents may need to face various constraints such as unemployment, inability to support the dependents, depression and social insecurities.

Way Forward

As the world tries to subsist, the pandemic ravages across the world. The Tamil Nadu government should create economic opportunities as prospects for labour migration are uncertain. However, with the pandemic the situation of shutdown workers got aggravated which will steer towards a 'vicious circle of decline, rather than a virtuous circle of growth' (Castles and Wise 2007). The present study implores the state to understand the migration and need of legal frameworks that need to be looked into and to prevent and regulate the recruiters and make sure the emigrant shutdown workers are safe from exploitation. Country and state-specific minimum wage together with enforced penalties for illegal recruiters should be implemented. It is also important that the extraordinary helping of these migrants through remittance in bolstering the economy and the need for granular data to design policies is adequate. The migrant crisis in the wake of the pandemic and lockdown demonstrated the shortcomings of existing data sources as they are outdated (Rajan, 2020). Also, programmes aimed to create awareness and intervention on global and regional levels are pertinent. Moreover, multilateral collaboration can be developed to support the UN's Sustainable Development Goals (SDGs) of promoting safe, orderly and regular migration.

Notes

1 https://www.ilo.org/global/publications/books/WCMS_652001/lang--en/index.htm
2 http://mea.gov.in/images/attach/NRIs-and-PIOs_1.pdf
3 https://www.bbc.com/news/world-asia-india-52555432

References

Brown, J. M., and Foot, R. (1994). Introduction: Migration—The Asian Experience. In J. M. Brown and R. Foot (Eds.), *Migration: The Asian Experience* (pp. 1–11). London: Palgrave Macmillan.

Boccagni, P., and Decimo, F. (2013). Mapping Social Remittances. *Migration Letters*, 10(1), 1–10.

Boillat, S., and Mähringer, J. (2020, September 16). COVID-19, Reverse Migration, and the Impact on Land Systems. Global Land Programme. https://glp.earth/news -events/blog/covid-19-reverse-migration-and-impact-land-systems

Castles, S., and Miller, M. (1998). *The Age of Migration: International Population Movements in the Modern World*. Hong Kong: Macmillan.

Castles, S. (2011). Migration, Crisis, and the Global Labour Market. *Globalizations*, 8(3), 311–324.

Chauvet, L., and Mercier, M. (2014). Do Return Migrants Transfer Political Norms to their Origin Country? Evidence from Mali. *Journal of Comparative Economics*, 42(3), 630–651.

Hadzic, D. (2020, March 30). European Union – Guidelines for Free Movement of Workers During Covid-19 Pandemic—KPMG Global. KPMG. https://home .kpmg/xx/en/home/insights/2020/03/flash-alert-2020-132.html

International Organization for Migration (IOM). (2020). Migration-Related Socioeconomic Impacts of Covid-19 on Developing Countries (Labour Mobility and Human Development) [Policy Brief]. International Organization for Migration (IOM). https://www.iom.int/sites/default/files/documents/05112020 _lhd_covid_issue_brief_0.pdf

IMF. (2020). Policy Responses to COVID-19. https://www.imf.org/en/Topics/imf -and-covid19/Policy-Responses-to-COVID-19

Khanna, A. (2020). Impact of Migration of Labour Force due to Global COVID-19 Pandemic with Reference to India. *Journal of Health Management*, 22(2), 181–191.

Lee, J. N., Mahmud, M., Morduch, J., Ravindran, S., and Shonchoy, A. S. (2021). Migration, Externalities, and the Diffusion of COVID-19 in South Asia. *Journal of Public Economics*, 193, 104312.

Marchant, N. (2021). Foreign Aid Hit a Record High Last Year. Here's what it means for the Global Pandemic Recovery. World Economic Forum. https://www .weforum.org/agenda/2021/04/foreign-aid-2020-covid-19-oecd/

Migration Data Portal. (2021, March 10). Migration Data Relevant for the Covid-19 Pandemic. Migration Data Portal. https://migrationdataportal.org/themes/ migration-data-relevant-covid-19-pandemic

Rajan, S. I. (Ed.). (2012). *India Migration Report 2012: Global Financial Crisis, Migration and Remittances*. Oxon: Routledge India.

Rajan, S. I. (2017). South Asia–Gulf Migration Corridor: An Introduction. In S. I. Rajan (Ed.), *South Asia Migration Report 2017: Recruitment, Remittances and Reintegration* (pp. 19–36). Oxon: Routledge India.

Rajan, S. I. (2018). Demography of Gulf Region. In M. Chowdhury, and S. I. Rajan (Eds.), *South Asian Migration in the Gulf* (pp. 35–59). London: Palgrave MacMillan.

Rajan, S. I. (2019). The Crisis of Gulf Migration. In C. Menjivar, M. Ruiz, and I. Ness (Eds.), *The Oxford Handbook of Migration Crises* (pp. 849–68). New York: Oxford University Press.

Rajan, S. I. (2020a). Migrants at a Crossroads: COVID-19 and Challenges to Migration. *Migration and Development*, 9(3), 323–330.

Rajan, S. I. (Ed.). (2020b). *India Migration Report 2020: Kerala Model of Migration Surveys*. Oxon: Routledge.

Rajan, S. I., D'Sami, B., and Raj, S. (2018). International Migration in Tamil Nadu: Results from the Tamil Nadu Migration Survey 2015. In S. Irudaya Rajan (Ed.), *India Migration Report 2017: Forced Migration* (pp. 249–260). Oxon: Routledge.

Rajan, S. I., and Zachariah, K. C. (2019). Emigration and Remittances: New Evidences from the Kerala Migration Survey 2018. Center for Development Studies Working Paper No. 483. Thiruvananthapuram.

Robinson, V. (1986). *Transients, Settlers and Refugees: Asians in Britain*. Oxford: Clarendon Press.

Wise, R. D., and Covarrubias, H. M. (2009). Understanding the Relationship between Migration and Development: Toward a New Theoretical Approach. *Social Analysis*, 53(3), 85–105.

World Bank Group and KNOMAD. (2020). COVID-19 Crisis Through a Migration Lens (Migration and Development Brief No. 32; p. 50). World Bank Group and KNOMAD.

Xiang, B., and Lindquist, J. (2014). Migration Infrastructure. *International Migration Review*, 48, S122–S148.

18 Understanding Economic Well-Being of the Elderly Return Migrants in India

Pinak Sarkar and Himanshu Chaurasia

Introduction

In recent decades a host of studies have immensely contributed to the domain of knowledge explaining the various facets of human mobility in India. These studies have enriched our understanding of the phenomenon of migration in India covering a wide range of aspects such as domestic migration patterns, migration trends across states, regional imbalances and migration, flow of domestic remittances, gains from migration both at the destination and origin, migrant's wage, and the socio-economic characteristics and circumstances which causes migration (Rogaly et al., 2001; Dholakia, 2006; Dubey et al.,2006; Joe et al. 2011; Roy and Debnath, 2011; Tumbe, 2011; Sarkar, 2014; Valatheeswaran, 2015; Khan, 2016. However, one aspect of migration which is neglected in the literature is the elderly return migration in India. This aspect of migration is very useful to understand the extent to which internal migration is rewarding in India for those who choose to return to the source or origin, also whether migration has any economic consequence, i.e. positive or negative among elderly return migrants.[1] For the elderly population, the positive economic consequence or economic success from migration is very important because it reflects the affordability in attaining medical care at old age, thus, can be linked to health and mental well-being at the old age. Overall the objective of this study is to specifically analyze the economic well-being of the elderly return migrants compared to the overall return migrants, and the non-migrants. And also to analyze the degree of relative advantage or disadvantage of the elderly return migrants in positioning themselves in the higher economic order in the wealth quintile.

Data and Methodology

The analysis is based on the Employment, Unemployment and Migration survey, July 2007–June 2008, NSS 64th round unit level data. Simple statistical tools are used in this study such as percentages, Odds-ratio analysis and Index of Relative Deprivation (RDI). The first objective compares

DOI: 10.4324/9781003315124-18

the economic well-being of the elderly return migrants in India, here, the percentage distribution of the monthly per capita consumption expenditure (MPCE) quintile classes for the elderly return migrants are compared with the all age return migrants' cohort and the non-migrant cohort. The second objective tries to examine the degree of relative advantage or disadvantage the elderly return migrants have to belong in the top quintile classes compared to the non-elderly return migrants using the Index of Relative Deprivation (RDI) which can also be interpreted as Index of Relative Advantage. The detailed methodology and mathematical derivation are explained in the appropriate subsection.

For analysis purpose, the elderly return migrants consists of those in the age group of 60 years and above age. Here the top two quintile classes Q4 and Q5 are referred as the top quintile classes.

Contextualizing Return Migration

In India, migration seems to be a rewarding and rational choice for the rural poor who migrate to urban areas, as it helps the migrants to come out of poverty (Joe et al., 2009: 2011). It is also observed in the Indian context that on average, a migrant worker earns higher wage than non-migrant/native workers (Khan, 2016). In a country like India, given the existence of regional disparity in development, it is obvious that people tend to move from the poorer regions/states to the richer regions/states (Sarkar, 2014). Overall migration takes place as a livelihood strategy which helps the migrants and the migrant households to come out of poverty. Livelihood strategy is often seen as a planned or deliberate attempts made by the households and family members to sustain, secure and improve the overall well-being and livelihoods. The choice is particularly based on the access to opportunities, assets, as well as ambitions of actors. Since these choices vary across different households and individuals, the livelihood strategy tends to be heterogeneous in nature. A livelihood mainly includes assets, capabilities/skills, along with both physical and social resources, to enhance means of living (Carney, 1998). According to Ellis (1998), livelihood strategy should not be viewed only from the income-generating perspective of households, it also comprises the social foundations, intra-household relationships, dealings and process of access to resources through the life cycle. Thus, it can be assumed that as migration is seen as a livelihood strategy, it is also quite likely that some migrants might choose to return to the place of origin after actualizing the gains from migration at the destination after staying for a particular length of time or duration of migration. As argued by Borjas (1999) a prospective migrant makes decisions based on the costs and benefits of relocating. A large number of migrants voluntarily return to their native, which suggests that the relative attraction of different places changes as an individual ages and gains experience. According to Reyes and Mameesh (2002), around half of migrants return to Mexico in under a year.

There are studies which try to determine return migration in India from a perspective of brain gain where return migration from western countries to the IT cities like Bangalore and Hyderabad brings back skill and also leads to transfer of knowledge and technology (Chacko, 2007).

Likelihood of Return Migration Pattern across Indian States

In this section, an attempt is made to evaluate the likelihood of return migration pattern across the Indian states using the Odds-ratio analysis. The odds ratios are a widely used descriptive statistic which indicates the measure of effect size and the likelihood of an event occurring to that of not occurring. In simple statistics, odds are calculated by taking the ratio of the probability of happening to that of not happening. Here, the odds are calculated on the basis of the ratio of occurrence to that of non-occurrence using the following formula:

$$Odds = \frac{Probability}{1 - Probability} \quad Or \, Odds = \frac{Occurrence}{1 - Occurrence}$$

$$Odds\,Ratio, ORxi = \frac{Oxi\,/(1 - Oxi)}{Oxr\,/(1 - Oxr)}$$

Where, ORxi= Odds Ratio of each data point I, Oxi / (1- Oxi) = Occurrence of each data point i to that of non-occurrence of I, Oxr/ (1- Oxr) = Occurrence of the reference point to that of non-occurrence.

Table 18.1 shows the likelihood or odds of return migration in the total migration stream across the Indian states with respect to All India as the reference category which is 1.00. The analysis also captures the stream differential pattern for both the rural and urban areas. One important observation which is made in the analysis is that Delhi has the highest likelihood of having return migration when compared to the all-India level and which is true for both the rural and urban areas with the Odds-ratio value of 5.27 and 2.71. The other states which have a higher likelihood of having return migrants compared to the all-India level in both the rural and urban areas are Himachal Pradesh, Kerala, Maharashtra, Tamil Nadu and Uttarakhand.

Comparison between the Non-migrant and the Return Migrant Population Cohort in the Wealth Quintile in Rural India

In this section, three groups of population cohorts, viz. non-migrant (NM), all age-return migrant (RM), and elderly return migrant (ERM) are considered for comparing and evaluating economic positioning in the wealth quintile. Figure 18.1 shows the quintile distribution of the NM and RM population cohorts in rural India. It is observed that the NM population is more dominated towards the lower quintile classes. However, when

Table 18.1 Odds-Ratio Likelihood of Return Migration across
the Major Indian States

Odds-Ratio
Return Migration across Indian States

Major Indian States	Rural	Urban	All
Andhra Pradesh	0.85	0.65	0.78
Bihar	1.87	0.74	1.72
Chhattisgarh	1.54	0.94	1.43
Delhi	5.27	2.71	2.66
Gujarat	1.16	0.85	1.03
Haryana	0.34	0.43	0.37
Himachal Pradesh	1.56	1.38	1.57
Jammu & Kashmir	0.42	1.14	0.55
Jharkhand	0.78	0.20	0.64
Karnataka	0.99	0.95	0.98
Kerala	1.77	1.70	1.76
Madhya Pradesh	0.74	1.08	0.84
Maharashtra	1.08	1.04	1.05
Orissa	0.74	0.64	0.74
Punjab	0.38	0.56	0.44
Rajasthan	0.48	0.44	0.47
Tamil Nadu	2.04	1.55	1.80
Uttarakhand	1.31	1.89	1.48
Uttar Pradesh	0.88	0.69	0.85
West Bengal	0.70	1.21	0.84
All India	1.00	1.00	1.00

Source: Calculated using unit level 64th round (2007–08) migration data.

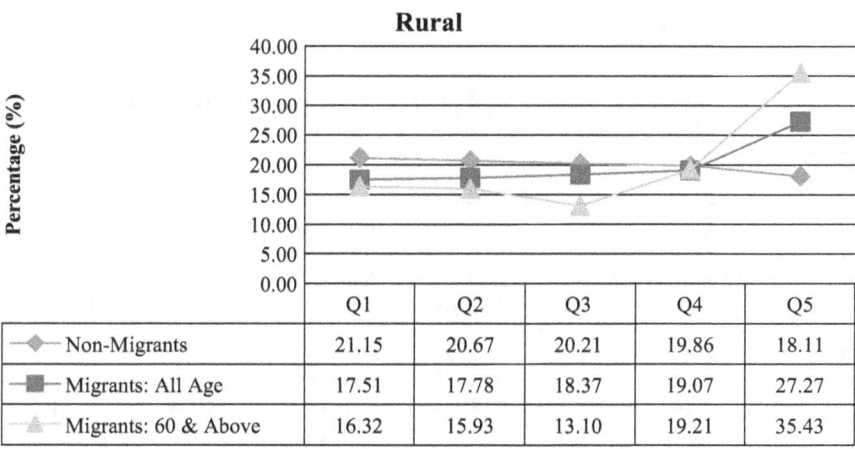

Rural

	Q1	Q2	Q3	Q4	Q5
Non-Migrants	21.15	20.67	20.21	19.86	18.11
Migrants: All Age	17.51	17.78	18.37	19.07	27.27
Migrants: 60 & Above	16.32	15.93	13.10	19.21	35.43

Figure 18.1 Quintile distribution of the NM and RM population cohorts in rural
India.

compared to the RM categories of all ages and elderly cohorts, it is interesting to observe that these RM population cohorts are more dominated in the higher quintile classes especially Q5. Further comparison between the two RM cohort shows that the elderly RM, i.e. 60 years and above age group have population dominance of 35.43 per cent which is much higher than the all age RM population cohort. This observation helps to conclude that the elderly return migrants are better situated in the wealth quintile compared to the all age RM and the NM population. The reason for such observation can be attributed to the factors that migration is a well-being strategy which brings economic stability and also helps the RM population to attain high economic well-being compared to the NM population, and also helps to have higher consumption not only in active life time but also at the old age.

Comparison of NM and RM Population across Educated and Socio-economic Groups in Rural India:

Table 18.2 shows the distribution of NM and RM cohorts in the wealth quintile for the illiterate and the literate population. Here too a very similar distributional pattern is observed like the previous section that NM population is more dominated towards the lower quintile classes whereas the all age RM and elderly RM are mostly dominated in the higher quintiles. When compared across the illiterate and literate categories it is observed that for obvious reasons the proportions of NM, all age RM and elderly RM are much higher for the literate migrants. But most importantly, the results are in accordance with the previous findings, for literate category the proportion of all age RM belonging in the Q5 is 41.28 per cent and for elderly RM is 71.85 per cent, whereas for illiterate category the proportion of all age RM belonging in the Q5 is 13.76 per cent and for elderly RM is 18.08 per cent.

Table 18.2 Distribution of NM and RM Population Cohort for Illiterate and Literate Groups in Rural Area

NM and RM Population Cohorts in Percentage (%)					
MPCE Quintile	*Illiterate*			*Literate*		
	Native/ NM	*RM All Age*	*RM Elderly*	*Native/NM*	*RM All Age*	*RM Elderly*
Q1	28.01	23.79	22.97	17.21	11.00	2.37
Q2	23.15	21.46	21.22	19.26	13.95	4.82
Q3	20.29	20.94	15.85	20.15	15.70	7.34
Q4	17.05	20.06	21.87	21.48	18.07	13.63
Q5	11.51	13.76	18.08	21.89	41.28	71.85
Total	100.00	100.00	100.00	100.00	100.00	100.00

Source: Calculated using unit level 64th round (2007–08) migration data.

Table 18.3 Distribution of NM and RM Population Cohorts for Social Groups in Rural Area

NM and RM Population Cohorts in Percentage (%)

MPCE Quintile	ST&SC			General Category		
	Native/ NM	RM All Age	RM Elderly	Native/ NM	RM All Age	RM Elderly
Q1	29.52	25.00	27.86	13.40	10.14	5.74
Q2	23.41	21.71	22.01	15.75	11.49	6.82
Q3	19.61	19.49	12.13	18.64	17.46	12.10
Q4	16.19	18.74	18.77	23.07	17.98	15.37
Q5	11.27	15.05	19.23	29.14	42.92	59.97
Total	100.00	100.00	100.00	100.00	100.00	100.00

Source: Calculated using unit level 64th round (2007–08) migration data.

Table 18.3 shows the distribution of NM and RM cohorts in the wealth quintile for the ST&SC and General category (Non-ST&SC) groups. Here too a very similar distributional pattern is observed like the previous section that NM population is more dominated towards the lower quintile classes whereas the all age RM and elderly RM are mostly dominated in the higher quintiles. When compared across the ST&SC and Others categories it is observed that the proportions of NM, all age RM and elderly RM are much higher for the general category population groups. But most importantly the results are in accordance with the previous findings. For general category, the proportion of all age RM belonging in the Q5 is 42.92 per cent and for elderly RM is 59.97 per cent, whereas ST&SC category the proportion of all age RM belonging in the Q5 is 15.05 per cent and for elderly RM is 19.23 per cent. Overall it is observed that for both the ST&SC and general category groups, the most economically better-off group is elderly RM followed by all age RM. Therefore, it can be argued that compared to non-migrants, the return migrants belong to a much higher position in the wealth distribution.

Comparison between the Non-migrant and the Return Migrant Population Cohort in the Wealth Quintile in Urban India

In this section, the same analysis is repeated for the population groups in urban India. Figure 18.2 shows the quintile distribution of the NM and RM population cohorts in urban India. It is observed that the NM population is more dominated towards the lower quintile classes. However, when compared to the RM categories of all ages and elderly cohort, it is interesting to observe that these RM population cohorts are more dominated in the higher quintile classes especially Q5. Further comparison between the two

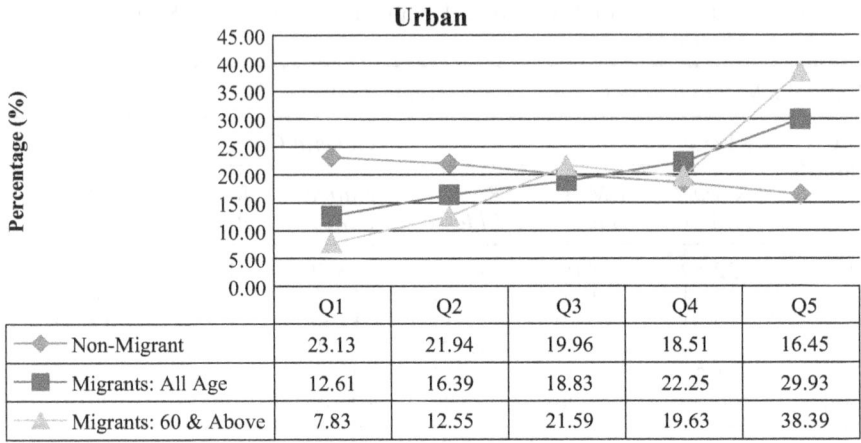

	Q1	Q2	Q3	Q4	Q5
Non-Migrant	23.13	21.94	19.96	18.51	16.45
Migrants: All Age	12.61	16.39	18.83	22.25	29.93
Migrants: 60 & Above	7.83	12.55	21.59	19.63	38.39

Figure 18.2 Quintile distribution of the NM and RM population cohorts in urban India.

RM cohorts shows that the elderly RM, i.e. 60 years and above age group have population dominance of 38.39 per cent which is much higher than the all age RM population cohort which is 29.93. This observation helps to conclude that the elderly return migrants are better situated in the wealth quintile compared to the all age RM and the NM population. The reason for such observation can be attributed to the factors that migration is a well-being strategy which brings economic stability and also helps the RM population to attain high economic well-being compared to the NM population, and also helps to have higher consumption not only in active lifetime but also at the old age.

Comparison of NM and RM Population across Educated and Socio-economic Groups in Urban India

Table 18.5 shows the distribution of NM and RM cohorts in the wealth quintile for the illiterate and the literate population. Here, too, a very similar distributional pattern is observed like the previous section that NM population is more dominated towards the lower quintile classes whereas the all age RM and elderly RM are mostly dominated in the higher quintiles. When compared across the illiterate and literate category it is observed that for obvious reasons the proportions of NM, all age RM and elderly RM are much higher for the literate migrants. But most importantly, the results are in accordance with the previous findings, for literate category the proportion of all age RM belonging in the Q5 is 35.79 per cent and for elderly RM is 50.53 per cent, whereas for illiterate category the proportion of all age RM belonging in the Q5 is 8.23 per cent and for elderly RM is 13.31 per cent.

Table 18.4 Distribution of NM and RM Population Cohorts for Illiterate and Literate Groups in Urban Area

NM and RM Population Cohort in Percentage (%)

MPCE Quintile	Illiterate			Literate		
	Native/ NM	RM All Age	RM Elderly	Native/ NM	RM All Age	RM Elderly
Q1	37.50	30.38	18.95	18.72	7.82	2.45
Q2	26.41	27.79	20.65	20.59	13.28	8.63
Q3	17.79	21.55	33.68	20.64	18.11	15.74
Q4	11.75	12.06	13.41	20.59	25.01	22.65
Q5	6.55	8.23	13.31	19.47	35.79	50.53
Total	100.00	100.00	100.00	100.00	100.00	100.00

Source: Calculated using unit level 64th round (2007–08) migration data.

Table 18.5 Distribution of NM and RM Population Cohorts for Social Groups in Urban Area

NM and RM Population Cohort in Percentage (%)

MPCE Quintile	ST&SC			General Category		
	Native/ NM	RM All Age	RM Elderly	Native/ NM	RM All Age	RM Elderly
Q1	34.47	19.10	13.11	14.09	5.20	2.37
Q2	25.06	19.15	14.69	16.92	10.67	10.14
Q3	20.74	22.44	34.36	19.40	16.33	14.85
Q4	12.76	22.08	14.77	23.46	25.20	21.25
Q5	6.97	17.23	23.07	26.14	42.59	51.39
Total	100.00	100.00	100.00	100.00	100.00	100.00

Source: Calculated using unit level 64th round (2007–08) migration data.

Table 18.5 shows the distribution of NM and RM cohorts in the wealth quintile for the ST&SC and general category groups. Here too, a very similar distributional pattern is observed like the previous section that NM population is more dominated towards the lower quintile classes whereas the all age RM and elderly RM are mostly dominated in the higher quintiles.

When compared across the ST&SC and Others categories it is observed that the proportions of NM, all age RM and elderly RM are much higher for the general category population groups. But most importantly, the results are in accordance with the previous findings. For general category the proportion of all age RM belonging in the Q5 is 42.59 per cent and for elderly RM is 51.39 per cent, whereas ST&SC category the proportion of all age RM belonging in the Q5 is 17.23 per cent and for elderly

RM is 23.07 per cent. Overall it is observed that for both the ST&SC and general category groups, the most economically better off group is elderly RM followed by all age RM. Therefore, it can be argued that compared to non-migrants, the return migrants belong to a much higher position in the wealth distribution.

Measuring the Degree of Relative Economic Advantage/ Disadvantage of Being Elderly RM compared to Other RM

In the previous section it is observed that the elderly RM are placed much higher in the wealth quintile compared to the all age RM and NM. In this context, it becomes interesting to analyze the extent of advantage or disadvantage faced by the elderly RM population cohort to be placed in higher quintile groups compared to the other RM. In this section, the other RMs are considered as those who are lesser than 60 years of age or non-elderly, according to the definition of this study; whereas the higher quintile groups are considered to be those who belong to the top two quintile classes, i.e., Q4 and Q5 combined. Here, the Index of Relative Deprivation (RDI) is used for the analysis. The mathematical formulation given by Jayaraj and Subramanian (2002) is followed as it is, but with some manipulation to fit it in the present study.

The Mathematical Formulation and Methodology of RDI

Following the methodology from Jayaraj and Subramanian (2002), where RDI was used to measure ailment prevalence rate (APR). They defined APR as the proportion of the number of ailing persons to the total population. The APR was thus decomposed as the weighted, i.e., population adjusted sum of the group-specific APRs as seen in the following equation:

$$APR = \sum_{i=1}^{n} \theta_i APR_i \ldots \tag{i}$$

Where, θ_i is the portion of a particular group i in the population; APR_i is the ailment prevalence rate of group i (undernutrition); and i represents the number of such groups (ranging from $i = 1, 2, 3 \ldots, J$).

In this particular section, an attempt is made to use this mathematical formulation to identify the extent of relative disadvantage or advantage faced by elderly return migrants in India. In this section, the purpose is to examine the extent to which elderly return migrants have any possible advantage/disadvantage in attaining a higher position in the wealth quintile, and here it is termed as Top quintile rate (TQR), similar to that of the APR. Here, for a given population, TQR is the ratio/proportion of the number of elderly return migrants belonging to the top quintile classes in the total return migrant population in both the rural and urban areas of the Indian states. For the empirical analysis, the top two wealth quintile representing the highest 40 per cent of the return migrant population, i.e., the aggregate of Q4 and Q5 is considered as top quintile group for calculating TQR. Here, the original APR equation (i) is replaced with the new TQR equation (ii). Thus, the TQR is decomposed as the weighted, i.e., population adjusted sum of the group-specific TQRs as seen in the equation:

$$TQR = \sum_{i=1}^{n} {}_i TQR_i \tag{ii}$$

Where, θ_i is the portion of a particular group i in the population; TQR_i is the share of the elderly return migrant population belonging to the top quintile classes of group i; and i denotes the number of groups (ranging from i = 1, 2..., J). In this study the groups are based on migrant age, i.e., elderly (60 years of age and above) and the others (less than 60 years of age).

Rearranging the equation (ii) provides the contribution (ω_i)of each group to the total TQR. In other words, ω_i is the share of the ith group in the top quintile classes (TQR).

$$\omega_i = \frac{\theta_i TQR_i}{TQR} \tag{iii}$$

Thus, RDI follows the concept of equity or equal in relative sense. Here, a state of zero relative deprivation is assumed if the influence of group i in TQR is equivalent to its population share, i.e., $\omega_{i\,=\,}\theta_i$ Under this condition there is neither advantage or disadvantage. Thus, group i will be relatively disadvantaged in acquiring higher economic position if the share of $\omega_{i\,<\,}\theta_i$ and relatively advantaged if the share of $\omega_{i\,>\,}\theta_i$ this can be written as follows:

$$\partial_i = \frac{\omega_i - \theta_i}{\theta_i} \tag{iv}$$

To normalize ∂_i , it is divided by ∂_i^{max}, to arrive at the maximum value that these deviations can attain. From (iv) it is evident that ∂_i is maximum when ω_i attains its maximum value (ω_i^{max})for any given θ_i. To derive the value ω_i^{max} equation (iii) is expressed in an alternative form as

$$\omega_i = \frac{\dfrac{n_i}{n} \times \dfrac{\alpha_i}{n_i}}{\dfrac{\alpha}{n}} = \frac{\alpha_i}{\alpha} \tag{v}$$

Where, n_i is the population of group i and n is the aggregate population, therefore $n_i / n_i = \theta_i$ and α_i is the number of migrants in the top quintiles in group i and hence $\alpha_i / n_i = TQR_i$. From (v) it follows that ω_i is maximized when α_i is at maximum. Note that α_i attain the maximum value of α if $n_i > \alpha_i$ and the maximum value of n_i when $n_i < \alpha_i$, that is

$$\omega_i^{max} = 1 ... \forall n_i \geq \alpha \tag{vi-i}$$

$$\omega_i^{max} = \frac{\theta_i}{APR} ... \forall n_i < \alpha \tag{vi-ii}$$

Since, the maximum values of ω_i is defined, the ∂_i^{max}, can be now defined as follows:

$$\partial_i^{max} = \frac{1}{\theta_i} - 1 ... \forall n_i \geq \alpha \tag{vii-i}$$

$$\partial_i^{max} = \frac{1}{APR} - 1 ... \forall n_i < \alpha \tag{vii-ii}$$

Finally, the normalized value of the RDI is given by

$$\partial_i^* = \frac{\partial_i}{\partial_i^{max}} = \frac{\omega_i - \theta_i}{1 - \theta_i} ... \forall n_i \geq \alpha \tag{viii-i}$$

$$\partial_i^* = \frac{\partial_i}{\partial_i^{max}} = \frac{\omega_i - \theta_i}{\theta_i} \times \frac{APR}{1 - APR} ... \forall n_i < \alpha \tag{viii-ii}$$

Equation (viii) finds an easy and interesting interpretation in the sense that, a group is said to be relatively disadvantaged whenever ∂_i^* is positive and is recognized relatively advantaged whenever ∂_i^* is negative.

However, in the empirical literature, RDI is mostly used in a rather simplistic formulation as follows:

$$RDI = \frac{(C_i - S_i)}{(c_i \; max - S_i)}$$

Where C_i is ω_i and S_i is θ_i. (Where i=1...n; c_i max = S_i / AD if S_i < AD and c_i max = 1 if S_i > AD; Where, AD = Σ Si*DCi. Here, DCi is the ith group of a specific characteristic (incidence), and Ci is the share of ith group in total migrants of same characteristics. Si is the share of the ith group of migrant in total migrant population. Ci max is the maximum contribution that the ith group can make; AD is the average incidence.

Table 18.6, shows the RDI of being elderly RM compared to others (non-elderly) RM in rural areas for illiterate, literate and social groups across the major India states. For ST&SC RM cohort it is observed that in 12 out of 20 selected states, the elderly RM have an advantage compared to the non-elderly RM to belong to the top quintile class, i.e., aggregate of Q4 and Q5,

Table 18.6 The RDI of Being Elderly RM Compared to Others RM in Rural India

RDI of being Elderly RM vs. Others RM (Non-elderly)

Major Indian States	ST&SC	General Category	Illiterate	Literate
Jammu & Kashmir	–0.289	–0.132	–0.302	–0.085
Himachal Pradesh	–0.355	–0.013	–0.249	–0.104
Punjab	–0.237	–0.044	–0.017	–0.163
Uttaranchal	1.020	–0.205	–0.343	–0.240
Haryana	0.583	0.015	0.017	0.067
Delhi	–0.046	0.000	–0.122	–0.018
Rajasthan	0.592	–0.457	–0.218	–0.139
Uttar-Pradesh	–0.034	–0.331	–0.312	–0.273
Bihar	–0.962	–0.247	–0.706	–0.884
West-Bengal	0.632	–0.758	0.234	–1.264
Jharkhand	1.020	0.000	–0.939	0.000
Orissa	–3.324	–1.705	–2.384	–0.650
Chhattisgarh	0.150	–0.206	0.091	0.918
Madhya-Pradesh	0.464	0.128	0.399	–1.523
Gujarat	–0.026	–0.026	–0.093	–0.072
Maharashtra	–0.236	–0.048	0.228	–0.578
Andhra-Pradesh	–0.185	–0.346	–0.185	–0.353
Karnataka	1.020	0.570	–0.187	–0.203
Kerala	–0.319	–0.070	–0.386	–0.142
Tamil-Nadu	–0.062	0.322	–0.129	–0.741
All India	–0.114	–0.253	–0.195	–0.436

Source: Calculated using unit level 64th round (2007–08) migration data.

also at the all-India level, the RDI value shows relative advantage with the value of –0.114.

Similarly, for general category, illiterate and literate RM cohort the elderly RM shows an advantage compared to the non-elderly RM to belong to the top quintile class with RDI value of –0.253, –0.195 and –0.436. However, for states with some categories with 0.000 RDI value reflects that there is neither advantage of disadvantage for the groups to belong to top quintile classes.

Table 18.7, shows the RDI of being elderly RM compared to others (non-elderly) RM in urban areas for illiterate, literate and social groups across the major India states. For ST&SC RM cohort it is observed that 10 out of 20 selected states have relative advantage, two states show neither advantage or disadvantage, however the all-India RDI value shows relative disadvantage with +ve value of 0.019. On the other hand, similar to the rural areas, for general category, illiterate and literate RM cohort the elderly RM in the urban area shows advantage compared to the non-elderly RM to belong to the top quintile class with RDI value of –0.074, –0.444 and –0.204.

Table 18.7 The RDI of Being Elderly RM Compared to Others RM in Urban India

RDI of being Elderly RM vs. Others RM (Non-elderly)				
Major Indian States	*ST&SC*	*Others*	*Illiterate*	*Literate*
Jammu & Kashmir	−0.644	−0.132	1.020	−0.415
Himachal Pradesh	−0.006	0.195	−1.664	0.133
Punjab	−4.474	−0.094	−0.470	−0.570
Uttaranchal	−6.105	0.069	0.970	−0.353
Haryana	0.000	−0.091	0.000	0.658
Delhi	1.020	−0.073	0.653	−0.297
Rajasthan	−0.593	0.386	0.559	0.012
Uttar– Pradesh	1.020	−0.377	−3.123	−0.119
Bihar	1.020	0.651	1.020	0.844
West Bengal	0.107	−0.306	−0.502	−0.351
Jharkhand	1.020	0.000	0.000	1.020
Orissa	1.020	−0.101	0.986	−0.890
Chhattisgarh	0.000	−0.176	1.020	0.231
Madhya– Pradesh	−0.790	0.211	0.295	−0.436
Gujarat	−0.279	0.139	1.020	−0.024
Maharashtra	−0.332	0.035	−1.852	0.047
Andhra Pradesh	0.360	−0.282	−0.385	−0.012
Karnataka	0.000	−0.361	−1.068	−0.396
Kerala	−1.336	−0.209	1.020	−0.419
Tamil-Nadu	−0.061	−0.268	1.020	−0.322
All India	0.019	−0.074	−0.444	−0.204

Source: Calculated using unit level 64th round (2007–08) migration data.

However, for states with some categories with 0.000 RDI value reflects that there is neither advantage or disadvantage for the groups to belong to top quintile classes.

Discussion

Migration as a phenomenon is always seen as a well-being strategy to enhance economic benefit to the migrant households and also to the individual migrants. Human mobility is not restricted to or by any particular group of homogenous people but is taken up as a livelihood strategy by heterogeneous groups, i.e., both literate and illiterate, poor and reach, people with endowments and without endowments, skilled and unskilled etc. Similarly, the migration strategy whether to take up a short duration migration/temporary migration/seasonal migration or long-term migration brings different levels of economic well-being to different categories of migrants. One way to understand economic gains from migration is to evaluate the extent to which migration serves as a rational decision in the long run or life cycle especially for those who choose to return to the place of origin.

In this empirical study, it is observed that migration is a rational choice as it helps the migrants to achieve upward economic mobility in the source region compared to the non-migrant population. Also, from the analysis it can be argued that migration also helps to achieve better economic position even at the old age, as the elderly return migrants are better placed in the wealth quintile compared to the all-age return migrants and non-migrants across various states and migrant groups.

Note

1 According to the NSSO, those migrants who had reported that the present place of enumeration was UPR any time in the past was considered as return migrant.

References

Borjas, J. G. (1999). Immigration and welfare magnets. *Journal of Labour Economics, 17*(4), 607–637.

Carney, D. (1998). *Sustainable rural livelihoods: What contribution can we make?* London: Department for International Development.

Chacko, E. (2007). From brain drain to brain gain: Reverse migration to Bangalore and Hyderabad, India's globalizing high teach cities. *Geo Journal, 68*(2 and 3), 131–140.

Dholakia, R. H. (2006). Regional imbalance under federal structure: A comparison of Canada and India. *Vikalpa, 31*(4), 1–8.

Dubey, A., Palmer-Jones, R., & Sen, K. (2006). Surplus labor, social structure and rural to urban migration: Evidence from Indian data. *The European Journal of Development Research, 18*(1), 86–104.

Ellis, F. (1998). Household strategies and rural livelihood diversification. *The Journal of Development Studies, 35*(1), 1–38.

Jayaraj, D., & Subramanian, S. (2002). Child labor in Tamil Nadu in the 1980s: A preliminary account of its nature, extent and distribution. *Economic and Political Weekly, 37*(10), 941–54.

Joe, W., Samaiyar, P., & Mishra, U. S. (2009). *Migration & urban poverty in India. Some preliminary observations* (CDS Working Paper No. 414). Trivandrum: Centre for Development Studies.

Joe, W., Samaiyar, P., & Mishra, U. S. (2011). On examining migration-poverty nexus in urban India. In S. I. Rajan (Ed.), *India migartion report 2011: Migration, identity and conflict* (pp. 236–256). New Delihi: Routledge India.

Khan, M. I. (2016). Migrant and non-migrant wage differentials: A quintile decomposition analysis for India. *The Indian Journal of Labor Economics, 59*(2), 245–273.

Reyes, B. I., & Mameesh, L. (2002). Why does immigrant trip duration vary across US Destinations? *Social Science Quarterly, 83*(2), 580–593.

Rogaly, B., Biswas, J., Daniel, C., Abdur, R., Kumar, R., & Sengupta, A. (2001). Seasonal migration, social change and migrants rights, lessons from West Bengal. *Economic and Political Weekly, 36*(49), 4547–4558.

Roy, N., & Debnath, A. (2011). Impact of migration on economic development: A study of some selected state. *International Proceedings of Economics Development & Research (IPEDR)*, 5(1), 198–202.

Sarkar, P. (2014). An analysis of inter-state quantum migration in India: An empirical validation of the 'push-pull framework' and gains from migration. *Indian Journal of Labor Economics*, 57(3), 267–281.

Tumbe, C. (2011). *Remittances in India: Facts & issues* (Indian Institute of Management Working Paper No. 331). Bangalore: Indian Institute of Management.

Valatheeswaran, C. (2015). International remittances and household expenditure patterns in Tamil Nadu. *The Indian Journal of Labor Economics*, 58(4), 631–652.

19 Emerging Relationship between Migration and Development in West Bengal

Jyoti Parimal Sarkar

Introduction

The process of migration whether internal or international is a very complex one and it has been discussed and theorised upon by the researchers for a long time. It is expected that migration has also brought about changes in all fields of human activity in West Bengal. Geographically, it constitutes only 2.8 per cent of the total land area of India and the population of West Bengal constitutes 7.54 per cent of India in 2011. The initial industrial development, especially jute industries on the banks of the Hugli river, attracted a large number of migrant labourers in West Bengal mainly from Bihar, Odisha and Uttar Pradesh. It was a centre of 'Trade and Commerce' in Eastern India. It attracted migrants from far off places like Gujarat, Rajasthan, Punjab and South Indian states. In the pre-independence era, the highest growth rate was observed in the decade of thirties (1931–41) with 22.9 per cent, the growth in urban population was even more remarkable, having a growth rate of 63.7 per cent and 32.5 per cent in the years 1931–41 and 1941–51, respectively. It shows that during the last phase of British rule, Calcutta–Howrah–Hugli and their surrounding urban areas were the centres of attraction for the migrant population resulting in abnormally high growth in the population of West Bengal.

Besides, the inflow of 'internal' migrants from neighbouring states, West Bengal has also received thousands of 'international' migrants, especially, from East Bengal (presently, Bangladesh). Thus, the immigrants from East Bengal (East Pakistan/Bangladesh) as well as the migrants from other states have brought about a change in the nature of growth and development of West Bengal, which has ultimately affected its social, political and economic dimensions. Therefore, it is felt necessary to study linkage between 'migration' and diversified 'development' in the state to help the policymakers take an appropriate strategy for development.

DOI: 10.4324/9781003315124-19

Level of Development: Socio-Economic Indicators for Districts of West Bengal

An analysis of per capita incomes of districts from the time point 1980–81 to 2010–11 shows that districts like Kolkata, Darjeeling, Howrah, Burdwan, 24 Parganas and Hugli are at the top. A composite index of development in agriculture, industry, economic infrastructure and social sector consisting of five indicators each has been calculated for districts of West Bengal using the technique of principal component analysis (PCA). Based on mean PCA values, districts having PCA above the mean value were identified as developed districts (Table 19.1).

It is observed that Burdwan, Howrah, Hugli and Nadia were continuously included into the 'high' category of agriculture development. The lopsided and biased development of the state in favour of Kolkata is evident in the case of industrial development, economic infrastructure and social sector. The adjacent districts such as Hoara, Hugli, Nadia and 24 Parganas being a part of the Kolkata agglomeration have also qualified as developed districts in terms of infrastructure facility in industrial and economics and social infrastructural sector. Post-liberalisation, low developed districts did qualify as high developed districts which means that the government has been successful in developing infrastructure facilities in the dry western part of West Bengal, i.e. Bankura, Birbhum and Medinipur. Darjeeling, a hilly district, also qualifies as a developed district in economic and social infrastructural development. However, the performance of the other districts in the social sector was better than that observed in the developmental pattern of 'economic infrastructure sector' pointing at the developmental efforts of the governments in the state.

Thus, the levels of development of different districts of West Bengal vary widely in various socio-economic spheres. This variation in the levels of development in different sectors of districts has affected the pattern of migration of the people within the state as well as across the state boundaries as the people seek improvement in their standards of living.

Overall Trend and Pattern of Migration in West Bengal

Firstly, the trend patterns of 'internal' and 'international' migrations into West Bengal have been analysed based on data collected from different volumes of Census of India. The mobility of people in West Bengal had declined remarkably over the three decades during 1971, 1981 and 1991 and before improving in the last two decades. But still the level of migration is lower than the level in 1961 (Table 19.2).

Similar pattern has been observed in case of male and female both in rural and urban areas except for rural female migrants. It has increased over this period from 44.4 per cent in 1961 to 52.9 per cent in 2011. By analysing 'types of migration' by the administrative distance criterion in the Census of

Table 19.1 Identification of Levels of Development in Various Sectors

Sectors	1970–71	1980–81	1990–91	2000–01	2010–11
Agricultural sector[1]	Burdwan, Birbhum, Howrah, Hugli, Nadia, Murshidabad	Burdwan, Nadia, Howrah, Hugli, 24-Parganas	Burdwan, Birbhum, Howrah, Hugli, Nadia, 24 Parganas	Burdwan, Birbhum, Howrah, Hugli, Bankura Nadia, 24 Parganas	Burdwan, Birbhum, Hugli, Howrah Nadia, 24 Parganas, Medinipur
Industrial sector	Burdwan, Darjeeling, Howrah, Hugli, Nadia Kolkata	Darjeeling, Birbhum, Burdwan, Nadia, Hugli, Kolkata	Darjeeling, Birbhum, Burdwan, Kolkata	Darjeeling, Birbhum, Hugli, Kolkata	Darjeeling, Birbhum, Puruliya, Medinipur, Kolkata
Economic infrastructure	Burdwan, Darjeeling, Howrah, Hugli, Nadia, Kolkata	Darjeeling, Birbhum, Burdwan, Nadia, Hugli, Kolkata	Darjeeling, Birbhum, Burdwan, Kolkata	Darjeeling, Birbhum, Hugli, Kolkata	Darjeeling, Birbhum, Puruliya, Medinipur, Kolkata
Social sector	Darjeeling, Nadia, Puruliya, Hugli, Bankura, Medinipur, Kolkata	Darjeeling, Howrah, Puruliya, Bankura, Kolkata, Birbhum, Medinipur	Darjeeling, Howrah, Puruliya, Hugli, Bankura, Medinipur, Kolkata	Darjeeling, Howrah, Bankura, Kolkata	Darjeeling, Howrah, Hugli, Bankura, Kolkata

Source: Author's calculations.

Table 19.2 Sex-Wise Percentage of Migrant Population in Both Rural and Urban Areas of West Bengal (1961–2011)

Year	Total			Rural			Urban		
	P	M	F	P	M	F	P	M	F
1961	37.06	30.24	45.61	31.61	19.53	44.41	53.92	58.02	48.08
1971	30.01	22.36	37.93	27.56	17.38	38.37	37.96	38.94	36.65
1981	29.59	19.92	40.20	26.11	12.94	40.03	39.25	38.03	40.74
1991	26.27	15.50	38.01	25.23	11.20	40.15	29.00	26.34	32.09
2001	30.76	18.03	44.40	28.39	11.73	45.92	36.88	33.79	40.34
2011	35.88	21.34	51.19	33.65	15.36	52.85	40.66	34.08	47.62

Sources: Migration Tables of West Bengal, D-I table, Census of India, 1961, 1971, 1981, 1991, 2001 and 2011.

Note: P = Persons; M = Male; F = Female

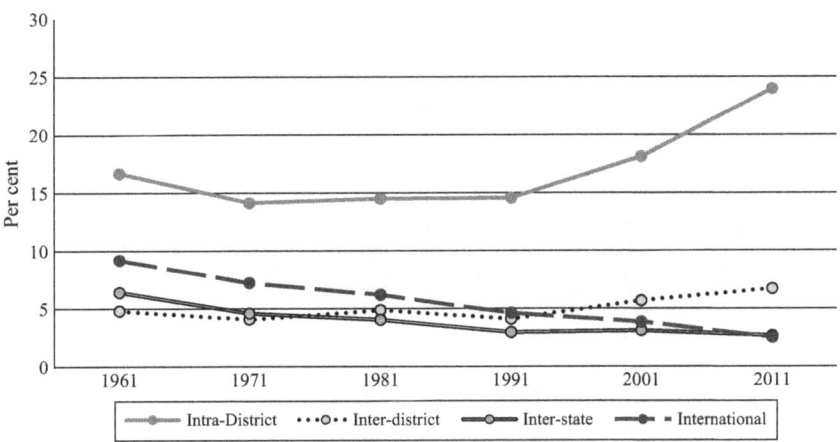

Figure 19.1 Classification of total migrant population in West Bengal by place of birth (POB): 1961–2011.

Sources: Migration Tables of West Bengal, D-I table, Census of India, 1961, 1971, 1981, 1991, 2001.

India for West Bengal, it is observed that the increase in mobility after the 1990s can be mainly attributed to the increase in mobility within the state (Figure 19.1). The flow of 'internal migrants' from other states has declined over the years. It also justifies observation by Dyson and Visaria, 2004.

Distributional Patterns of Internal Migration: District-wise

Internal migration comprises three types of migration inflows, viz., intra-district migration, inter-district migration and inter-state migration. We have analysed the mobility of 'inter-district' and 'inter-state' migrants across districts as presented below in detail (Figures 19.2 and 19.3).

Figures 19.2 and 19.3 reveal that the concentration of both 'inter-state' and 'inter-district' migration was in the developed districts (Table 19.1). Nearly 40 per cent of inter-district migrants resided in the five developed districts, Burdwan, Hugli, Howrah, 24 Parganas and Nadia of the state. Districts were ranked according to the percentage of 'male' and 'female' migrants separately and presented (Table 19.3). The numbers suggest that there were different patterns of inflow of migrants for males and females, and their ranks vary widely between males and females. However, the contrast in ranks based on the proportion of male and female migrants has made it clearer that 'male' migration, which is more economic in nature, has a better relationship with the level of development of these districts.

However, there was a little variation in the ranking positions, Kolkata continued to be at the top in case of 'inter-state' migration at all time points, but it held the top position in case of 'inter-district' migration only in 1961.

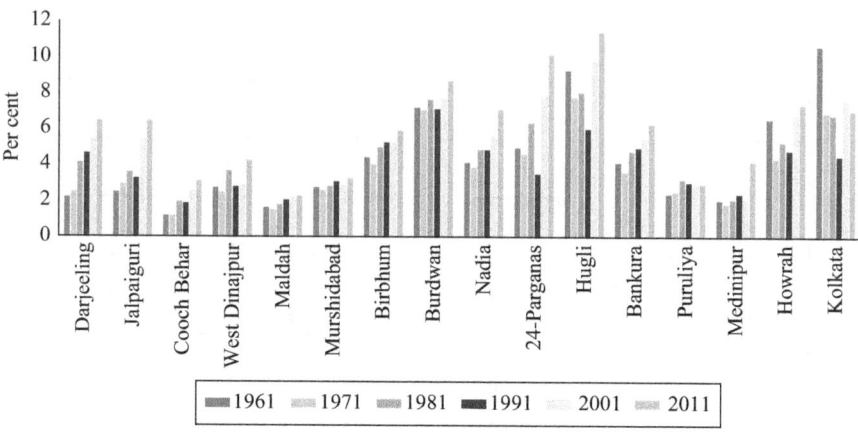

Figure 19.2 Percentage of inter-district migrant population (place of birth) in districts of West Bengal: 1961–2011.

Source: Migration Tables (D-I) of West Bengal, Census of India, 1961, 1971, 1981, 1991, 2001 and 2011.

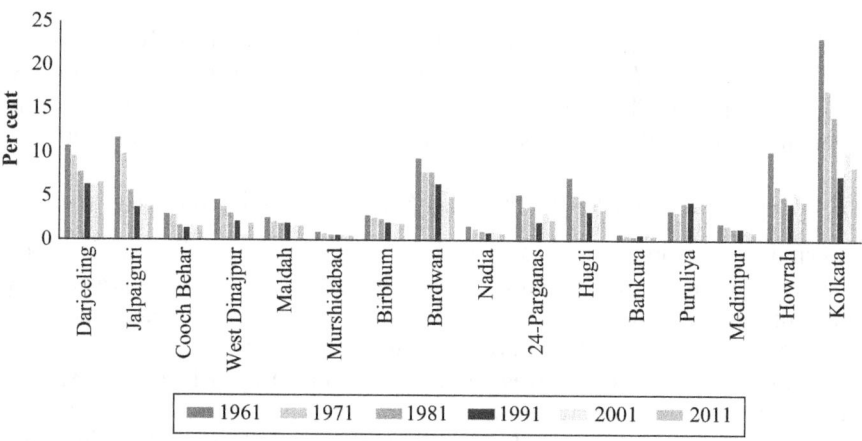

Figure 19.3 Percentage of inter-state migrant population (place of birth) in districts of West Bengal: 1961–2011.

Source: Migration Tables of West Bengal, D-I table, Census of India, 1961, 1971, 1981, 1991, 2001, 2011.

Darjeeling and Jalpaiguri districts, which are the hilly districts in the northern part of West Bengal, occupied high positions in terms of receiving 'inter-state' migrants especially due to the tourism and hotel industry and the presence of tea plantation and its related industry. However, due to continuous fall in tea prices internationally in the recent years, the industry has been facing a crisis which has led to the closure of many tea plantations or abandonment by the private managements (West Bengal Human

Development Report, 2004). This may explain the fall in the proportion of inter-state migrants in the district of Darjeeling and Jalpaiguri.

Kolkata occupied the first position in case of 'inter-state' migration for males for all the census years and for females till the 1981 census and again in 2001. The ranks based on the proportion of 'inter-state' male migration in districts of the state appear to correspond better with the level of development (Table 19.1) than the ranks based on the proportion of 'inter-district' male migration pointing to the stronger economic motive in case of 'inter-state' males (Tables 19.3 and 19.4).

Reasons for Migration (Inter-district and Inter-state Types)

The analysis of 'reasons for migration' for 'inter-district' and 'inter-state' types of migrants, respectively, confirm that 'work/employment' was the dominant reason for the males, whereas 'marriage' was the dominant reason for the females to migrate. This phenomenon was more prominent for 'inter-state' male migrants. It is confirmed that a greater proportion of males migrated for 'work/employment' purposes in case of 'inter-state migration' than that was in case of 'inter-district migration'(Figures 19.4 and 19.5).

One out of two 'inter-state' male migrants and one out of three 'inter-district' male migrants moved for 'work/employment' purposes. On the other hand, 'marriage' was the most dominant reason for female migration in case of both 'inter-state' and 'inter-district' categories of migration. More females have migrated for 'marriage' purposes in the 'inter-district' category of migration (3 out of 5 females in 1981 and 3 out of 4 females in 1991 and 2 out of 3 females in 2001 and 2011) than that of 'inter-state' category (1 out of 2 females, roughly). It means that non-economic factors were the more dominant reasons in case of intra-state migrants than inter-state migrants.

Characteristics of Migration

'Landholdings' is also an important determinant for measuring the economic status of the migrants (Figure 19.6). A detailed analysis of the data shows that mobility rate was very high in case of males, who were landless, and it declined systematically with increase in landholdings possessions.

It can be observed that the percentage of migrants in educational levels during 2007–08 shows that besides high migration among the illiterates; the percentage of migration is high in 'primary and middle' as well (Figure 19.7). In fact, in urban areas, maximum migrants in West Bengal have educational attainment of up to 'primary and middle school'. Also, it is observed that the male migrants with a higher level of education ('graduates and above') have preferred to migrate to urban areas rather than rural areas. The difference between male and female literacy is high at 11.15 per cent (Chattoraj & Chand, 2015).

Table 19.3 Percentage of Inter-district Migrant Population (Place of Birth) in Districts of West Bengal (1961–2011)

Districts	Males						Females					
	1961	1971	1981	1991	2001	2011	1961	1971	1981	1991	2001	2011
Darjeeling	10	9	5	2	5	4	14	14	10	7	10	10
Jalpaiguri	9	7	8	5	7	7	13	11	12	12	9	8
Koch Bihar	16	16	13	16	12	14	16	16	15	16	13	14
West Dinajpur	8	10	7	10	10	10	11	12	13	14	14	12
Maldah	14	14	15	14	13	15	15	15	16	15	16	16
Murshidabad	12	13	14	13	15	13	9	9	11	9	12	13
Birbhum	7	8	10	9	9	9	6	5	4	4	7	7
Burdwan	3	2	3	1	4	5	3	2	2	1	2	2
Nadia	6	6	9	8	8	8	7	7	7	6	6	5
24 Parganas	5	4	2	6	2	1	8	8	6	11	4	3
Hugli	2	3	4	4	3	2	1	1	1	2	1	1
Bankura	11	11	11	11	11	11	5	6	3	3	3	4
Puruliya	13	12	12	12	14	16	10	10	9	10	11	15
Medinipur	15	15	16	15	16	12	12	13	14	13	15	11
Howrah	4	5	6	7	6	6	4	4	5	5	5	6
Kolkata	1	1	1	3	1	3	2	3	8	8	8	9

Sources: Migration Tables of West Bengal, D-I table, Census of India, 1961, 1971, 1981, 1991, 2001 and 2011.

Table 19.4 Percentage of Inter-State Migrant Population (Place of Birth) in Districts of West Bengal (1961–2011)

Districts	Males						Females					
	1961	1971	1981	1991	2001	2011	1961	1971	1981	1991	2001	2011
Darjeeling	4	2	2	2	3	2	3	3	4	3	3	2
Jalpaiguri	3	3	5	6	6	6	2	2	5	5	5	5
Koch Bihar	9	9	11	10	9	10	13	10	13	12	10	12
West Dinajpur	8	8	8	8	13	8	8	6	6	9	16	9
Maldah	12	12	12	12	12	11	11	11	10	8	9	10
Murshidabad	15	15	15	16	16	16	15	15	15	16	14	15
Birbhum	10	11	10	11	10	9	9	8	7	7	8	8
Burdwan	5	4	3	3	4	4	4	4	2	2	4	4
Nadia	11	13	13	14	11	13	14	14	14	15	13	14
24 Paraganas	7	7	7	7	7	7	10	12	11	13	12	11
Hugli	6	6	6	5	5	5	7	9	9	10	7	7
Bankura	16	16	16	15	15	15	16	16	16	14	15	16
Puruliya	13	10	9	9	8	12	6	5	3	1	2	1
Medinipur	14	14	14	13	14	14	12	13	12	11	11	13
Howrah	2	5	4	4	2	3	5	7	8	6	6	6
Kolkata	1	1	1	1	1	1	1	1	1	4	1	3

Sources: Migration Tables of West Bengal, Census of India, 1961, 1971, 1981, 1991, 2001, 2011.

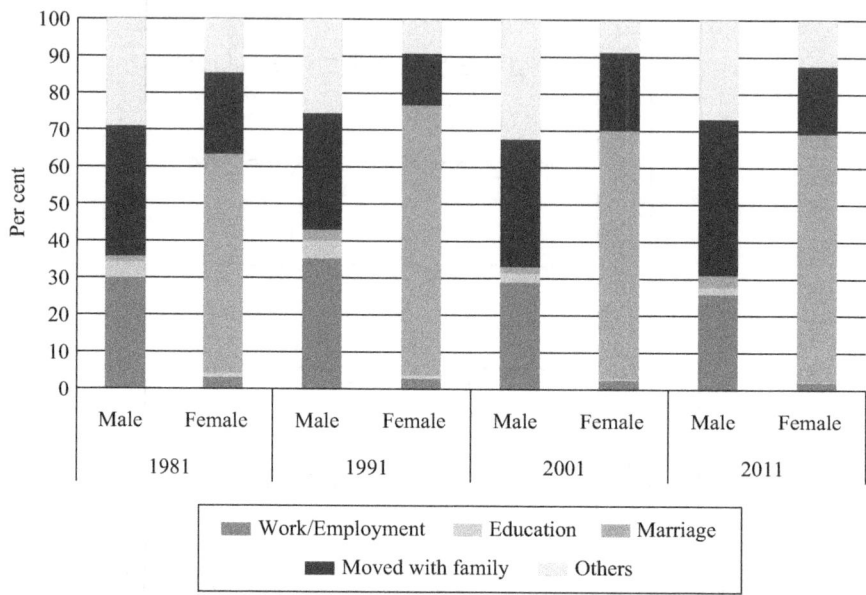

Figure 19.4 Reasons for inter-district (ID) migration in West Bengal, 1981–2011.
Source: Migration Tables, D-3, West Bengal, Census of India; 1981, 1991, 2001 and 2011.

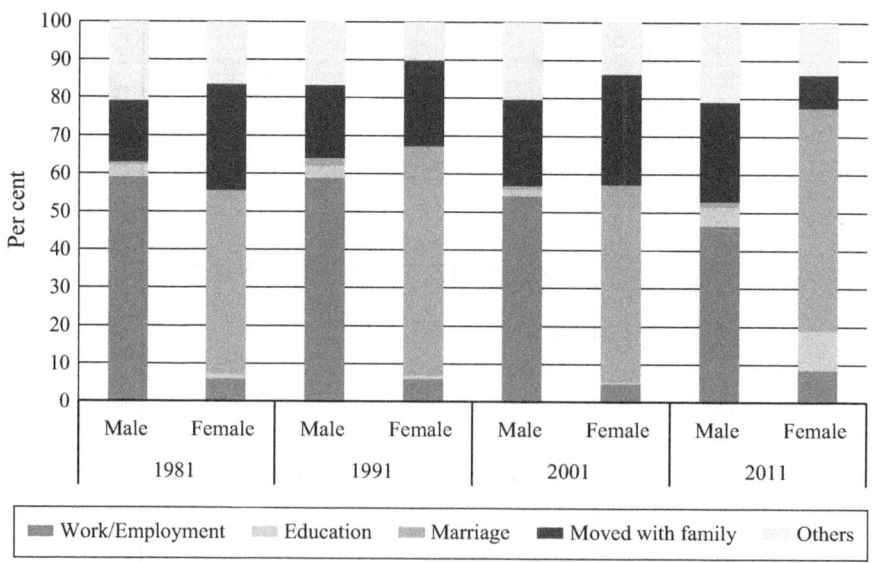

Figure 19.5 Reasons for inter-state (IS) migration in West Bengal, 1981–2011.
Source: Migration Tables, D-3, West Bengal, Census of India; 1981, 1991, 2001 2001 and 2011.

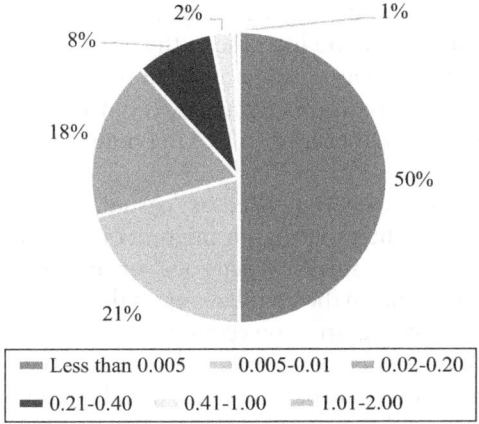

Figure 19.6 Percentage of migrants based on landholding in West Bengal, 2007–08.
Source: Computed from unit-level data of the 64th Round of NSS.

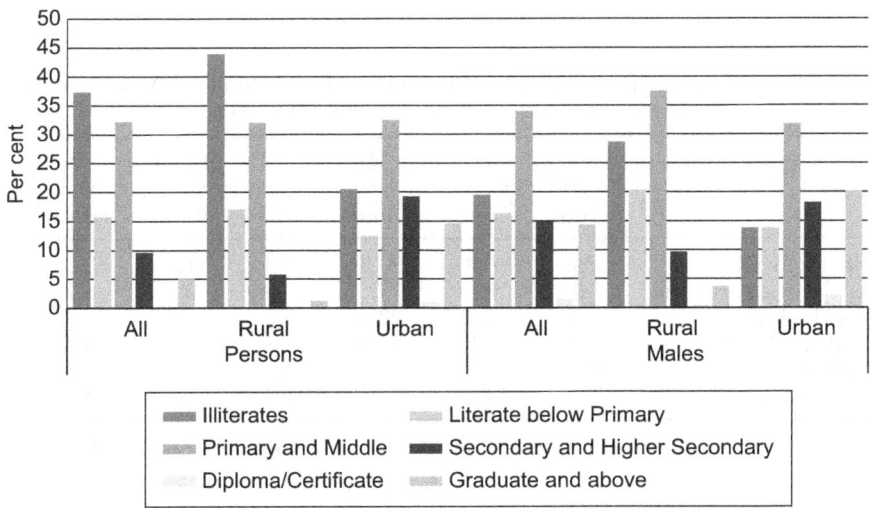

Figure 19.7 Percentage of migrants in different educational levels in West Bengal, 2007–08.

Source: 64th Round of NSS Report No. 533: Migration in India: July 2007–June 2008.

While the level of education of the migrants explains the supply side of the migrants, employment growth of an economy explains the demand side of the migrants. Post-liberalisation, especially during the period between 2004–05 and 2009–10, West Bengal witnessed the highest growth in non-agricultural employment compared to all other states in India (Chowdhury

& Chakraborty, 2016). It also witnessed the highest growth in manufacturing employment albeit in the informal sector. In fact, a significant increase in casualisation of workers in rural West Bengal and increase in the dominance of self-employment activities in the urban areas with a concomitant stagnation in regular salaried employment in urban areas was observed (ibid.). This is also reflected in the usual principal activities status of the migrants in both rural and urban areas (Table 19.5).

The migrants in rural West Bengal are mostly engaged as 'casual labour' followed by 'self-employed' category. On the other hand, migrants in urban areas are mostly either engaged in 'regular waged/salaried jobs' or are 'self-employed'. A larger presence of male migrants in the 'regular wage/salary earning' category reflects the positive impact of migration on economic status. The dominance of self-employment besides 'regular wage/salaried jobs' of male migrants is also noticeable. As male migrants in urban areas are unable to find productive paid employment, they engage themselves in self-employment.

Next, classification of migrants according to social groups (i.e., ST, SC, OBC and 'others' categories) and percentage of migrants among these social categories (Table 19.6), revealed that rate of migration was highest in SC

Table 19.5 Percentage Distribution of Migrants by Usual Principal Activity Status for Different Categories in West Bengal (2007–08)

Usual Principle Activity Status	Persons		Males		Females	
	Rural	Urban	Rural	Urban	Rural	Urban
Self-employed	3.8	6.4	24-.1	14.8	1.9	2
Regular waged/salaried	0.8	8.1	7.2	20.4	0.2	1.7
Casual labour	4.4	3.4	22.0	8.3	2.7	0.8
Total employed	9.1	17.8	53.3	43.5	4.9	4.5
Unemployed	0.5	7.3	3.8	19.7	0.2	0.8
Not in labour force	90.2	74.8	42.7	36.8	94.6	94.5

Source: 64th round of NSS Report No. 533: Migration in India: July 2007–June 2008.

Table 19.6 Percentage of Migrants in Different Social Groups in West Bengal (2007–08)

Social groups	Persons			Males			Females		
	All	Rural	Urban	All	Rural	Urban	All	Rural	Urban
ST	5.9	5.3	0.6	3.7	2.5	1.2	6.3	5.8	0.5
SC	28.6	22.3	6.3	26.0	13.5	12.5	29.0	23.9	5.1
OBC	7.7	5.8	1.9	7.4	2.7	4.7	7.7	6.3	1.4
Others	57.8	38.2	19.6	62.8	19.9	42.9	56.9	41.6	15.3

Source: Computed from unit-level data of 64th round of NSS.

category after 'others' category in case of total population, total male and total female and also in both rural and urban areas. On the other hand, ST was the least mobile social group overall and it had comparatively higher mobility in rural areas. In fact, rural areas had a greater overall mobility than that was in urban areas for all social groups. This holds true in case of female migration also for social groups. But in case of male migration, greater mobility is observed in urban areas compared to rural areas for all the social groups.

To sum up, we can say that mostly migrants are characterised by land-lessness or low landholding, illiterate or educated up to primary and middle school and major reasons are work and education, reflecting the fact that in-migration in West Bengal is used as a better livelihood strategy.

NSS data pertaining to 'monthly per capita consumption expenditure' (MPCE) of both rural and urban migrants/households, separately, is presented in Figure 19.8. We have observed that the migration rate (i.e., percentage of migrants) was lower in lower 'monthly per capita expenditure (MPCE)' classes, which actually increases steadily with the increase in income ranges. Thus, the highest migration rate was observed in the highest MPCE class in both rural and urban areas. Similar trend is observed in the case of male migrants also. The above observation is not clinching evidence that economically better off people are more likely to migrate to avail new economic opportunities elsewhere, since reported expenditure levels reflect post-migration situation (Kundu and Sarangi, 2007).

If we combine the above two sections of migration rates among various 'MPCE' classes and 'landholdings' classes, we can conclude that migration has had a positive impact on living conditions of migrants. The migrants predominantly belonged to 'landless' and 'marginal landholdings' classes

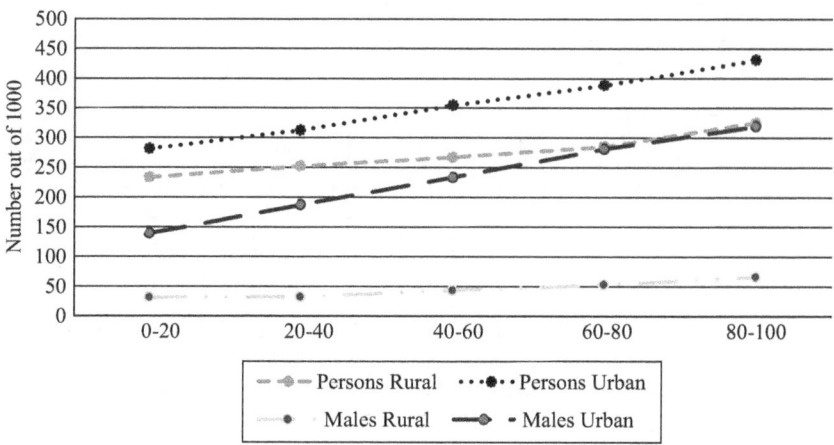

Figure 19.8 Migration rates for rural and urban in across MPCE Quintile Classes.
Source: 64th Round of NSS Report No. 533.

and they might have improved their economic status by belonging to higher MPCE classes after migration (i.e., in post-migration period) than non-migrants. Also, the larger presence of male migrants in the 'regular wage/salary earning' category explains the higher presence of male migrants in higher MPCE classes.

A broader division of population into 'poorest', 'relatively poor', 'middle class' and 'rich' categories has further strengthened our earlier observations that migrants were better off as compared to non-migrants. A larger proportion of male and female migrants were in 'middle class' and 'rich' categories than that were for non-migrants which means that migrants are economically better off than non-migrants.(Figure19.9).

After discussing development and migration separately, we have examined the linkage between migration and development in the state. Exploration of relationship in terms of socio-economic parameters pertaining to four sectors' development and 'inter-state' migration is presented in Table 19.7 (a) and (b) showing that 'industry', 'economic infrastructure' and 'social' sectors had significant relationship with inter-state migration at all time points.

On the other hand, agriculture showed statistically insignificant relations at all time points. Thus, it has brought to the fore fact that 'inter-state migration is closely linked with development of socio-economic infrastructure facilities rather than only with 'economic/income reason'. Table 19.7 (b) shows that 'inter-state male migrants' had maintained better relationship with all sectors' development. Strong and stable relationship was observed in industry and social sectors and relationship is significant.

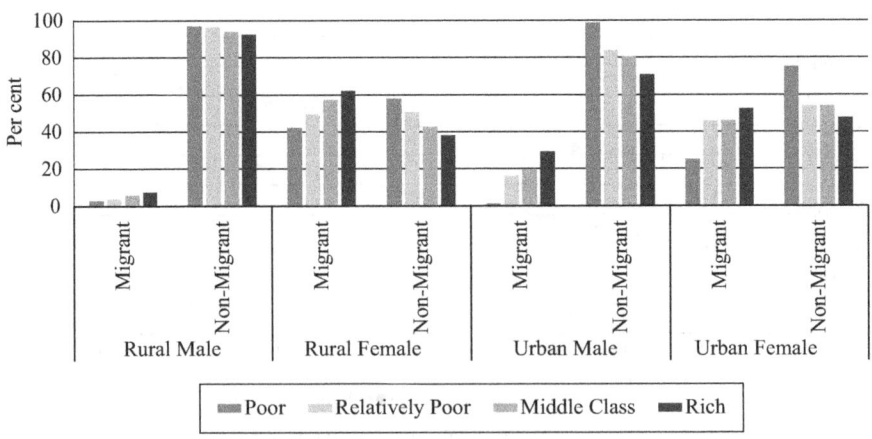

Figure 19.9 Distribution of migrants and non-migrants in different economic status in rural and urban areas in West Bengal, 2007–08.

Source: Computed from unit-level data of 64th round of NSS.

Table 19.7 (a): Coefficient of Correlation (r) between Inter-State Migration and Sectoral Indices of Development of Districts for 1971–2011

Census Year	Sectoral Indices of Development (PCA)			
	Agriculture	Industry	Economic Infrastructure	Social Sector
1971	0.37	0.67 (3.38)*	0.84 (5.20)*	0.67 (3.34)*
1981	0.42	0.80 (4.98)*	0.73 (4.03)*	0.72 (3.89)*
1991	0.34	0.57 (2.54)*	0.64 (3.13)*	0.65 (3.22)*
2001	0.43	0.69 (3.61)*	0.71 (3.82)*	0.81 (5.09)*
2011	0.24	0.53 (2.32)*	0.45 (1.87)**	0.77 (4.46)*

Source: Author's calculations.

Note: * indicates the value of t-statistic is significant at 5% level of significance.** indicates the value of t-statistic is significant at 10% level of significance.

Table 19.7 (b): Coefficient of Correlation (r) between Inter-state Male Migration and Sectoral Indices of Development of Districts for 1971–2011

Census Year	Sectoral Indices of Development (PCA)			
	Agriculture	Industry	Economic Infrastructure	Social Sector
1971	0.48 (1.99)**	0.73 (4.01)*	0.75 (4.31)*	0.58 (2.69)*
1981	0.57 (2.47)*	0.83 (5.64)*	0.75 (4.28)*	0.75 (4.21)*
1991	0.59 (2.63)*	0.57 (2.61)*	0.51 (2.22)*	0.51 (2.23)*
2001	0.56 (2.45)*	0.74 (4.18)*	0.73 (3.98)*	0.83 (5.64)*
2011	0.47 (1.95)*	0.66 (3.30)*	0.45 (1.89)**	0.82 (5.39)*

Source: Author's calculations.

Note: * indicates value of t-statistic is significant at 5% level of significance. ** indicates value of t-statistic is significant at 10% level of significance.

In fact, in the case of the social sector, the relationship with inter-state migration grew stronger over years as the value of correlation coefficient increased from 0.48 per cent in 1971 to 0.82 per cent in 2011. On the other hand, economic infrastructure showed a strong relationship with inter-district migration, but its relationship grew weaker as coefficient of correlation declined from 0.75 per cent in 1971 to 0.45 per cent in 2011. Also, inter-state male migration showed a statistically significant positive relationship with agricultural infrastructural development. Initially the agriculture sector in terms of infrastructural development showed a significant relationship at 10 per cent level of significance that had improved to 5 per cent level of significance for the next benchmark years. It has vindicated that 'inter-state' migration, particularly male migration, has strong relationship with economic development in terms of socio-economic development indices for districts of West Bengal.

This explains the fact that besides employment as a criterion for decision, migrants also take into consideration various socio-economic and infrastructural development factors such as transport and communication, banking facility, electricity, education and health facilities in decision-making. This can also mean that migration is not an individual decision but family-oriented decision (Stark, 1984).

Like inter-state migration, inter-district migration had also good relationship with all sectors except the social sector from 1991 onwards and the economic infrastructure sector in 1991 and 2011{Table19.8 (a)}. The relationship between inter-district migration and agriculture improved over the years. However, inter-district male migration maintained better relations with all sectors.

The coefficient of correlation (r) varied between 56 to 68 per cent for agriculture sector in case of 'inter-district male' migration [Table19.8 (b)] whereas, 'r' value varied between 47 to 59 per cent in case of 'inter-state male' migration [Table 19.8 (b)]. Thus, it can be said that the agriculture sector had a better relationship with inter-district male migration than inter-state male migration. The fact that the rural density of population had increased from 371 in 1971 to 761 in 2011 has not left enough space for migrant workers. Besides, the explanation for the lack of relationship between agricultural development and migration for both inter-state and inter-district migrants can be due to the dominance of flow of seasonal migrants to the agricultural sector which is not captured in the official data (Rogaly et al., 2001). However, it can be said that male migration (in both inter-state and inter-district) had better relationship with the level of district development than that was in case of overall 'inter-state' and 'inter-district' migrations which include women also. Thus, these observations have further proved that male migrants are more closely linked with level of development of region rather than those observed in case of overall migrants, which includes women. The implication of this phenomenon is that besides employability, distance also

Table 19.8 (a): Coefficient of Correlation (r) between Inter-District Migration and Sectoral Indices of Development of Districts for 1971–2011

Census Year	Sectoral Indices of Development (PCA)			
	Agriculture	Industry	Economic Infrastructure	Social Sector
1971	0.58	0.55	0.55	0.51
	(2.55)*	(2.49)*	(2.48)*	(2.24)*
1981	0.80	0.52	0.50	0.44
	(4.80)*	(2.28)*	(2.51)*	(1.85)**
1991	0.71	0.39	0.29	0.27
	(3.65)*	(1.56)	(1.15)	(1.05)
2001	0.81	0.53	0.46	0.39
	(5.02)*	(2.35)*	(1.96)**	(1.57)
2011	0.76	0.57	0.04	0.22
	(4.23)*	(2.62)*		

Source: Author's calculations.

Note: * indicates value of t-statistic is significant at 5% level of significance.** indicates value of t-statistic is significant at 10% level of significance.

Table 19.8 (b): Coefficient of Correlation (r) between Inter-District Male Migration and Sectoral Indices of Development of Districts for 1971–2011

Census Year	Sectoral Indices of Development (PCA)			
	Agriculture	Industry	Economic Infrastructure	Social Sector
1971	0.58	0.67	0.72	0.65
	(2.55)*	(3.36)*	(3.92)*	(3.16)*
1981	0.68	0.66	0.56	0.53
	(3.35)*	(3.27)*	(2.51)*	(2.36)*
1991	0.56	0.72	0.66	0.71
	(2.43)*	(3.84)	(3.29)*	(3.73)*
2001	0.62	0.69	0.59	0.56
	(2.82)*	(3.54)*	(2.73)*	(2.53)*
2011	0.60	0.52	0.09	0.36
	(2.69)*	(3.03)*	(0.34)*	

Source: Author's calculations.

Note: * indicates value of t-statistic is significant at 5% level of significance.** indicates value of t-statistic is significant at 10% level of significance.

plays an important role in migration flow. In case of inter-district migration, it has been found that the flow of such migration is mostly from contiguous districts. So, the need for social development in destination weakens as short distance helps in compensating for the disadvantage in case of inter-district migrants.

District-Wise Distribution of International Migration

Besides inflow of 'internal' migrants from neighbouring states, West Bengal also received thousands of 'international' migrants, specially from East Pakistan (Bangladesh), immediately after the partition of erstwhile Bengal province in 1947. Actually, during the Indo-Pak War of 1971, which is also known as the War of Independence of Bangladesh, about one crore people were driven out from East Pakistan, or they fled to India to escape bloody repression of Pakistani soldiers and took shelter in India as refugees (Turner, 2006). Even by a conservative estimate, about 5,00,000 Bangladeshis had come to reside in West Bengal between 1971 and 1981 (Samaddar, 1999). It is natural that cross-border migrants would prefer to settle themselves in border areas until they find suitable alternatives.

West Bengal had 19 districts, out of which ten are bordering districts along Bangladesh, covering a total international border of 4,096 kilometres long (Nanda, 2005). It can be observed that a still higher number of migrants prevailed in bordering districts (Figure 19.10). The growth rates during the first decade after partition of Bengal in 1947 shows an abnormally high growth rate in bordering districts. The bordering districts of

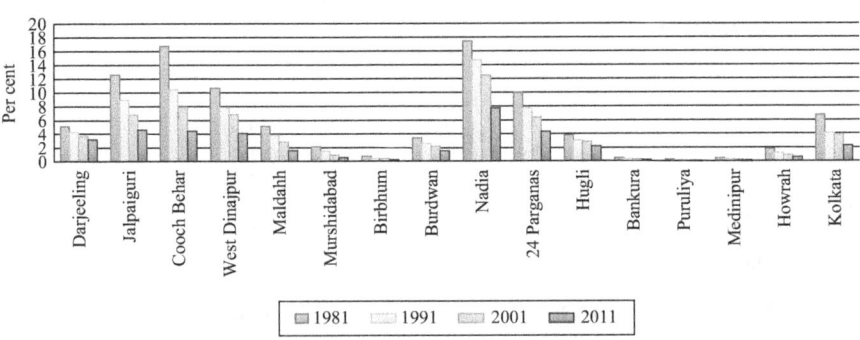

Figure 19.10 Percentage of immigrants from Bangladesh in districts of West Bengal: 1981–2011. *Note:* As per Census of 2011, there were 19 districts after the bifurcation of 3 districts, viz., 24 Parganas, Midnapur and West Dinajpur. In fact, West Bengal is now divided into 23 districts, which includes the newly formed Alipurduar, Kalimpong, Jhargram and the splitting of the former Burdwan district into East Burdwan and West Burdwan.

Sources: Migration Tables of West Bengal, D-I table, Census of India, 1991, 2001 and 2011.

Table 19.9 Results of Regression Equation for Decennial Growth Rates in Population of Districts in West Bengal, 1961–2011

Years	β_0	β_1	β_2	R^2
1961–1971	19.97	6.146E^{-7}	11.09	0.48
	(5.65)	(0.54)	(3.49)*	
1971–1981	18.13	1.284E^{-7}	9.70	0.52
	(6.56)	(0.18)	(3.73)*	
1981–1991	21.47	-2.977E^{-7}	6.230	0.33
	(8.24)	(-0.54)	(2.47)*	
1991–2001	13.65	6.615E^{-9}	8.26	0.55
	(6.34)	(0.02)	(4.02)*	
2001–2011	11.76	-6.81E^{-08}	4.92	0.24
	(4.68)	(-0.19)	(1.98)**	

Source: Author's calculations

Note: Figures in parentheses are the calculated values of t-statistic.
Crtical value of 't' at 5 per cent level of significance with 13 d.f. is 2.16.
* and ** indicates significance at 5 per cent level and 10 per cent level of significance, respectively.

Jalpaiguri, Cooch Behar and Nadia had very high growth rates. The lowest growth rate of 8.48 per cent was in Kolkata during this decade. Thus, to examine whether bordering districts have a tendency to grow at a faster rate than a non-bordering district, we have run regression equation taking decadal 'population growth rates' in districts as independent variable and 'population size' of district in the base year and a dummy variable (D) for bordering districts as explanatory variables and presented in Table 19.9.

The regression results show that bordering districts in West Bengal had higher population growth rates than was observed in non-bordering districts. If two districts are of the same population size, then a bordering district had grown at 11.09 percentage points higher than a non-bordering district during the decade of the 1960s (1961–71). During the 1990s (1991–2001) population in bordering districts grew at 8.26 percentage points higher than that was in non-bordering districts. The magnitude further came down to 4.92 in the last period of 2001–11. The probable reason for explaining higher growth rates in bordering districts could be that more people might have migrated from neighbouring Bangladesh and settled down in these bordering districts resulting in higher population growth rates. Again, international migrants in West Bengal did not have any relation with the sectoral development of districts. As stated earlier, 'safety and security' of their lives were their main concern (Table 19.10).

The international migrants (mainly, Bangladeshis) have settled down in border districts irrespective of their level of development as 'safety' and 'security' of their lives appears to be main concerns to them.

Table 19.10 Coefficient of Correlation (r) between International Migration and Sectoral Indices of Development of Districts for 1971–2011

Census Year	Sectoral Indices of Development (PCA)			
	Agriculture	Industry	Economic Infrastructure	Social Sector
1971	N.A.	N.A.	N.A.	N.A.
1981	-0.09	-0.30	-0.04	-0.18
1991	-0.18	-0.10	-0.14	-0.14
2001	-0.26	-0.06	-0.05	-0.06
2011	-0.15	-0.10	-0.24	-0.05

Source: Author's calculations.

Conclusion

Analysing the type of migration in West Bengal showed that over the study period inter-state migration has been replaced by inter-district migration. Nearly 40 per cent of inter-district migrants resided in five districts of West Bengal, namely Burdwan, Hugli, Howrah, 24 Parganas and Nadia. These districts were either industrially or agriculturally developed districts. The picture becomes clearer when 'male' migration, which is presumably more economic in nature, appears to have a better relationship with the level of development of districts. Besides economic reasons, 'distance' also acts as an important factor for inter-district migration as it was observed that most districts (except Kolkata and Darjeeling) received a higher proportion of inter-district migrants from their contiguous districts. It has been observed that the concentration of 'inter-state' migration was in developed districts of West Bengal. Proportion of inter-state migrants was also higher in the same districts as was in case of inter-district migrants. Darjeeling and Jalpaiguri districts, which are hilly districts in northern part of West Bengal, have occupied high ranks in terms of receiving 'inter-state' migrants though it has lost their pre-eminence in recent times due to the closure of several of its tea gardens. Bordering districts of West Bengal, sharing a border with Bangladesh, has been home to a larger proportion of international migrants. Nadia district has received the highest proportion of immigrants from Bangladesh. However, over the period of the study, a steady decline in international migration has been observed in West Bengal. Mostly the migrants are characterised by landlessness and lower level of education (education up to secondary). Males migrate for economic reasons like 'employment' and they prefer urban areas of economically developed districts of West Bengal.

After examining all relationships between various types of migration and development of different socio-economic sectors of districts in West Bengal through correlation analysis, it has been found that there is a strong linkage between socio-economic development of a district and migration.

Agriculture development appears to have a weaker relationship with migration which can be either due to high density of rural population or nature of migration of agricultural workers, who are seasonal or circular in nature and so are not captured by the official data. Thus, these findings have supported the 'developmentalists' modernisation theory (i.e., economic development attracts the migrants) and have also, to some extent, validated the 'modernisation theory' in case of West Bengal. Over the period of the study, social sector development has been becoming strongly correlated with male inter-state migration compared to male inter-district migration. Finally, international migration in West Bengal had no relation with any types of sectoral development at the district level.

Acknowledgements

This chapter is part of the PhD thesis submitted to Jawaharlal Nehru University, New Delhi. I am thankful to Professors Anuradha Banerjee and Deepak Kumar Mishra for their support and guidance.

Note

1 As there is no cultivable land in the district of Kolkata, West Bengal, we have considered the remaining 15 districts for the analysis of development in this sector.

References

Chattoraj, K. K., & Chand, S. (2015). Literacy trend of West Bengal and its differentials: A district level analysis. *IOSR Journal of Humanities and Social Science (IOSR-JHSS)*, 20(9), 1–19.

Chowdhury, S., & Chakraborty, S. (2016). Employment growth in West Bengal: An assessment. Institute of Development Studies Kolkata, Working Paper-52, 1–41.

Development and Planning Department. (2004). Human Development Report of West Bengal. Government of West Bengal, Kolkata.

Dyson, T., & Visaria, P. (2004). Migration and urbanization, retrospect and prospects. In T. Dyson, R. Cassen, & L. Visaria (Eds.), *Twenty first century India* (pp. 108–129). New Delhi: Oxford University Press.

Kundu, A., & Sarangi, N. (2007). Migration, employment status and poverty: An analysis across urban centres. *Economic and Political Weekly*, 42(4), 299–306.

Nanda, A. K. (2005). Emigration from Bangladesh to India. *Asian and Pacific Migration Journal*, 14(4), 487–500.

Rogaly, B., Biswas, J., Coppard, D., Rafique, A., Rana, K., & Sengupta, A. (2001). Seasonal migration, social change and migrants' rights: Lessons from West Bengal. *Economic and Political Weekly*, 36(49), 4547–4559.

Samaddar, R. (1999). *The marginal nation: Transborder migration from Bangladesh to West Bengal*. New Delhi: Sage Publication.

Sarkar, J. P. (2010). Cross-border migration in developing countries. In S. Irudaya Rajan (Ed.), *Governance and labour migration: India migration report 2010*. New Delhi: Routledge, 113–133.

Stark, O. (1984). Migration decision making: A review article. *Journal of Development Economics, 14*, 251–259.

Turner, B. (2006). *The statesman's yearbook 2006*. New York: Palgrave Macmillan.

20 Migration, Remittances and Welfare

A Study of Ratnagiri District of Rural Maharashtra

Bhupesh Gopal Chintamani

Introduction

Income imbalances amongst the countries and also within the countries have been very much prevalent throughout the world. The role played by international remittances in bridging the income dispersion of the households within countries, both at the micro and macro level, is of paramount importance. At the macro level, impact of remittances on the country's macroeconomic indicators like growth rate of gross domestic product (GDP), exchange rate stability, import and export deficit, etc. have well been documented (Nayyar,1994; Jadhav, 2003;Ratha, 2003; Chami et al., 2005;Gupta, 2006;Ratha and Mohapatra, 2007; Mallick, 2008; Singh and Hari, 2011;Guha, 2013a). On the other hand, some studies at the level of single and multiple countries suggest that remittances reduce poverty dynamics in the recipient countries (Adams and Page, 2003; Adams, 2004; Adams and Page, 2005; Muhammad and Ahmed, 2009; Ahmed et al., 2010; Day, 2015). According to the World Bank (2021) report, India received remittances to the tune of $83 billion which is the highest within all the recipient countries. In India, Kerala receives the maximum share of inward remittances; which has resulted in higher per capita income and also dramatically altered the consumption patterns of the state. All the aforementioned facts have earned the state an alternative name as remittance state(Kannan and Hari, 2002; Zachariah and Rajan, 2007; 2010; Rajan and Zachariah, 2010; 2019)

The economic impact of remittances on the overall well-being of Kerala has driven the study to inquire about such micro-level impacts in the state of Maharashtra which is the second-largest remittance-receiving state as of today (RBI, 2018). According to Taylor (1999) choice of emigration might be a decision taken by the individual members, but other household features like the number of members in the household, socio-economic conditions also play an essential role in the decision-making of the out-migrants. Extensive studies have been undertaken to understand the impact of remittances on the states of Kerala, Punjab, Goa, Gujarat, Andhra Pradesh, and Bihar by (Zachariah et al., 2002a; 2002b; Zachariah et al., 2003;

DOI: 10.4324/9781003315124-20

Sasikumar and Hussain, 2007; Kapuria, 2018; Kaur, 2018; Parida et al., 2015; Guha,2013b; Mohanty et al., 2014; Dey, 2015; Chintamani, 2017).

Data and Methodology

As mentioned in the NSSO report 64th round report 2007–08 (NSSO, 2010), the Ratnagiri district reports a very high proportion of out-migration. The study has carried out a pilot survey, visited all Block Development Officers (BDO), Panchayat Officers (PO), and Directorate of Economics and Statistics (DES) office for understanding the data sufficiency for the sample collection. It has used census 2011 enumeration data to randomly select blocks based on the lottery method. From each selected block, five villages and within each village, ten emigrants and non-migrant sample households were randomly selected. The snowball method had been used for identifying household level sample units and finalized with the listing schedule with specified conditions.

Socio-economic Profile of Out-migrants of Ratnagiri District of Rural Maharashtra

The Ratnagiri district performs much better in the level of economic development indicators such as educational attainment, gender sex ratio, and child sex ratio. According to Gogate (1991), the region is well connected to the flow of immigrants to gulf countries and dominated by Muslim households overall.

Household Characteristics

In total, 180 sample households have been interviewed, out of which 82 households are from Guhagar and 98 households are from Dapoli. In the selected sample villages, in total (including Guhagar and Dapoli) 50.56 per cent of sample households come under the OPEN category, 37 per cent in OBC group, and the remaining belong to NT, SC, and SC groups (Table 20.1). It has also been noticed that a small percentage of sample households belong to other social groups such as Schedule Caste (SC) (5 per cent), Nomadic Tribes (NT) (3.89 per cent), and Schedule Tribes (ST) (3.33 per cent). The social group representation suggests that NT, SC, and ST groups have also migrated internationally, which has not been seen earlier.

Though, they are significantly less in number when compared to other social groups in participated survey respondents; it is expected to increase in the coming years. Overall, it confirms that international migration is high among OPEN and OBC social groups while another social group such as NT, SC, and ST carries less number of migrants.[1]

The structure of the family is almost identical across both types of sample households. Further, of the total number of respondent categories, 46

Table 20.1 Sample Households Representation as per Social Groups

Household Social Group	Guhagar Tehsil	Dapoli Tehsil	Total	Migrant	Non-Migrant
Open	44 (53.66)	47 (47.96)	91 (50.56)	48 (54.55)	43 (46.74)
OBC	27 (32.93)	40 (40.82)	67 (37.22)	32 (36.36)	35 (38.04)
NT	1 (1.22)	6 (6.12)	7 (3.89)	3 (3.41)	4 (4.35)
SC	6 (7.32)	3 (3.06)	9 (5.00)	2 (2.27)	7 (7.61)
ST	4 (4.88)	2(2.04)	6 (3.33)	3 (3.41)	3 (3.26)
Total	82 (100.0)	98 (100.0)	180 (100.0)	88 (100.0)	92 (100.0)

Source: Authors' calculation based on field survey (2018–19). Note: Parenthesis considered to be percentages.

Table 20.2 Sample Household Basic Characteristics in the Sample Groups

Primary Information of Household	Migrant Household		Non-Migrant Household	
	Count	Percent	Count	Percent
Gender (Respondent)				
Male	29	33.0	53	57.6
Female	59	67.0	39	42.4
Family Type				
Join	66	72.72	69	75.0
Nuclear	24	27.27	23	25.0
Gender (Head of Household)				
Male	38	43.2	75	81.5
Female	50	56.8	17	18.5
Age-old members above 60 years				
Yes	45	51.1	37	40.2
No	43	48.9	55	59.8
Children (Age 0-6) composition				
Yes	28	31.81	19	20.7
No	60	68.18	73	79.3
Religion				
Hindu	25	28.4	21	22.8
Muslim	58	65.9	64	69.6
Buddhism	5	5.7	7	7.6
Total	88	100.0	92	100.0

Source: Authors' calculation based on field survey (2018–19).

per cent are male and 54 per cent are female. In the case of sample households of migrants, 33 per cent are male and 67 per cent are female and in the case of non-migrant, 58 per cent are male and 42 per cent are female (Table 20.2). These results indicate that a large number of female-headed households exist over the total sample and also follows only for a migrant household. Table 20.2 represents the gender head of the household categorized according to the status of migration.

This result supports the argument that female-headed households are more in number only in the migrant household and males are predominant in non-migrant households. The members in the household whose age is above 60 years old are captured as 51 per cent in the migrant household as compared to 40 per cent in a non-migrant household. Therefore, it can be concluded that the rise in the number of old age members leads to more remittances being sent by the migrant. Moreover, children under the age group of 0 to 6 years have occupied one-third proportion in the total sample household.

Descriptive Statistics of Sample Household

The discussion of the household-related descriptive statistics has been presented in Table 20.3. The mean size of the household is almost the same among migrant and non-migrant households in the two tehsils of Ratnagiri district.

However, there are minor differences in the mean size of households between migrant (4.49) and non-migrant (5.13) households, in Guhagar (4.38 and 5.31) and most likely to be the same in Dapoli (4.58 and 4.98). There is a slight difference in the age of the head of the household (53.61 years) in migrant and (51.50 years) in the non-migrant household; also a lower level split between the mean age of the respondent (46.64 years) in migrant and (44.11 years) in the non-migrant household. Thus, the above-mentioned variables (result) are more or less similar among control (non-migrant) and non-control (migrant) sample households. The mean annual income of the household without remittances for a sample of migrant households is ₹73,563 whereas for Guhagar ₹75,400 and Dapoli ₹72,407; for non-migrant households, it is ₹1,26,969 whereas for Guhagar ₹1,06,733 and Dapoli ₹1,43,968. It shows that the annual income of non-migrant households is far ahead and is approximately double that of migrant household income without remittances. Thus, annual income with remittances in the migrant household compared to the non-migrant household is substantially higher and almost double; in the case of Guhagar, it is more than double. Thus, results indicate that inward remittances increases the share of income of migrant households compared to non-migrant household income.

Result signifies that remittances do not only improve household income but also change other paradigms at the household level which would indirectly benefit the rural market dynamics (changing aspect of demand). In response to the most preferred income source of the family, the data suggests that remittance income (87 per cent) is the only most desired source of income among migrant households, in Guhagar (89 per cent) and Dapoli (85 per cent). Non-agricultural income remarkably stands as the second most favored source of income (25 per cent) for migrant households, in Guhagar (26 per cent) and Dapoli (25 per cent). However, agricultural income was stated as the least source of income (11 per cent), and in Guhagar (6 per cent) and Dapoli (15 per cent). The non-agricultural income comprises income from the business, trading, SME, salary, etc., and agriculture income comprises wage income. However, it is observed that the result of

Table 20.3 Descriptive Statistics of Sample Household

Remittance receiving household characteristics	Gubagar Tehsil (40)		Dapoli Tehsil (48)		Total (88)	
	Mean	SD	Mean	SD	Mean	SD
Household size	4.38	2.00	4.58	1.44	4.49	1.72
Age of the respondents	45.75	12.53	47.38	16.25	46.64	14.62
Age of the head of households	50.95	15.13	55.83	13.48	53.61	14.38
Annual income without remittance	75,400.00	33600.45	72407.41	77781.72	73563.64	63878.00
Annual income with remittance	2,25,295.00	1,18,727.54	2,07,645.83	1,00,544.98	2,15,668.18	1,08,896.55
Annual expenditure of household	1,52,364.50	96,454.44	1,39,959.38	62,990.45	1,45,598.07	79,703.39

Non-remittance receiving household characteristics	Gubagar Tehsil (42)		Dapoli Tehsil (50)		Total (92)	
	Mean	SD	Mean	SD	Mean	SD
Household size	5.31	1.41	4.98	1.19	5.13	1.29
Age of the respondents	43.07	13.17	44.98	9.54	44.11	11.32
Age of head of the household	50.02	12.43	52.74	10.83	51.50	11.60
Annual income of the household	1,06,733.33	40,200.80	1,43,968.00	55,288.22	1,26,969.57	52,171.47
Annual expenditure of the household	89,741.19	22,682.34	99,849.32	34,959.91	95,234.74	30,257.84

Source: Authors' calculation based on field survey (2018–19).

the non-migrant household is completely different where their most favored source of income is agricultural income and non-agricultural income is the second most important preference. It is also experienced that some of the household income is fully dependent on remittances.

Demographic Profile of Migrant (Emigrant)

International remittances have been an essential part of driving economic growth in India. The demographic and socio-economic characteristics of the migrant household have a fundamental element to incorporate remittances character among recipient households (Sisenglath, 2009; Sil, 2011).

Age Representation of Expatriate

Previous studies have emphasized that youth among all age groups in the household get attracted to emigration (Sil, 2011;Singh, 2011). It is observed that the government never encourages its citizens to out-migration, but immigration policy restriction probably leads to illegal expatriates from home countries (Khadria and Meyar, 2013).

Table 20.4 evaluates that before migration, young age among all individuals is higher, which is more than 20 per cent in the categories of 21–25 years of age followed by 26–30 and 31–35 years of age group. Similarly, the present age of migrants is higher in the category of 35–40 years of age and 40–45 years of age group. Young age individuals up to the category of 35-year age constitute 80 per cent, before migration wave where it constitutes only 30 per cent after migration status. On the other hand, middle aged and old age migrants under the age group of 36–55 years constitute 20 per cent of the migration wave before migration and 70 per cent after migration status.

Over the years, the age group status of out-migrants reveals that the present mean age of the expatriate is only 39 years of age as compared to 29 years of age before out-migration. The study finding is in-line with the

Table 20.4 Age of Expatriates Before and After Migration

Age Before Migration	Frequency	Percent	Cumulative Percent	Age after Migration	Frequency	Percent	Cumulative Percent
18–20	9	10.2	10.2	18–20	0	0.0	0.0
21–25	22	25.0	35.2	21–25	3	3.4	3.4
26–30	21	23.9	59.1	26–30	13	14.8	18.2
31–35	18	20.5	79.5	31–35	10	11.4	29.5
36–40	14	15.9	95.5	36–40	25	28.4	58.0
41–45	3	3.4	98.9	41–45	17	19.3	77.3
46–50	1	1.1	100.0	46–50	9	10.2	87.5
50–55	0	0.0	0.0	50–55	11	12.5	100.0
Total	88	100.0	Mean = 28.94	Total	88	100.0	Mean = 39.49

Source: Authors' calculation based on field survey (2018–19).

previous study's results (Sil, 2011; Singh, 2011; Guha 2013b). Finally, we may conclude that 80 per cent of the migrants belong to the young age group before migration and 70 per cent of migrants belong to the middle and old age group after migration.

Marital Status of Expatriates

The profile of migrant marital status before and after has been presented in the Figure 20.1. Significant proportions of migrants are unmarried before migration, and a substantial per cent of them got married after the migration process. It has been observed that 47 per cent of out-migrants are married and 53 per cent are unmarried migrants before migration in the overall sample (migrant) household. After the migration process, it has been observed that marital status has changed and increased up to 86 per cent among out-migrant individuals in the total sample (migrant) household. These findings are more consistent with the earlier studies of (Guha, 2013b,Sil, 2011; Nayar, 2002).

Family Status of Expatriates

Figure 20.2 suggests that 57 per cent of migrant households are headed by females, including left behind wives (27 per cent) and left behind mothers (30 per cent), and 43 per cent by males . In the total sample, a higher number of a household headed by females indicates female autonomy in migrant households. Further, female decision autonomy has improved and played a major role in household spending and non-spending choices. The above finding matches with some previous studies (Guha, 2013b; Sasikumar and Hussain, 2007; Sil, 2011, etc.).

It is also noticed that in the out-migrant profile, there is no female migrant so far in the study area, which is different from existing studies such as Kerala, Punjab, Gujarat migrant perseverance of female subordinates

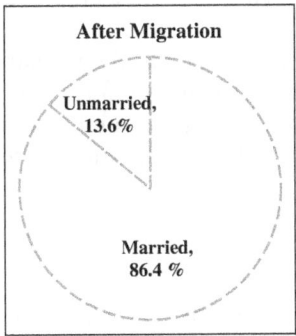 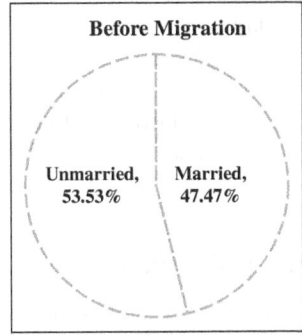

Figure 20.1 Marital status of migrants.

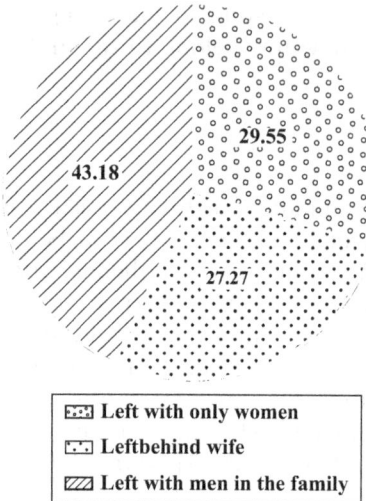

Figure 20.2 Family status of migrants.

(Zachariah and Rajan, 2007; Kapuria, 2018:Kaur, 2018; Guha, 2013b, Chintamani, 2017).

Education Status of Expatriates

The previous studies point out that having a low education level and higher expectations somehow assists the migrant individual to take a prominent decision for migration and sending remittances to their households. It is found from Figure 20.3 that the majority of the migrants had a secondary level of schooling (53.4 per cent). In the case of the Guhagar it was (63 per cent) and Dapoli (40 per cent). The second-most level of education attainment is the higher secondary level with 21.6 per cent. For Guhagar it was (11 per cent) and for Dapoli it was (30 per cent).

However, the third-most level of education is understood in the primary level of schooling (13.5 per cent), whereas Guhagar consists (14.3 per cent) and Dapoli (17.5 per cent). Finally, graduation and above type of education is seen to be 11.4 per cent, whereas for Guhagar (11.4 per cent) and Dapoli (12.5 per cent).

Present Destination of Migrants

Figure 20.4 below shows those out-migrant destination countries from Ratnagiri, where it is observed that the selected region favors Middle East countries as a traditional destination for migration. From the destination it is clear that none of the immigrants from Middle East countries have taken

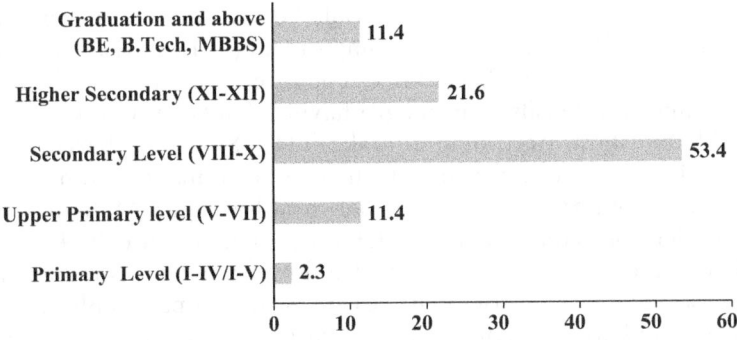

Figure 20.3 Education status of migrants.

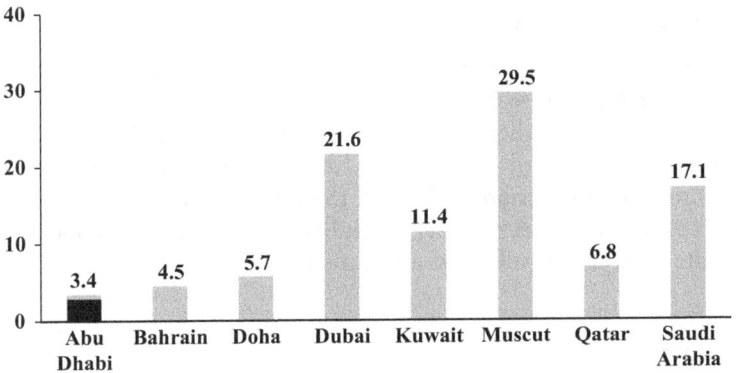

Figure 20.4 Destination of migrants from sample households.

permanent or resident citizenship, which suggests these migrants will come back to their home country after their work visas get expired. The destination chosen by the migrant also helps in forming formidable relationships with these countries for the home country.

Further, it is observed that among the GCC countries, Oman (Muscat) is the most favored country followed by United Arab Emirate (UAE) (comprising Abu Dhabi and Dubai), Kingdom of Saudi Arabia, and Kuwait, etc., for the expatriate from Dapoli and Guhagar tehsils at Ratnagiri. An interesting fact to know is that UAE and Oman are the most favored destinations for Guhagar immigrants, whereas UAE, Saudi Arabia are the most favored destinations for Dapoli immigrants among GCC countries. Currently, a substantial change in the form of emigration policy has been made by the Ministry of Overseas and Indian Affairs (MOIA), Government of India, to provide social security to the migrants in the host country. The existing out-migrant cluster suggests a cultural, religious, and traditional factor that is very much traceable for Muslim individuals. Thus, it indicates that the present set of skills occupied by out-migrants could be a reason that they immigrate only to these GCC countries. According to RBI (2018), India received the largest remittance inflow from GCC countries. Hence, Dapoli and Guhagar are important tehsils of Ratnagiri having significant international migrants in Maharashtra. According to Prakash (1998) and Zachariah and Rajan (2015), Kerala is fully dependent on remittance money from GCC countries: likewise, our analysis suggests that rural Ratnagiri, Maharashtra is partly dependent on remittances from GCC countries (Figure 20.4). It is expected that in the coming year, emigrant inflow from rural Ratnagiri is expected to rise to GCC countries. The reason is the strong establishment of new refineries and power plant planned projects by states and investment from these GCC countries in the respective projects, which might lead to improving labor bonding among these countries.

Occupation Structure of Expatriates

The detailed analysis of occupation structure before and after has been discussed and presented in Figure 20.5.

Figure 20.5 reveals that there is a substantial shift from being unemployed to becoming employed workmen. Also, there is a significant large-scale jump in unskilled expatriates. Overall, the falling cases of semi-skilled human resources and forceful increase in skilled manpower is a good sign compared to the occupation status of migrants before migration.

Mode of Transfers

Table 20.6 displays that young migrants send more money than money sent by longer stayed migrants. In the present study, money transferred through banking services (48 per cent) was observed to be the most preferred root

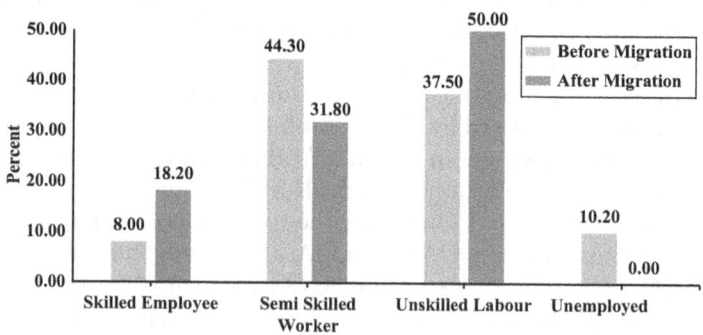

Figure 20.5 Occupation structure of migrants.

of transfer among all kinds of transfers. Money transferred through Non-resident Rupee Account (NRI A/c) (23 per cent) for the recipient household recorded to be the second-most choice of migrants. Further, Money Transfer Operator (MTO) (16 per cent) is seen to be the third favorite route of transfer. Automated Teller Machine (ATM) (5 per cent) is the last course of action in the mode of payment, however, money carried personally by an individual migrant is very minimal (8 per cent) in general Table 20.5.

Surprisingly, there is no mode of transfer through relatives, draft or cheque, and post office deposits. A few years ago, the Konkan division is known as the "money ordered economy" because several migrants households received money from their migrants through post office services (the most favored source) followed by the draft, cheques, and visiting relatives, which has declined at present. The technological improvement in the banking system has changed the route of transfer payment and the reduction in the transaction cost led using formal channels by the migrants. Subsequently, it has been observed that a substantial amount of inward inflow is now operated via the formal route (90.9 per cent). In the past, informal sources of remittance transfer like "hundi" or "hawala" networks have been one of the preferred ways. The informal person is an agent who delivers money at the doorstep of the recipient household. It is a less time-consuming process compared to the banking sector. Of the sample, 34 per cent of households revealed that they receive goods in kind. Goods sent by migrants include electronic items,

Table 20.5 Mode of Transfer Information

Particulars	Frequency	Percent	Cumulative
Mode of transfers			
Direct bank A/c	42	47.7	47.7
Automated Teller Machine	5	5.7	53.4
Money Transfer Operator (MTO)	14	15.9	69.3
NRI bank A/c	20	22.7	92.0
Money send to relative	0	0.0	00.0
Daft/cheque	0	0.0	00.0
Post office	0	0.0	00.0
Carried by migrant	7	8.0	100.0
The preferred source of income			
Formal	80	90.9	90.9
Informal	8	9.1	100.0
Any transferred through informal			
No	83	94.3	94.3
Yes	5	5.7	100.0
Received in kind of goods			
Yes	30	34.1	34.1
No	58	65.9	100.0
Total	88	100.0	100.0

Source: Authors' calculation based on field survey (2018–19).

ornaments, jewelry items, perfume, and biscuits, etc. It all expresses the need of migrant households which get fulfilled with various means of exchange, including money and non-money market of transfers by an expatriate.

Impact of Remittance on Various Types of Expenditure using MANOVA

Methodology

The chapter also captures the remittance association with the select baskets of household expenditures. Thus, univariate regression analysis has been performed separately for food, education, and health expenditure which shows a positive and significant relationship with the dependent (remittance) variable. Further multivariate analysis of variance (MANOVA) test[2] has been carried out for the same variables to understand the essence of univariate results. Thus, independent and dependent are replaced with (categorical variable) three groups of households and a select basket of household expenditure (food, education, and health). Three groups of households are international remittance recipient households (IREM), domestic remittance recipient households (DOREM), and non-receiving remittance households (NIREM). The idea is to check if there are any statistical differences between household groups on combinations of selected expenditure of the household.[3]

Results and Discussion

In the multivariate tests, it has focused on the "Wilks Lambda" test of statistics to determine whether the one-way MANOVA was significant or not. However, the significance value of $P = 0.000$, which implies $P < 0.05$. Therefore, we can conclude that given types of household expenditure depend on types (categories) of households, they belong ($P < 0.05$) as per results.[4] To determine whether the dependent variable differs from the independent variable, the next between-household effects illustrate what types of household have a statistically significant effect on all the three dependent variables ($P < 0.05$). However, food is significant at 1 per cent level of significance, and health and education are significant at 5 per cent level of significance. Health expenditure becomes highly significant compared to education expenditure. About the dependent variable of food, education, and health expenditure, they are our test hypothesis, as follows for multiple comparisons of Tukey's HSD post-hoc test.

Multiple Comparison of Hypothesis

1. There is no mean difference between the household groups on food spending.
2. There is no mean difference between the household groups on health spending.

3. There is no mean difference between the household groups on education spending.

Table result indicates multiple comparisons of mean scores of health, education, and food, where there are statistically significant differences between the NIREM and IREM household (P<0.05) and between DOREM and IREM household (P<0.05), but not between the NIREM and DOREM household (P>0.05). In the case of *food expenditure*, there are statistically significant differences between the mean group of NIREM and the mean group of IREM (P=0.000 < 0.05), and between-group DOREM and group IREM (P=0.007 < 0.05), but there are no statistically significant differences between group NIREM and group DOREM (P=0.492 > 0.05). Similarly, for the **health expenditure**, the mean group NREM has statistically significant differences between the group IREM (P=0.006<0.05) and between group DOREM and group IREM (P = 0.015<0.05), but there is no statistically significant difference between group NIREM and group DOREM (P=0.957>0.05). But, in the case of **education expenditure**, the mean group NIREM has statistically significant differences between group IREM (P=0.069<0.10), and between group DOREM and group IREM (P=0.059<0.10), but there is no statistically significant difference between group NIREM and DOREM (P=0.891>0.10).[5]

Hence, food and health expenditure are significantly at a 5 per cent level (P = 0.05), but education expenditure significant at 10 per cent (P = 0.10), which suggests that education is comparably less effective than health and basic food expenditure.

Conclusion

The present chapter has examined socio-economic characteristics of emigrants and has also tested welfare effects of remittances in the households with the use of different sets of household expenditures. The findings of the study are as follows. First, analysis revealed that emigration has been dominated by Muslim households in total, and social groups of NT, SC, and ST have witnessed their participation in the process of emigration, which was new in the records. Second, significantly large amounts of remittances in the total income of migrant households suggest an improved expenditure pattern in the households that boost rural market dynamics. Thus, inward remittances are the first preference of income for emigrant households in total. However, agriculture and fisheries (Macchi) are a prime source of occupation for non-migrant households. Third, the analysis spotted no female emigrant from the studied region. A momentous shift from unemployed to employed status has been recorded from the pre and post-occupation structure of the emigrant. It also pointed out that Oman (Muscat) is the most favored country amongst the GCC. Improved banking system

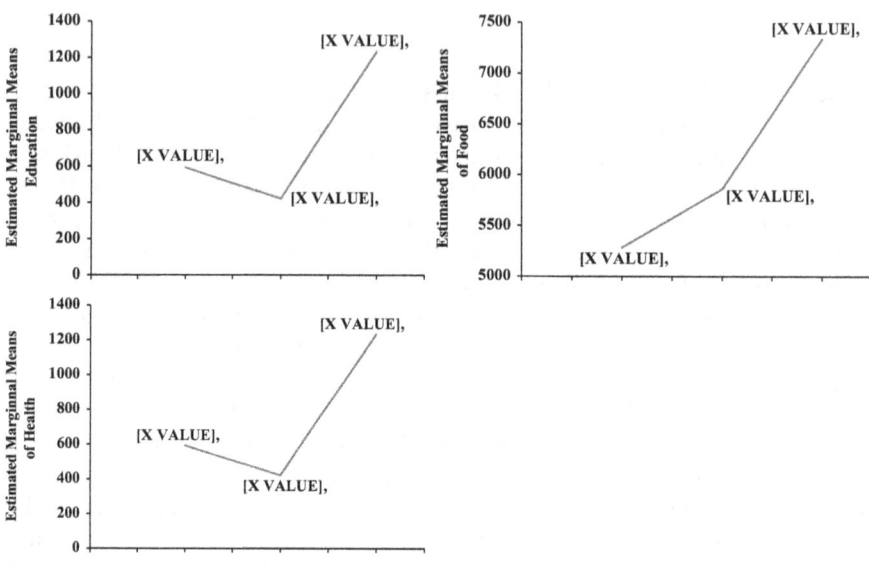

Figure 20.6 Expenditure pattern of the group of households on education, health, and food spending.

increased formal operation of money transfers where direct transfers top NRI account underlined first position. It notes that migrants of Ratnagiri have substantially shifted their money transfer mechanism through banking mode instead of the post office method of transfer.

Finally, overall, it has been found that remittance is utilized more on health and education than consumption expenditure and the study suggests that health expenditure has a crucial component compared to education expenditure among sample households. Moreover, test results have revealed that food and health expenditure are significantly at a 5 per cent level ($P = 0.05$), but education expenditure is significant at 10 per cent ($P = 0.10$), which suggests education is comparably less effective than health and basic food expenditure. Thus, the study concludes that emigrants avail fruitful and bulk of income for respiratory consumption and investment at the rural households which rise welfare and uplift sample households at the end.

Acknowledgements

This paper is a part of the PhD thesis titled "The Economic Aspects of Remittances in India: Post Liberalization" where the author has conducted a primary study in the villages of Dapoli and Guhagar tehsil of Ratnagiri district of rural Maharashtra, India.

Notes

1 In case of ST, it shows higher percentage of out-migrant profile because the percentage has been calculated based on total members in the sample household in specified groups, where the total member representation is minimal.
2 The multivariate analysis of variance (MONOVA) test of statistics performed using SPSS.24 software has been used.
3 MANOVA is helpful to understand the non-parametric test which deals with the Wilks Lambda test of the statistic (Nicola Crichton pp.331)
4 To undergo with the Tukey's HSD post-hoc test within MONOVA, we need three categories of independent variable. Hence, we have created one more group among non-remittance as domestic remittance household (DOREM) which is irregular and inconsistent, has small number within non-remittance household. However, there is no difference in domestic remittance and non-remittance household and such category gives more understanding with graph of Tukey average effect.
5 Among all selected expenditure, food and health is significant at 5 per cent level of significance and education is significant at 10 per cent level of significance.

References

Adams, Jr., R. H. (2004). Remittances and poverty in Guatemala. Available at SSRN 625295.

Adams, R. H., & Page, J. (2003). *International migration, remittances, and poverty in developing countries*. Policy Research Working Paper; No. 3179. Washington: World Bank Publications.

Adams, Jr., R. H., & Page, J. (2005). Do international migration and remittances reduce poverty in development countries? *World Development, 33*(10), 1645–1669.

Ahmed, V., Sugiyarto, G., & Jha, S. (2010). Remittances and household welfare: A case study of Pakistan. Working Paper No.149. *Asian Development Bank.* Tokyo.

Chami, R., Fullenkamp, C., & Jahjah, S. (2005). Are immigrant remittance flows a source of capital for development? IMF Staff Papers, 52(1), Washington, DC: IMF.

Chintamani, B. G. (2017). A study on remittances and development outcomes evidence from India. *GRFDT, 3*(9), 32.

Dey, S. (2015). Impact of remittances on poverty at origin: A study on rural households in India using covariate balancing propensity score matching. *Migration and Development, 4*(2), 185–199.

Gogate, S. (1991). Impact of migration to the Middle East on rural Ratnagiri. *Konkan New, 6*(2), April-June 2014.

Gupta, P. (2006). Macroeconomic determinants of remittances: Evidence from India. *Economic and Political Weekly, 41*(26), 2769–2775.

Guha, P. (2013a). Macroeconomic effects of international remittances: The case of developing economies. *Economic Modelling, 33*, 292–305.

Guha, P. (2013b). Migrants' private giving and development: Diasporic influences on development in central Gujarat, India (No. id: 5594).

Jadhav, N. (2003, October). Maximising developmental benefits of migrant remittances: The Indian experience. In Joint Conference of DFID-World Bank, London.

Kannan, K. P., & Hari, K. S. (2002). Kerala's gulf connection: Emigration, remittances and their macroeconomic impact, 1972–2000. Centre for Development Studies Working Paper No. 328.

Kapuria, S. (2018). International migration from Punjab and challenges for governance. *Punjab University Research Journal of Art*, *XLV*(1), 1–19.

Kaur, A. P. (2018). International migration and impact of remittances on left behind wives: A case study of the doaba region of Punjab. In S. I. Rajan, & N. Neetha (Eds.), *Migration, gender and care economy* (pp. 103–123). Delhi: Routledge.

Khadria, B., & Meyer, J. B. (2013). Restructing Innovation Systems in India through Migartion. *Migration and Development*, *2*(2), 213–236.

Mallick, H. (2008). Do remittances impact the economy?: Some empirical evidences from a developing economy. Center for Development Studies Working Paper No. 407.

Mohanty, S. K., Dubey, M., & Parida, J. K. (2014). Economic well-being and spending behaviour of households in India: Does remittances matter? *Migration and Development*, *3*(1), 38–53.

Muhammad, M., & Ahmed, J. (2009). Dynamic impact of remittances on economic growth: A case study of Pakistan. *Forman Journal of Economic Studies*, *5*(2009 January–December), 59–74.

Nayyar, D. (1994). *Migration, remittances and capital flows.* New Delhi: Oxford University Press.

Nayyar, D. (2002). *Cross border movements of people.* WIDER Working Papers (1986–2000) 2000/194. Helsinki: UNU-WIDER.

NSSO. (2010). Employment and unemployment situation in India 2007–08. NSS Report No. 531, NSS 64th round.

Parida, J. K., Mohanty, S. K., & Raman, K. R. (2015). Remittances, household expenditure and investment in rural India: Evidence from NSS data. *Indian Economic Review*, *50*(1), 79–104.

Prakash, B. A. (1998). Gulf migration and its economic impact: The Kerala experience. *Economic and Political Weekly*, 33(50), 3209–3213.

Rahta, D. (2003). Workers' remittances: An import and stable source of external development finance. Global Dvelopment Finance 2003, Striving for Stability in Development Finance, 157–175.

Rajan, S. I., D' Sami, B., & Raj, S. S. A. (2015). Tamil Nadu migration survey 2015. Center for Development Studies Working Paper No. 472.

Rajan, S. I., & Zachariah, K. C. (2010). Remittances to Kerala: Impact on the economy. Middle East Institute. http://www.mei.edu/content/remittances--kerala--impact--economy. Published February 2, 2010. Accessed December 7, 2017.

Rajan, S. I., & Zachariah, K. C. (2019). Emigration and remittances: New evidences from the Kerala migration survey, 2018. Center for Development Studies Working Paper No. 483.

Ratha, D., & Mohapatra, S. (2007). *Increasing the macroeconomic impact of remittances on development.* Washington, DC: Development Research Group, World Bank.

Reserve Bank of India (RBI). (2018). Globalizing people: India's inward remittances. RBI bulletin. Retrieved from https://rbidocs.rbi.org.in/rdocs/Bulletin/PDFs/1AR_14112018071B947 4B5D74DDC91FC8AA015C5A360.PDF

Sasikumar, S. K., & Hussain, Z. (2007). *Migration, remittances, and development: Lessons from India.* New Delhi: VV Giri National Labour Institute.

Sil, M. (2011). International remittances and its impact on households and village development: A comparative study of Gujarat and Kerala states, India. Ph.D. Thesis, Tata Institute of Social Sciences, Mumbai.

Singh, P. (2011). Dynamics of international migration from rural Punjab a case study of Hoshiarpur and Kapurthala districts. http://hdl.handle.net/10603/121652

Singh, S. K., & Hari, K. S. (2011). *International migration, remittances and its macroeconomic impact on Indian economy.* IIMA Working Papers WP2011-01-06, Indian Institute of Management Ahmedabad.

Sisenglath, S. (2009). *Migrant worker remittances and their impact on local economic development.* Geneva: International Labour Organization.

Taylor, E. J. (1999). The new economics of labour migration and the role of remittances in the migration process. *International Migration, 37*(1), 63–88.

Zachariah, K. C., & Irudaya Rajan, S. (2007). Migration, remittances and employment: Short-term trends and long term implications. Centre for Development Studies Working Paper No. 395.

Zachariah, K. C., & Irudaya Rajan, S. (2012). Inflexion in Kerala's Gulf connection: Report on Kerala migration survey 2011. Center for Development Studies Working Paper No. 450.

Zachariah, K. C., & Irudaya Rajan, S. (2015). Dynamics of emigration and remittances in Kerala: Results from the Kerala migration survey 2014. Centre for Development Studies Working Paper No. 463.

Zachariah, K. C., Mathew, E. T., & Irudaya Rajan, S. (2003). *Dynamics of migration in Kerala: Dimensions, differentials, and consequences.* Hyderabad: Orient Blackswan.

Zachariah, K. C., Prakash, B. A, & Irudaya Rajan, S. (2002a). Gulf migration study: Employment, wages and working conditions of Kerala emigrants in the United Arab Emirates. Center for Development Studies Working Paper No. 326.

Zachariah, K. C., Prakash, B. A, & Irudaya Rajan, S. (2002b). Working in Gulf: Employment, wages and working conditions. In K. C. Zachariah, K. P. Kannan, & S. Irudaya Rajan (Eds.), *Kerala's Gulf connection: CDS studies on international labour migration from Kerala state in India* (pp. 129–198). Thiruvananthapuram: Centre for Development Studies.

Zachariah, K. C., & Rajan, S. I. (2010). Stability in Kerala emigration: Results from the Kerala migration survey 2007. In S. I. Rajan (Ed.), *India migration report 2010* (pp. 85–112). New Delhi and Oxford: Routledge.

21 Drivers of Economic and Social Change

The Impact of Indian Labour Migration to the Gulf

Shibinu S.

Introduction

Worldwide, there were 281 million international migrants in 2020 up from 258 million in 2017, 248 million in 2015, 220 million in 2010, 191 million in 2005 and 173 million in 2000. The United States, Germany, Saudi Arabia, Russia, the United Kingdom and the United Arab Emirates (UAE) remained the top six migrant destination countries. India is slated as the top origin country with the largest emigrant population in the world (nearly 18 million people) and the top receiver of international remittance with an estimated US$ 83 billion annually (World Bank, 2021; International Organization of Migration, 2022). India to the United Arab Emirates (over 3 million), the third largest corridor in the world, comprises mainly of labour migrants. Other corridors of India are the United States and Saudi Arabia (World Bank, 2020). In Kerala, large-scale emigration to the GCC countries, namely Bahrain, Kuwait, Oman, Qatar, Saudi Arabia and the UAE, have a history of more than 50 years (Rajan, Varghese and Jayakumar, 2010a; 2010b; Rajan, 2015, 2016; Rajan and Zachariah, 2019).

The mobility from Kerala was due to high deprivation in the region both economically and socially. For individuals who move, the excursion quite often involves penances and vulnerability which run from the enthusiastic expenses of division from families and companions to high financial charges (Zachariah, Mathew and Rajan, 2001a; 2001b; Rajan, 2014). Migrants have to pay most of the travel costs on their own (Zachariah, Prakash and Irudaya Rajan, 2002; Sivakumar and Rajan, 2022). This increases the liability position of the family even before migration. If the agent does not provide congruous documents and a work permit, then the migrant is expatriated immediately from the Gulf. A unique characteristic of migration to the Gulf countries is that it is contract migration. If the contract agreements are violated, then remittances will be lower and violators face rigorous imprisonment. Even if all these conditions are satisfied, the problem of remittance management within the origin could be a problem. In spite of all this, an average Keralite worker chooses to emigrate.

DOI: 10.4324/9781003315124-21

With this background, the chapter examines to illuminate the research questions on what has been the socio-economic consequences of emigration and how it is liable to affect the demographic changes in Kerala households using the Kerala migration surveys (Rajan and Zachariah, 2011; 2017; 2019)

Socio-economic Consequences of Emigration: A Snapshot

Why do people (choose to) leave their homes? Several studies have been carried out in Kerala by researchers at both the micro and the macro level. There is evidence that migration decision is a complex process that depends on many factors, such as migration governance system, skill transfer, or personal characteristics, such as age, gender, and educational background (Mathew and Nair, 1978). In a study published in 1994, Nair presents that the households that receive remittances have improved their standard of living by raising the levels and quality of consumption (Nair, 1994). Prakash (1998) observed that emigration has reduced the pressure of unemployment on the Kerala economy as about 40 per cent of the migrants were unemployed at the time of migration. Zachariah, Mathew and Rajan (1999; 2000) found that majority of the migrants were from relatively poorer families; unskilled or semi-skilled workers with educational attainment of matriculation or below; unemployed young men, aged below 35 at the time of migration. Kerala has received a significant flow of remittances since the early 1980s, when it was equivalent to 10 per cent of the Net State Domestic Product (NSDP), and the savings rate had been significantly high since the early 1990s. People saved what they have not consumed in the form of financial or non-financial assets, mainly for house construction, investment in gold, fixed deposits and share markets (Zachariah, Mathew and Rajan, 2003; Zachariah and Rajan, 2001; Rajan, 2021, Shibinu, 2016; 2021).

Data Source and Methodology

The study uses the data from the Kerala Migration Survey (KMS), 2016, undertaken by the Centre for Development Studies, as a follow-up study of KMS 2011 to examine the change in the quality of life due to migration at household as well as individual levels (Zacharia and Rajan, 2011; 2012; Rajan, 2010). Apart from looking at the overall scenario of the state, special focus is laid on three districts in the state, Thiruvananthapuram, Ernakulam and Malappuram for this research. Thiruvananthapuram is the state capital and ranked third in terms of the number of emigrants, while Malappuram is the highest migration pocket of Kerala and Ernakulum, the most urbanized district, and the financial capital of Kerala (Rajan and Zachariah, 2017).

A standard of living index was constructed to compare the living standards of the Gulf migrant and non-migrant households, employing the same method used in the National Family Health Surveys (NFHS). The variables used for constructing the index are ownership of house, size of land, type of house, cooking fuel, assets of consumer durables such as car, taxi, computer, internet, refrigerator, microwave oven, TV, mobile and landline, DVD player and monthly income of households. All these variables were added by giving a standard weight for each variable. Based on the mean and standard deviation, it is re-coded as Lower Class (below (Mean − SD)), Lower Middle Class (between (Mean − SD)) and Mean), Middle Class (between (Mean + SD) and Mean) and Upper Class (above Mean + SD). Bivariate analysis was carried out to assess the effect of migration on the socio-economic characteristics of the Gulf migrant and non-migrant households.

Socio-economic Profile of Gulf Migrants: Pre- and Post-emigration Phase

The study focused on the socio-economic living conditions of the Gulf-migrant and non-migrant households. For this, we took into consideration the social, demographic and economic characteristics of the Gulf migrants during the pre and post-migration phases. The socio-economic profiles of non-migrants were also analyzed. In order to investigate inequality, a comparison of the living conditions was made between Gulf and non-Gulf migrant households. The social and demographic characteristics selected for the analysis are: age, sex, marital status, family type, household headship, education and religion. A comparison of the economic characteristics of the same group has also been attempted to analyze the economic impact. The economic characteristics are household size, working members in the household, remittance, standard of living index, savings, investments and asset holdings. A technical analysis was done to investigate the inequality between Gulf migrant households and non-migrant households and finally, the impact of migration.

Majority of the Gulf emigrants are males. The proportion of females among the Gulf emigrants is 9.2 per cent. Ernakulam has the highest proportion of female Gulf migrants (22 per cent) followed by Thiruvananthapuram (16.6 per cent). The study found that youth form the major proportion of migrants to the Gulf from Kerala. About 59 per cent of males and 53 per cent of females fall under the age group 20–39 years. Gulf migrants are, of course, much younger at the time of emigration. The average age at the time they emigrated was 25.6 years. Females were younger than males at the time of migration (21.4 and 26.1 years, respectively). Malappuram has a higher proportion of younger Gulf migrants than the other two districts, with most of them having migrated before the age of 30. Some of the Gulf migrants are accompanied by their families, including children and older persons.

Duration of stay of majority of the male Gulf migrants is 6 to 10 years whereas for female Gulf migrants, it is 2 to 5 years (see Table 21.1) About one-fourth of the Gulf migrants stay abroad for 11 to 20 years. More than 10 per cent of the Gulf migrants have gone abroad recently and their

Table 21.1 Average Duration of Stay in Gulf by Gender

	Male	Female	Total
<1 year	11.3	6.7	10.8
2–5 years	16.0	38.7	18.1
6–10 years	32.4	25.3	31.8
11–20 years	24.0	26.7	24.3
21+years	16.3	2.7	15.0

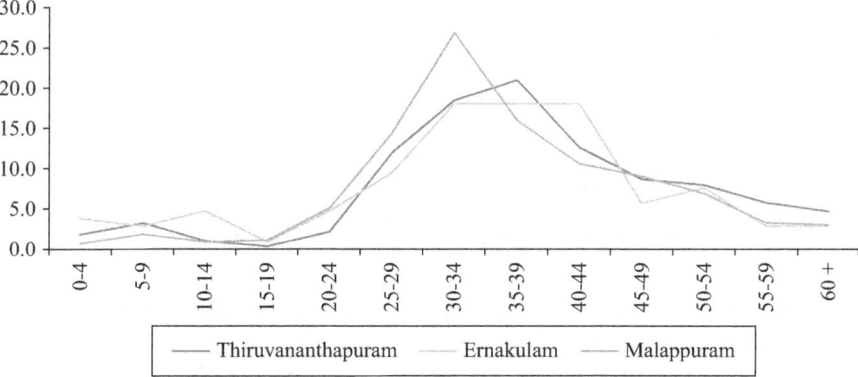

Figure 21.1 Age composition of Gulf migrants by three districts.

duration of stay is less than one year. The average years of stay in the Gulf countries are the highest among the Gulf migrants from Malappuram and Thiruvananthapuram (11 years), while for Ernakulam, it is 10 years (see also Figure 21.1). Early migration and long duration of stay in the destination countries are the unique characteristics of Gulf migrants from Malappuram. Duration of stay has an impact on the socio-economic outcome of the households in the origin countries.

Looking at the distribution by religion, it is found that the majority of the Gulf migrants from Thiruvananthapuram are Hindus (62 per cent) whereas in Ernakulam, Christians comprise the highest number (49.5 per cent). As expected, Muslim Gulf migrants dominate in Malappuram (86.3 per cent). Gender disparity by religion can be observed among the Gulf migrants. Among Christians, 23.1 per cent are female, which is the highest among all the three religious categories (Figure 21.2). Among Muslims, 94.3 per cent of the migrants are male. Females among Christians are more empowered to go abroad than those in the other two religious groups.

Most of the Gulf migrants are espoused. The proportion of unmarried women Gulf migrants is the highest in Thiruvananthapuram and Ernakulam (31.5 per cent and 31.2 per cent respectively). Largest number of male and

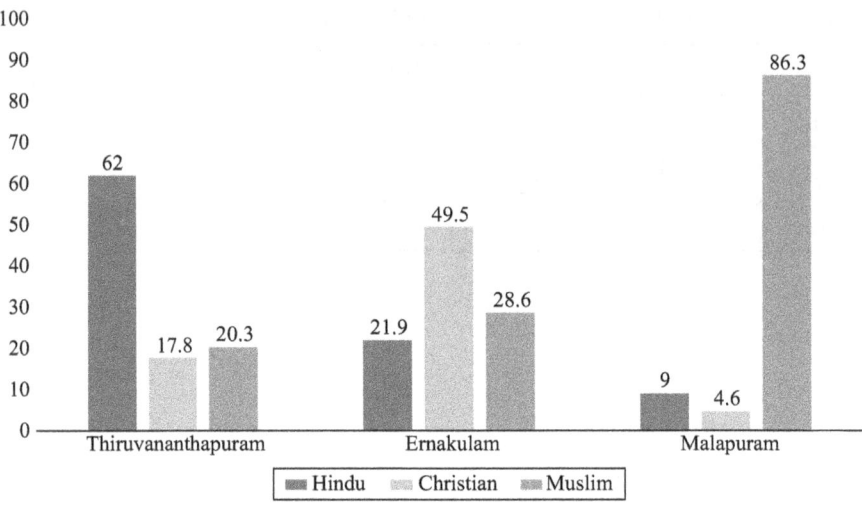

Figure 21.2 Religious distribution of Gulf migrants by districts.

female emigrants in the separated category is also from Ernakulam (2.3 per cent and 2.3 per cent, respectively).

It is noteworthy that about 1.3 per cent of the female Gulf migrants from Malappuram are widows. Though the practice of female migration is predominantly lower in Malappuram on religious grounds, this is a unique story revealed by the data.

The district-wise educational profile of the Gulf migrants, revealed that migrants from Ernakulam had higher educational qualifications (61 per cent), followed by Thiruvananthapuram (51.8 per cent). Migrants in Malappuram were more likely to have secondary or below level of education (73.1 per cent). Male migrants are more likely to complete secondary level education (30.6 per cent), while female migrants are more likely to have a graduate degree or above (46.7 per cent). About 15 per cent of the male Gulf migrants have completed the higher secondary level and 15 per cent have done certificate courses (Figure 21.3).

Analysis of the pre and post-occupational status shows significant differences in the case of certain job categories like agriculture, accountancy, teaching and business. In the case of professionals, nurses have experienced no change in their occupation. About 88 per cent of engineers found the same job in the destination country while about 12 per cent of them were under-employed. Many of the professionally or technically qualified Gulf migrants ended up in occupations other than what they were promised in their job contract. This might be the reason for the large and increasing number of unsuccessful migration stories reported from different parts of the state (Table 21.2).

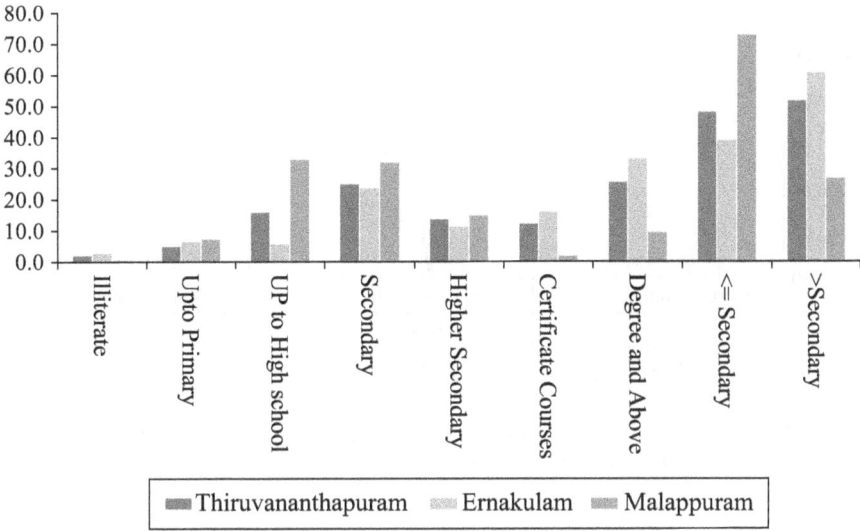

Figure 21.3 Educational .level of Gulf migrants by districts.

Table 21.2 Main Occupation of Gulf Migrants before and after Migration

Before Migration	Per cent	After Migration	Per cent
Agriculture	11.1	Salesman	20.8
Salesman	10.8	Motor vehicle driver	7.8
Motor vehicle driver	9.0	Others	7.0
Peon	7.1	Engineer	6.0
Engineer	6.3	Accountant	4.8
Others	5.3	Peon	4.6
Construction worker	4.0	Manager	3.7
Painter	3.7	Construction worker	3.5
Cook	2.9	Business	2.7
Accountant	2.7	Storekeeper	2.4
Teacher	2.7	Electrician	2.1
Business	1.9	Painter	2.1
Carpenter	1.8	Mechanic	2.0
Manager	1.8	Nurse	1.9

Among the Gulf countries, the major destination country for Keralites is Saudi Arabia, followed by the United Arab Emirates (UAE). About 43.2 per cent of Gulf migrants are in Saudi Arabia followed by UAE (37.2 per cent) and Qatar (6.7 per cent). The major attraction of these two countries is the increased demand for unskilled labourers in the construction industry and oil fields. About 91.1 per cent of the total male emigrants prefer to go to Gulf countries while only 60 per cent females do. The migration from Kerala to Middle East countries is male dominated. About 40.5 per cent of

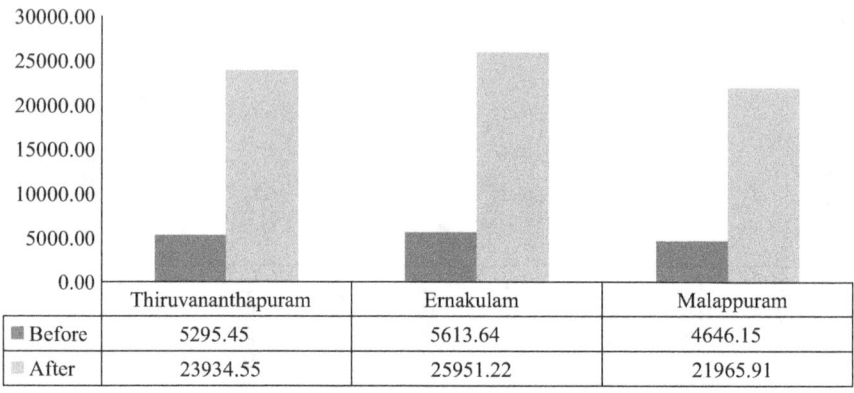

	Thiruvananthapuram	Ernakulam	Malappuram
■ Before	5295.45	5613.64	4646.15
▨ After	23934.55	25951.22	21965.91

Figure 21.4 Average monthly income of Gulf migrants during the pre- and post-migration phase by districts (in Rs.).

female emigrants prefer to go to other countries such as the United States, the United Kingdom or Canada.

The average monthly income of the Gulf migrants prior to migration is more or less similar in Thiruvananthapuram and Ernakulam. Similar drifts are also seen in the post-migration phase in all three districts. This deviation in income (Figure 21.4) may be the after-effect of differences in the achievement of education of Gulf migrants at the district level. However, a five-fold increase in income can be seen in all the three districts as a result of migration (Figure 21.4).

Remittance and Cost of Migration

Household remittances are the remittances received by family members of the migrant households. Remittances are calculated in this study with the help of a raising factor (weight) which is obtained by taking the quotient of estimated Census households for 2016 and the sample households. Household remittances for districts are multiplied by the raising factor to obtain the household remittances. Most of the household remittances were received by the households as regular periodic remittances. Malappuram received the largest remittance of Rs. 2,283 crores, followed by Thiruvananthapuram (Rs. 1,462 crores) and Ernakulam (Rs. 556 crores). Though the monthly income of the Gulf migrants from Ernakulam is high, their remittance is low. This may be because they save their income in some other mode either in the Gulf or foreign banks. Most of the low-skilled Gulf migrants are from a fragile economic background. To improve their family welfare, they are compelled to send a sizeable proportion of their income back as remittances. This may be the reason for higher remittances in the case of Malappuram.

The socio-economic characteristics of Gulf migrant households revealed the private costs and benefits of migration. Malappuram has the highest number of Gulf migrants, receives the largest amount of remittances, and has the lowest average cost of migration. A real disparity is observed between the standard of living of the Gulf migrant and non-migrant households. However, in the case of savings, investment and consumption, there is no valid variation between these households. So, it can be concluded that nowadays the demonstration effect is very evident in Kerala. Earlier studies on migration from Kerala have indicated that inequality has fallen. The increased wages in Kerala have also boosted this effect.

Loans taken by the Gulf migrant households are mainly utilized for purchasing or constructing houses. About 12 per cent Gulf migrant households have utilized the loans for wedding/dowry purpose. About 6 per cent Gulf migrant households utilized the loan for emigration expenses. About 44 per cent of Gulf migrant households in Ernakulam utilized the loan for the construction or purchase of houses (Table 21.3). This is partly associated with increased cost of construction prevailing in the urban centres.

The main dream of any migrant is to have a good home. This is evident from the landscape throughout Kerala. Also, loans utilized for educational purposes are comparatively high in the Gulf migrant households of Ernakulam. Loans taken for marriage purposes are high in Gulf migrant households of Malappuram, followed by Thiruvananthapuram. Loans availed for meeting the emigration expenses in Malappuram are comparatively smaller because of the prevalence of the 'chain migration' process, which means, majority of the migration happened through friends and relatives rather than recruitment agencies.

Table 21.3 Utilization of the Loan Taken by the Gulf Migrant Households

	Thiruvananthapuram	Ernakulam	Malappuram
Purchase of land	2.1	0.0	3.3
Purchase of agricultural equipment	2.8	0.0	16.7
Investment in business	2.8	0.0	0.0
Purchase of house (including construction)	35.2	43.8	33.3
Purchase of vehicles or Household durables	8.3	6.3	3.3
Educational purpose	7.6	12.5	0.0
Medical purpose	6.9	6.3	6.7
Wedding/dowry	12.4	6.3	13.3
Emigration expenses	6.2	6.3	3.3
Other	15.9	18.8	20.0
Total	100.0	100.0	100.0

Social Impacts of Migration

Generally, if the head of the household has migrated, a female member takes up the position as the head of the household. Non-migrant households are more likely to be male-headed households. When comparing the Gulf migrant households, it is found that around half of the households are headed by females. In other words, women do 'double-shifts' or 'double-days' which means they work for their husbands too. Though it is a dual task to look after their children as well as other family members, the economic status of their households and their dignity within the family and relatives circle considerably improved following the emigration of a family member.

Average family size of households in Thiruvananthapuram and Ernakulam is four, irrespective of their migration status. But the average family size of the non-migrant households in Malappuram is five. There are more single members in the non-migrant households compared to the Gulf migrant households. However, in Malappuram, more migrant households have more than five members than non-migrant households.

Females are more educationally qualified than males, irrespective of their household composition. In Thiruvananthapuram, more than 71 per cent young male members of the Gulf migrant households have secondary or higher levels of education while in Ernakulam, 88 per cent have acquired the same. A greater proportion of the members of Gulf migrant households in Ernakulam (41.4 per cent) have higher educational qualifications (degree and above) compared to their counterparts in non-migrant households (28.2 per cent). Malappuram has a different approach towards higher education. Compared to the other two districts, the number of degree holders is fewer among both types of households. However, members of non-migrant households in this district have better educational status compared to those in the Gulf migrant households (Table 21.4).

Migration of youth from the household usually is seen to increase the number of older people living alone. In our study, we have considered

Table 21.4 Educational Level of Family Members in the Age Group 20–49 by Households and Three Districts, 2016

Districts	Educational Level	Male		Female	
		Gulf-Migrant HH	Non-Migrant HH	Gulf-Migrant HH	Non-Migrant HH
Thiruvananthapuram	<10th Class	28.0	29.0	20.2	26.8
	>=10th Class	71.4	69.4	79.8	70.8
Ernakulam	<10th Class	12.1	19.9	4.2	18.6
	>=10th Class	87.9	79.5	95.8	81.1
Malappuram	<10th Class	47.4	39.9	37.1	36.6
	>=10th Class	52.3	58.6	62.6	61.5

Table 21.5 Percentage Distribution of Older Person Households, 2016

Type of HH	Trivandrum		Ernakulam		Malappuram	
	Gulf Migrant HH	Non-migrant HH	Gulf Migrant HH	Non-migrant HH	Gulf Migrant HH	Non-migrant HH
Non-aged HH	92.5	88.8	91.9	91.2	98.5	96.9
Aged HH	7.5	11.2	8.1	8.8	1.5	3.1

Table 21.6 Percentage Distribution of Households with Adult Male Members, 2016

Type of HH	Trivandrum		Ernakulam		Malappuram	
	Gulf Migrant HH	Non-migrant HH	Gulf Migrant HH	Non-migrant HH	Gulf Migrant HH	Non-migrant HH
Male Absent	30.8	8.2	27.0	4.6	20.0	4.4
Male Present	69.2	91.8	73.0	95.4	80.0	95.6

households consisting of only members aged 60 and above, as aged households. It is seen that there is a higher number of aged households as the non-migrant households than Gulf emigrant households across the three districts (Table 21.5).

Emigration from Kerala is mainly male dominated. This could often lead to households with no adult members, which would increase the burden on the women in the left behind households. The study shows that the proportion of households with no adult males present is significantly higher in the Gulf migrant households compared to the non-migrant households (Table 21.6).

Economic Impacts of Migration

Though the standard of living index includes the type of house and household amenities for its construction, it is significant to analyze it separately to find the economic impact of migration among non-migrant and Gulf migrant households. The quality of houses varies sharply among the Gulf migrant and non-migrant households. About 46 per cent of migrant households have a luxurious or very good house while 31per cent of the non-migrant households have such quality houses (Table 21.7). About one-fifth of the non-migrant households have poor or kutcha houses. Gulf migrant households are less likely to have poor or kutcha houses. Thiruvananthapuram has the highest proportion of poor or kutcha houses. It is interesting to note that though Malappuram has the highest proportion of Gulf migrants, there is a larger number of luxurious or very good houses in Ernakulam (55.6 per cent) followed by Thiruvananthapuram (46.1 per cent).

Table 21.7 Percentage Distribution of Type of Houses by the Households, 2016

	Gulf Migrant HH	Non-migrant HH
Luxurious or Very Good	45.9	31.0
Good	46.4	48.5
Poor or *Kutcha*	7.8	20.5
Total	100.0	100.0

Household amenities possessed by the households are a major indicator of the economic impact of migration. One out of four Gulf migrant households owns a four-wheeler. Possession of a motor car is 6.8 points higher for Gulf migrant households than non-migrant households in Malappuram. It is interesting to note that though most Gulf migrant households possess mobile phones and an internet connection, the picture is not too bad among the non-migrant households. When it comes to possessing a refrigerator, there is a big gap between Gulf migrant and non-migrant households (Table 21.8).

A feasible option to study the direct impact of economic indicators on the households is the construction of the standard of living index. Here, the index is grouped at four levels. Clearly, non-migrant households fall in the lower level of living standard category, whereas Gulf migrant households are skewed towards the higher level or middle level of living standards. Thus, clear evidence of the disparity in the standard of living of the Gulf migrant and non-migrant households is demarcated.

Average total investment in Gulf migrant households is Rs. 11,70,000 and that in non-migrant households is Rs. 11,30,00. It is found that though the investment is positively skewed to migration, its indirect effect shadowed the non-migrant households. There is not much variation between investments of Gulf migrant and non-migrant households. This trend can be seen in savings and consumption also. Though Gulf migrant households lead the position, the disparity is negligible.

Average total savings of Gulf migrant households is Rs. 14,132 and that of non-migrant households is Rs. 13,322. Thus, it can be inferred that migration has a direct impact on the migrant households and an indirect impact on the non-migrant households. Mean consumer expenditure of the Gulf migrant households for a month is Rs.12,380 while it is Rs. 10,990 for non-migrant households. Due to the increase in income over the period among Gulf migrant households, their monthly consumption expenditure was also high compared to non-migrant households. The migrant households incurred higher expenditure on food, clothing, education, fuel, light, travel, entertainment and medical expenses.

Investment among Gulf migrant households is high in Thiruvananthapuram while it is high among non-migrant households in Ernakulam. Since

Table 21.8 Possession of Household Amenities by Type of Households, 2016

	Thiruvananthapuram			Ernakulam			Malappuram		
	Non-migrant HH	Gulf Migrant HH	Gap	Non-migrant HH	Gulf Migrant HH	Gap	Non-migrant HH	Gulf Migrant HH	Gap
Motor car	18.2	23.0	4.8	20.2	25.0	4.8	13.2	20.0	6.8
Taxi/truck/lorry	3.1	5.9	2.8	6.3	1.4	-4.9	4.5	4.0	-0.5
Motor cycle/scooter	44.6	47.1	2.5	57.1	66.7	9.6	31.1	42.0	10.9
Telephone	22.3	33.3	11	44.1	52.8	8.7	21.9	43.0	21.1
Mobile phone	89.4	96.6	7.2	87.7	95.8	8.1	88.8	93.3	4.5
Television	88.4	96.1	7.7	94.2	97.2	3.0	84.3	87.3	3.0
MP3/DVD/VCD	27.6	50.0	22.4	51.1	65.3	14.2	16.3	18.3	2.0
Refrigerator	56.7	84.8	28.1	64.9	81.9	17.0	35.9	57.3	21.4
Computer/laptops	21.3	24.0	2.7	26.0	41.7	15.7	11.6	18.7	7.1
Microwave oven	5.5	6.4	0.9	13.8	18.1	4.3	2.2	4.0	1.8
Internet connection	14.3	17.6	3.3	18.7	23.6	4.9	2.5	3.3	0.8

Table 21.9 Standard of Living of Gulf Migrant and Non-migrant Households, 2016

		Gulf Migrant HH	Non-migrant HH
Thiruvananthapuram	Lower class	5.9	19.6
	Lower middle class	37.3	41.2
	Middle class	36.3	18.9
	High class	20.6	20.3
Ernakulam	Lower class	0.0	6.8
	Lower middle class	30.6	42.8
	Middle class	37.5	29.1
	High class	31.9	21.4
Malappuram	Lower class	3.7	17.5
	Lower middle class	54.0	63.5
	Middle class	31.7	13.2
	High class	10.7	5.7

Table 21.10 Income Utilization Pattern by Type of Households, 2016

		Mean	Standard Deviation
Savings	Non-migrant HH	13,321.8	10,057.1
	Gulf migrant HH	14,131.6	10,255.5
Consumption	Non-migrant HH	10,990.0	11,258.5
	Gulf migrant HH	12,379.8	13,094.4
Investment	Non-migrant HH	1,13,4004.2	5,79,728.8
	Gulf migrant HH	1,17,4879.4	6,03,027.6
Health Expenditure	Non-migrant HH	6,176.3	3,237.4
	Gulf migrant HH	6,690.3	3,267.4
Education Expense			
Thiruvananthapuram	Non-migrant HH	15,454.6	5,581.8
	Gulf migrant HH	16,166.5	5,935.0
Ernakulam	Non-migrant HH	15,139.7	5,989.3
	Gulf migrant HH	16,322.6	6,979.1
Malappuram	Non-migrant HH	11,186.4	4,792.1
	Gulf migrant HH	11,543.9	4,401.6

Ernakulam is the financial capital of Kerala, more non-migrant households are likely to invest in businesses and other areas. Consumption expenditure among the Gulf migrant households is higher in Ernakulam compared to the other two districts. Savings are higher among the Gulf migrant households of Malappuram and Ernakulam compared to those in Thiruvananthapuram.

The Gulf migrant households spend more money on marriages, other ceremonies and on durable goods and other major areas like health and education. The study considered the hospitalization charges for health expenses. Most of the Gulf migrant households accessed private hospitals for their treatments. Utilization pattern of education reveals that Ernakulam incurred higher expenditure on education compared to the other two districts.

The number of dependents is higher in Gulf migrant households compared to non-migrant households which is the highest in Malappuram. Unemployment rate is high among the family members of Gulf migrant households compared to non-migrant households and is higher in Thiruvananthapuram compared to the other two districts. In the Gulf migrant households, most family members are women and children who are outside the labour force. So, it is not surprising that the proportion of the members in these households in the working group is lower compared to those in the non-migrant households.

Conclusions

A good number of Keralites have migrated to Gulf countries in quest of fortune. These emigrants are mainly semi-skilled/unskilled young men with a low level of education, having moved temporarily, leaving behind their families in order to accumulate wealth for their households. In one among five Gulf migrant households, migration has changed the headship of the family in favour of females.

The living condition of migrant households has changed substantially through the inflow of foreign remittances. A good share of these households has perceived improvement in terms of the economic status of their households. Good quality houses, costly household durables and other luxury items can be seen more among Gulf migrant households. The extent of improvement, however, largely varies according to the emigrant's duration of stay abroad. The longer the duration of stay abroad the better the economic status of the native household. The consumption expenditure is higher in a Gulf migrant household than in a non-migrant household. Consumption expenditure among the Gulf migrant households is higher in Ernakulam compared to the other two districts. In conclusion, for the economic and social change, there is a direct impact of migration on the migrant households and an indirect impact on the non-migrant households.

References

International Organization for Migration. (2022). *World migration report 2022*. Geneva: International Organization for Migration.

Mathew, E. T., and Nair, G. P. R. (1978). Socio-economic characteristics of emigrant's households: A case study of two villages in Kerala. *Economic and Political Weekly, 13*(28), 1141–1153.

Nair, G. P. R. (1994). *Migration of Keralites to the Arab world, Kerala's economy: Performance, problems and prospects*, ed. B. A. Prakash. New Delhi: Sage Publication.

Prakash, B. A. (1998). Gulf migration and its economic impacts: The Kerala experience. *Economic and Political Weekly, 33*(50), 3209–3213.

Rajan, S. I. (2010). *India migration report 2010: Governance and labour migration.* New Delhi: Routledge.

Rajan, S. I., Varghese, V. J., and Jayakumar, M. S. (2010a). Looking beyond the emigration act 1983: Revisiting the recruitment practices in India. In S. I. Rajan (Ed.), *Governance and labour migration: India migration report 2010* (pp. 251–287). New Delhi: Routledge.

Rajan, S. I., Varghese, V. J., and Jayakumar, M. S. (2010b). Overseas recruitment in India: Structures, practices and remedies. Centre for Development Studies (Thiruvananthapuram) Working Paper No. 421.

Rajan, S. I., and Zachariah, K. C. (2011). Impact of emigration and remittances on Goan economy. In S. I. Rajan (Ed.), *India migration report 2011* (pp. 295–316). New Delhi: Routledge.

Rajan, S. I. (Ed.). (2014). *India migration report 2014: Diaspora and development.* Oxon: Routledge.

Rajan, S. I. (2015). Migration and development: The Indian experience. In G. P. Freeman, and N. Mirilovic (Eds.), *Handbook on migration and social policy* (pp. 137–161). Northampton, MA: Edward Elgar Publishers.

Rajan, S. I. (Ed.). (2016). *India migration report 2016: Gulf migration.* New Delhi: Routledge.

Rajan, S. I. (2021). *India migration report 2020: Kerala model of migration surveys.* New York: Routledge.

Rajan, S. I., and Zachariah, K. C. (2017). Kerala migration survey 2016: New evi-dences. In S. I. Rajan (Ed.), *India migration report 2017: Forced migration* (Chapter 8, pp. 289–305). New Delhi: Routledge.

Rajan, S. I., and Zachariah, K. C. (2019). Emigration and remittances: New Evidences from the Kerala migration survey, 2018. Centre for Development Studies Working Paper No. 483. Thiruvananthapuram, Kerala.

Shibinu, S. (2016). Socio-economic dynamics of Gulf migration: A panel data analysis. Unpublished, University of Kerala, India.

Shibinu, S. (2021). Socio-economic dynamics of Gulf migration: A panel data analysis. Chapter 6. In S. IrudayaRajan (Ed.), *India migration report 2020: Kerala model of migration surveys* (pp. 120–135). New York: Routledge.

Sivakumar, P., and Irudaya Rajan, S. (Eds.). (2022). *Sustainable development goals and migration.* New Delhi: Routledge.

World Bank. (2020). COVID-19 crisis through a migration lens. Migration and Development Brief No. 32. World Bank, Washington.

World Bank. (2021). Resilience: Covid-19 crisis through migration lens. Migration and development brief 34. World Bank, Washington.

Zachariah, K. C., and Irudaya Rajan, S. (2001). Migration mosaic in Kerala: Trends and determinants. *Demography India, 30*(1), 137–165.

Zachariah, K. C., Mathew, E. T., and Irudaya Rajan, S. (2003). *Dynamics of migration in Kerala: Dimensions, differentials and consequences.* Hyderabad: Orient Longman.

Zachariah, K. C., Mathew, E. T., and Rajan, S. I. (1999). Impact of migration on Kerala's economy and society. Working Paper No. 297. Thiruvananthapuram: Centre for Development Studies.

Zachariah, K. C., Mathew, E. T., and Rajan, S. I. (2000). Socio-economic and demographic consequences of migration in Kerala. Working Paper No. 303. Thiruvananthapuram: Centre for Development Studies.

Zachariah, K. C., Mathew, E. T., and Rajan, S. I. (2001a). Impact of migration on Kerala's economy and society. *International Migration, 39*(1), 63–88.

Zachariah, K. C., Mathew, E. T., and Rajan, S. I. (2001b). Social, economic and demographic consequences of migration in Kerala. *International Migration, 39*(2), 43–72.

Zachariah, K. C., Prakash, B. A., and Irudaya Rajan, S. (2002). Working in Gulf: Employment, wages and working conditions. In K. C. Zachariah, K. P. Kannan, and S. Irudaya Rajan (Eds.), *Kerala's gulf connection: CDS studies on international labour migration from Kerala state in India* (pp. 129–197). Thiruvananthapuram: Centre for Development Studies.

Zachariah, K. C., and Rajan, S. I. (2011). Inflexion in Kerala's Gulf connection: Report on the Kerala migration survey 2011. Working Paper No. 450. Thiruvananthapuram: Centre for Development Studies.

Zachariah, K. C., and Rajan, S. I. (2012). *Kerala's Gulf connection, 1998–2011: Economic and social impact of migration.* New Delhi: Orient Blackswan.

Index

Aadhaar 310, 311, 313
ability 52, 61, 63, 146, 152, 154, 157, 164, 168, 231
abnormally 349, 366
abroad 1, 2, 5–7, 10–12, 14, 18, 21, 22, 31, 40, 43, 49, 56, 74–76, 78, 81, 82, 86, 106, 108–12, 114–19, 121–23, 132, 140, 151, 152, 156–58, 161, 168–70, 173, 175, 176, 178–87, 190, 193, 196, 198, 202, 204, 206, 209, 216, 221–23, 275, 329, 330, 390, 391, 401
absence 57, 98, 103, 147, 163, 237, 244, 247, 260, 272, 301, 307
abuse 49
accident 247, 250, 255, 307, 328
accommodation 50, 68, 77, 78, 140, 171, 176, 180, 183, 256, 258, 308, 323, 328
accreditation 43, 46, 51–53, 55, 129, 156, 170, 194
acquisition 51, 211, 224
ActionAid 307
advertisement 323, 324
AED 47, 50, 53, 55
AFD-WB 288
Afghanistan 237
Africa 14, 15, 26, 33, 52, 85, 100, 121, 130, 131, 133–39, 158, 184, 185, 196, 226, 227, 230, 234, 236–38, 242, 287, 321
aged-care 24
ageing 12, 13, 55, 108, 124, 155
agreement 38, 39, 55, 65, 128, 131, 142, 147, 149, 150, 155, 160–62, 164, 240, 257, 266
Alappuzha 291, 292, 294
anti-discrimination 131
Anti-immigrant 236

APR 342–44
ARC 130
ARHC 313, 314
ASEAN 24, 128–30, 144, 147, 161
Asia 11, 24, 43, 44, 55, 56, 85, 86, 105, 106, 119, 161, 162, 207, 226, 230, 234, 236, 238, 242, 245, 259, 260, 262, 267, 287, 310, 321, 332
asylum-seekers 240
ATM 381
Australia 13–17, 19–22, 26, 33, 38, 52, 53, 55, 124, 125, 132–38, 142, 143, 153, 154, 162, 177, 179, 198, 200, 201, 230, 242, 287
Austria 95, 124, 125
Au-Yeung 227
Awas 308, 313
ayurveda 152, 200
AYUSH 152, 200

baby-boom 25
Bahrain 247, 248, 250, 259, 321, 325, 379, 388
Bangalore 180, 336, 347, 348
Bangladesh 206, 236, 349, 366–69
BDO 372
Belgium 92, 93, 95, 97, 98, 125, 140, 159, 318
Bengal 152, 153, 310, 337, 346, 347, 349, 350, 352–62, 364, 366–69
Berkeley 11, 83, 85
Bihar 218, 273, 277, 305, 310, 312, 337, 345, 346, 349, 356, 357, 371
Bloomington 195
BMC 229
BOCW 315
Bombay 2, 3, 203
brain-drain 163, 192
Brazil 133–36, 138

Britain 52, 89, 206, 333
Bulgaria 95

Cairo 242
calamities 301, 303
California 11, 83–85
Cambridge 105, 224, 225, 227, 303
Canada 23, 25–36, 38–42, 52, 53, 88,
    124, 125, 132–38, 153, 165, 177,
    198, 200, 201, 347, 394
care 12, 14, 16, 18, 23, 24, 27, 28, 33,
    35, 36, 40, 41, 43, 44, 47, 48, 55–58,
    61–68, 70, 73, 75, 77–83, 85, 88, 96,
    98, 102, 103, 106–8, 115, 118, 121,
    123, 127, 139, 140, 144–47, 151,
    152, 155, 160, 162, 163, 165–69,
    171–75, 177, 178, 180, 183, 188,
    190–92, 194, 195, 197, 206–8,
    211, 217, 228, 242, 250, 268, 308,
    334, 386
caregivers 21, 22, 88, 151, 153, 154,
    166, 238
Caribbean 128, 321
CARIM-India 105
CBT 180
CC 288
CCCPR 36, 41
CECA 144–46, 148, 149
census 13, 22, 293, 305, 306, 316, 318,
    350, 352–58, 363, 365, 366, 368,
    372, 394
CEPA 145, 148
CGFNS 16
CHH 266
Chhattisgarh 277, 337, 345, 346
Chicago 83
Chile 38, 125
CIMS 260
CMDS 119
cohort 335, 336, 338–42, 344, 345
Columbia 30, 31, 34, 38, 40, 228
COMCAD 105
conflict 11, 232, 237, 239, 347
Constitution 22, 63, 75, 78, 124,
    269, 270, 278, 280, 283, 309, 314,
    319, 331
contiguous 366, 368
COPS 28, 29
corridor 54, 87, 89, 95, 96, 99, 102–4,
    135, 226, 231, 332, 388
covid 100, 140, 209, 210, 218, 221,
    223, 227, 258, 262, 328, 332
CPNRE 36
CPSO 34, 41

Croatia 95
CRRTs 179
CSA 40
CSOs 307, 308, 314–16
CSR 315
Cuba 133–36
CWDS 119
Cyprus 95

Dalits 86
daughter 6, 41, 70, 71
DC 243, 286, 288, 385–87
decolonization 234, 241, 321
Delhi 2, 11, 49, 85, 86, 119, 160, 161,
    164, 195, 196, 203, 207, 208, 218,
    224, 226, 228, 262, 303, 306, 309,
    318, 319, 336, 337, 345, 346, 369,
    370, 386, 387, 401–3
DEMIG 225
Demography 226, 332, 402
Denmark 93, 95, 104, 105, 124,
    125, 142
deportation 245
deprivation 223, 334, 335, 342,
    343, 388
DESA 209
de-stigmatisation 47
destination 2, 3, 9, 12, 13, 17, 19–22,
    26, 27, 39, 47, 51, 53, 64, 88, 95,
    102, 104, 122–24, 127, 132, 137–39,
    141, 142, 151, 152, 154–56, 159, 192,
    201, 205, 206, 210–14, 216, 219, 225,
    232, 237, 239, 244, 246–48, 250, 252,
    257, 259–61, 287, 307, 318, 321, 323,
    325, 327, 329, 334, 335, 366, 378,
    379, 388, 391–93
DFID 293
DHA 44, 52, 54, 55
DHCA 44, 54
diaspora 9, 10, 56, 245, 246, 249, 258,
    259, 261, 264, 321, 402
digital 143, 157, 173, 206, 315
Dirham 47
disaster 290, 291, 294, 302–4, 308
doctor 26, 42, 50, 59, 60, 65, 70, 76,
    176, 188, 200, 203, 207, 208
Doha 248, 250, 379
DOREM 382, 383, 385
dowry 6, 181, 395
DSGE 267
duality 57, 62, 167
Dubai 3, 9, 44, 45, 47, 48, 50–52,
    54–56, 140, 330, 379
Dutch 264, 267, 286, 287

EAC 128, 129
Ebola 210
EBSCO 83
EC 104, 203
ECG 168
ECNR 48
ECR 48, 49, 135, 138, 141, 159, 161, 203–5
ECSA-HC 158
Egypt 46
elderly 250, 334–36, 338–47
embassy 143, 324, 327
emergency 14, 20, 123, 257, 310
emigrant 56, 262, 322, 323, 328, 331, 376, 380, 383, 388, 397
E-Migrate 159
Emirates 43–45, 50, 55, 133–37, 247, 248, 250, 321, 324, 325, 387, 388, 393
Encyclopaedia 225
England 215, 225
Entrepreneurship 142, 143, 160
environment 5, 82, 158, 178, 179, 202, 211, 222, 290, 303
EPA 131, 149
EPAs 131
EQUINET 130
ERM 336
ESA 228
ESDC 28
ESI 308
ESIC 311, 314
Ethnographic 84
EU 87, 89, 90, 92, 93, 95, 96, 99, 102–6, 195
EUI 104, 105, 195
Europe 41, 59, 104, 105, 159, 195, 205, 221, 227, 230, 267
Eurostat 92–95, 104
exodus 58, 214, 306, 311, 316
Expatriation 250

female-headed 267, 280–82, 373
Fiji 15
Filipino 23, 131
Finland 125, 152
FMGE 202
France 25, 35, 38, 84, 88, 93–95, 124, 125, 133–36, 138, 154
FSUs 293, 294, 302
FTA 144, 147–50, 152, 160, 161

GCC 52, 89, 95, 200, 244, 247, 248, 252, 259, 260, 321, 323, 379, 380, 384, 388

GDP 291, 306, 371
Geneva 41, 42, 104, 105, 107, 159, 161, 162, 197, 206, 208, 226, 228, 229, 261, 303, 304, 318, 319, 387, 401
geography 11, 56, 88, 96, 226, 230, 242
Germany 90, 92, 96–100, 102–5, 123–25, 131–38, 140, 142, 153, 154, 201, 227, 287, 388
GH 168, 169
Ghana 131, 287
Globalization 226
GLP 332
GMC 138, 160
GC-UK 160
GMDAC 307
GNM 18, 64, 68, 69, 72, 78, 109, 168, 169, 194
Goa 371
grandparents 65, 115
gratuity 253, 254
Greece 95, 125, 288
GRFDT 385
Guatemala 287, 385
Gujarat 308–10, 312, 313, 318, 337, 345, 346, 349, 371, 377, 385, 387
gulf 1–4, 6–12, 19, 47, 48, 52, 55, 56, 100, 105, 108, 118, 119, 122, 132, 135, 138, 140, 141, 170–72, 179, 182–85, 192, 193, 200, 201, 236, 238, 241, 242, 244–47, 249, 250, 252, 253, 260–63, 320, 321, 328, 332, 372, 386–403

HAAD 44, 45, 54, 55
Harvard 224, 225
Haryana 218, 337, 345, 346
HAU 84
HDI 241
HDL 387
HDR 242
HDRP 242
health-workforce 160, 161
Helsinki 386
HFO 38
HHR 163, 215
Highly-Skilled 104, 105
Himachal 218, 336, 337, 345, 346
Hindi 118, 323
HMR 162
HOL 83, 242
homeopathy 200
hospital 2–5, 8–10, 18, 32, 47, 59–61, 64–78, 80, 110–15, 118, 145, 146,

148, 149, 158, 168–94, 200, 201, 218, 254, 255, 311
household-surveys 286
HP 25–28, 31, 36, 38, 39
HR 252
HRA 254
HSD 382, 385
HSS 162
HST 158
Hugli 349–51, 353, 354, 356, 357, 366, 368
Human Capital 225
Hungary 2, 6, 7, 10, 20, 21, 51, 52, 71, 95, 125
HWD 87, 90, 93, 97, 98, 101, 103
Hyderabad 262, 336, 347, 387, 402
hypothesis 117, 266, 271, 275, 282, 382

IBID 12, 23, 166, 167, 235, 360
ICCU 191
Iceland 93, 95
ICM 164, 195
ICU 170, 178, 179, 183–87, 189, 191
ID 16, 23, 83, 106, 159, 195, 196, 242, 358, 385
IDB 288
IDE-JETRO 109
Idukki 289–92
IEHP 38
IEHPs 201
IELTS 17, 116, 172, 177, 180
IEN 35, 36, 165
IENCAP 38
IFRC 289, 303
IGO 288
IGVET 143
IHDE 165, 166, 195
IHME 160
IIMAD 320
IJCEPA 161
IJE 85
IJNURSTU 84, 195
IJPP 226
IL 120
ILO 23, 88, 118, 127, 131, 151, 161, 244, 261, 307, 331
IMD 291, 292
IMF 264, 287, 288, 322, 332, 385
IMG 34, 318
IMI 225
inclusive 119, 307
index 15, 22, 162, 240, 305, 318, 321, 331, 334, 335, 342, 350, 389, 390, 397, 398

India–ASEAN 144, 147, 148
India-born 93
India–Canada 39, 89
India-EU 105, 195
India–EU 87, 89, 90, 92, 93, 102–4
India–Gulf 89, 135
India–Italy 99
India–Japan 145, 148
India–Korea 148
India-Kuwait 195
India–Malaysia 144, 146, 149
Indians-abroad 119
India–Singapore 145, 149
India-trained 33–36, 38, 99, 201
India–UAE 54
Indo-Gangetic-Brahmaputra 303
Indo-German 143
Indonesia 24, 131, 133–37, 147
inequalities 96, 235, 305, 307, 331
infection 223, 320
infiltration 193
infrastructure 1, 14, 140, 158, 290, 293, 333, 350, 351, 362–65, 368
in-migration 310, 361
Inquiry 83, 196, 225, 228
INR 19, 47, 55, 115, 118
insurance 171, 245, 255, 273, 287, 295, 296, 301, 307, 308, 312, 323
integration 24, 38, 48, 105, 106, 119, 130, 207, 248, 321
Interdisciplinary 303
internet 4, 224, 323, 390, 398, 399
IOM 56, 88, 105, 127, 209–11, 214, 224, 226, 228, 241, 307, 320, 332
IOSR 369
IOSR-JHSS 369
IPEDR 348
Iran 33, 35
Ireland 17–19, 23, 26, 33, 38, 52, 74, 88, 90, 92, 95–102, 104–6, 124, 125, 132–34, 136–38, 140, 159, 165, 177, 179, 180, 194, 201, 207
IREM 382, 383
IRPA 28, 35
ISAS 55
Israel 125
Italy 25, 90, 92–100, 102, 103, 105, 106, 125, 132–37, 142, 201
ITUC 305
IUTC 318
IZA 241, 287

Jakarta 24
Jalpaiguri 354–57, 366–68

Jamaica 124, 132
Jammu 337, 345, 346
Japan 23, 24, 109, 131, 138, 139, 142, 143, 145, 147, 149, 151, 153, 154, 159–61
Jeddah 248, 250
Jharkhand 277, 310, 337, 345, 346
JITCO 143
JOCN 106
JVEPA 147

Kannur 291, 292, 294
Karnataka 109, 152, 203, 289, 309, 321, 337, 345, 346
Kasaragod 290–92
Kashmir 289, 303, 337, 345, 346
Kenya 85, 196, 237
Kerala 1–6, 9, 11, 17, 18, 47, 53, 56, 64, 74, 77, 86, 88, 89, 99, 100, 105, 106, 108, 119, 135, 138, 140, 141, 152, 162, 167, 169, 181, 183, 184, 188, 192–94, 196, 201, 203, 204, 208, 215, 218, 228, 240, 246–51, 253, 255, 257–63, 273, 289, 290, 292–94, 301–3, 308, 318, 320, 321, 323, 332, 333, 336, 337, 345, 346, 371, 377, 380, 386–90, 393, 395, 397, 400–403
Kingdom 14, 15, 19, 23, 25, 26, 33, 35, 83, 87, 124, 125, 133–36, 160, 164, 195, 198, 200, 201, 207, 210, 215, 221, 379, 388, 394
KMS 248, 293, 389
KNOMAD 106, 264, 288, 333
Kochi 255
Kolkata 350, 351, 353–57, 366–69
Kollam 290–92, 294
Konkan 381, 385
Korea 144, 161, 238
Kottayam 6, 289, 291, 292
Kozhikode 289, 291, 292, 294
KSA 207
KSDMA 289, 293, 303
Kuwait 2, 3, 9, 164, 195, 247, 248, 250, 254, 259, 321, 325, 379, 388

Latvia 94, 95, 125
lawyer 185, 314
LBB 258
LDCs 122
Leadership 208
Lebanon 55
left-behind 232
LFP 264

Liberty 225
LICs 287
lifestyle 59, 60, 311
linguistic 154, 156
Lithuania 94, 95
lockdown 209, 219, 254, 258, 259, 306, 308, 309, 311, 313, 314, 318, 322, 330, 331
London 11, 84, 85, 104, 105, 119, 160, 196, 225, 227, 288, 331, 332, 347, 385
longitudinal 89
lottery 288, 372
LPNs 31, 32, 35, 36, 38
LTSSL 14
Lucknow 118, 206
Luxembourg 95, 125

MA 84, 145, 146, 148, 224, 225, 402
MADAD 247, 257
Madhya-Pradesh 345
Maharashtra 64, 167, 181, 186–88, 203, 218, 289, 303, 305, 309, 336, 337, 345, 346, 371, 372, 380, 384
maintenance 224, 260, 322, 323
Malappuram 290–92, 294, 389–401
Malayali 2, 6, 7, 10, 105, 171, 181, 183, 192, 193, 255
Malaysia 11, 133–39, 144, 146–48, 160, 161, 321
Maldives 18, 132, 201, 325
male-headed 267, 280–82, 396
mandatory 34, 189, 205, 245
manpower 158, 204, 207, 323, 380
MARD 203
Mauritius 321
MBAs 185
MBBS 199, 207, 379
MCCQE 34
MCI 198, 200, 208
MEA 105, 195, 330, 331
MED 158
medical-professionals 161
Medinipur 350, 351, 354, 356, 357, 366
Melbourne 20, 127, 128, 158, 162
MFA 244, 245, 258, 260–62
MH 71, 169–72
MICECA 160
MICs 287
midwifery 18, 64, 98, 109, 129, 162, 169, 194, 200, 206, 208
migration-poverty 347
Millennium 227

Mitigation 303
MNC 181
Mo 287
MoA 38
MOHAP 44–46, 55
MOIA 379
MoLE 308
MoU 38, 128, 131, 143, 151, 307, 318
MP 277
MPCE 335, 338, 339, 341, 361, 362
MPI 206
MPRA 287
MRA 13, 16, 20, 22, 38, 148–50
MSDE 142–44
MTO 381
Muslim 18, 110–14, 272, 326, 372,
    373, 380, 383, 391, 392
Myanmar 321, 325

NABH 170, 172, 178, 183, 194
NAFTA 38
narratives 59, 67, 69, 71–76, 79–81,
    168, 169, 171, 173–75, 181, 186,
    193, 240, 246, 248, 323, 331
NBER 225, 287
NCERT 305, 319
NCLEX-RN 36
NCNZ 23
NCR 218
NDMA 308
NEPAD 130
Nepal 206
NESB 55
Netherlands 93–95, 104, 105, 125,
    131, 140
NFHS 389
NGOs 307, 309, 313, 315, 316
NHS 89, 127, 128, 131, 132, 152, 198,
    199, 206
Nigeria 33, 325
NIREM 382, 383
NMIS 308
non-migrant 87, 90, 103, 272, 335,
    336, 339, 340, 347, 362, 372–74,
    376, 383, 389, 390, 395–401
non-resident 158, 201, 246, 247,
    262, 330
NORI 141, 203, 204
Norka 138, 142, 158, 247, 249, 260–62
Norka-roots 204, 246, 247, 254, 257,
    261, 262
NREGA 284, 300
NREM 383
NRI 381, 384

NRT 330
NSDC 143, 151
NSDP 389
NSH 258
NSS 200, 264, 268, 288, 334,
    359–62, 386
NSSO 316, 347, 372, 386
NT 145, 146, 148, 372, 373, 383
nurse 2, 4, 6–8, 10–12, 14, 16, 17,
    19–23, 26, 29, 31, 35, 36, 46, 47, 50,
    52, 58, 60–62, 64–79, 81–87, 91, 99,
    101, 103, 106, 108, 109, 112, 113,
    115, 117–19, 132, 139, 141, 149,
    153, 163–66, 168–96, 201, 203, 204,
    206–8, 212, 221, 225, 226, 228, 393
Nutrition 318
nutritionists 139
NY 23, 105, 106, 118, 243

OBC 110–14, 279, 281, 360, 372, 373
ODEPC 138, 140, 142, 158, 204
Odisha 153, 277, 307–10, 313, 349
oecd 12–15, 22, 24, 25, 40–42, 87,
    88, 90, 92, 93, 96–105, 108, 119,
    121–27, 132, 133, 135–37, 139, 159,
    162, 196, 198, 199, 201, 207, 209,
    214, 226, 227, 236, 241
OECDSTAT 26, 28, 33, 35, 40
OET 17
OMCAP 138, 158, 204
OMCL 138, 158, 204
on-job-training 214
Ontario 31, 33–36, 38, 40
Orissa 337, 345, 346
outflows 129, 132, 140–42
out-migrants 371, 372, 376, 377, 380
out-migration 129, 142, 190, 209,
    217–20, 223, 267, 277, 376
outreach 307, 317
overseas 12–14, 19, 22–24, 46, 48, 49,
    58, 74, 75, 78, 81, 108, 112, 114–17,
    122, 132, 140, 141, 152, 153, 155,
    158, 165, 169, 170, 173, 174,
    177–79, 181–93, 195, 198, 200, 201,
    204–7, 221, 224, 226, 232, 245, 264,
    320, 379, 402
OXFAM 303
Oxford 55, 206, 225, 227, 314, 332,
    333, 369, 386, 387
oxygen 210

PAHO 129, 158
pandemic 25, 27, 39, 48, 51, 87, 96,
    117, 139, 140, 159, 198, 202, 205,

209, 210, 217–19, 222, 223, 244–47,
    249–54, 256, 258–62, 294, 306, 308,
    312, 318, 320, 322, 328–32
paradox 76, 167
paralysis 312
Paris 24, 42, 105, 159, 226–28
PBB 64, 72, 168, 169
PCA 350, 363, 365, 368
PDNA 291, 302
peripheral 214
PF 257
PGE 323
Philadelphia 84
physicians 3, 26–34, 38–42, 47, 55,
    60, 61, 98, 122, 123, 130, 132, 139,
    162, 198, 201, 205
pilot 23, 118, 131, 372
Plumber 327
PMKY 152
POB 353
Poland 35, 88, 95, 125, 142
pollution 47, 63, 71
post-arrival 245
post-colonial 163, 215, 233, 234,
    239, 241
post-COVID 155
Post-emigration 390
post-flood 289, 293
post-independence 199, 241
pre-covid 28, 159, 209, 218, 220–22, 310
pre-departure 153
pre-pandemic 244, 247, 259, 260
PRH 210
PRID 206
progression 200, 221
Projection 28
propensity 114, 237, 268, 273, 284,
    285, 287, 385
prostitution 5, 80
PSI 88
PSV 52
psychiatry 146, 221
PTI 159, 161
Punjab 88, 100, 288, 337, 345, 346,
    349, 371, 377, 386, 387

Qatar 18, 19, 152, 247–50, 321, 325,
    330, 379, 388, 393
QCI 194
quarantine 245, 313
Quarterly 347
Quasi-experimental 287
Quebec 30, 31, 33, 34, 38, 153
quintiles 268, 338–41, 343

Rajasthan 309, 337, 345, 346, 349
ration 307, 308
RCEP 147, 152
RCPSC 34
RDI 334, 335, 342–46
recruitment 2, 8–10, 12–14, 23, 38,
    40, 42, 48, 49, 99, 101, 102, 122,
    123, 127, 128, 130–32, 138, 140–42,
    144, 150, 152, 153, 155, 157, 158,
    160–64, 170, 195, 201, 203–5,
    213–16, 226, 238, 258, 322, 323,
    332, 395, 402
re-emigrate 328, 329
refugees 209, 228, 232, 237, 238, 241,
    333, 366
rehabilitation 262, 293, 301
reintegration 128, 144, 155–57, 247,
    262, 322, 332
Re-migrate 250
remittance 264–73, 275, 276, 278, 280,
    281, 285–88, 331, 371, 374, 375,
    380–82, 384, 385, 388, 390, 394
remittance-based 276
remuneration 2, 21, 22, 25, 26, 32, 39,
    46, 59, 158, 189, 193, 244, 310
reproduction 44, 105, 256
reservation 221, 268, 272, 287
residency 16, 23, 36, 50, 51, 102, 138,
    199, 242
reskilling 53
respiratory 384
retirement 13, 25, 257
returnees 244, 246–50, 252, 253, 255,
    260, 262
return-migrant 245
Riyadh 248, 250
RM 336–42, 344–46
RMSE 277, 282, 285, 286
RMSE's 277
RNs 31, 32, 35, 38, 40
RPN 36, 37
RTAs 38
Russia 202, 388

Saudi 9, 18, 19, 33, 75, 138, 140, 152,
    201, 203, 207, 238, 247–50, 257,
    258, 321, 324, 325, 379, 388, 393
SD 375, 390
SDG 307
SEARO 58, 86
segregation 46, 61
self-employment 300, 360
senior-generation 71, 78, 79
SER 228

Seva 309
SF 118
SG 118
Sharjah 44, 52, 55
Shramik 308, 313
shutdown 320, 322–31
Singapore 132–37, 145, 148, 149, 160, 161, 201, 238, 262, 321, 325
Slovenia 95, 125
slums 310
SMC 312–14
SME 374
SOAS 288
Sociology 11, 84
Somalia 46, 237
SOPEMI 227
South-East 85, 86, 161, 207, 236, 242
South–North 231–34, 237
South-South 202, 230–43, 232, 237, 240, 242, 243
Spain 93–95, 125, 142
spillover 39
stakeholders 102, 142, 157, 246, 247, 257, 260, 261, 308, 315–17
stigma 4–7, 9, 47, 48, 75, 79–81, 175, 182, 186, 187, 192
stranded 245, 313, 322, 331
students 16, 22, 25, 30, 31, 40, 42, 60, 88, 104, 105, 108, 129, 172, 178, 187, 199, 202–4, 206, 224, 228, 291
Sub-Saharan 121, 227
Sudan 46, 100, 237
Switzerland 93, 119, 124, 125, 142, 318
Syria 46, 237

Tamil-Nadu 345, 346
tehsil 373, 375, 384
Thailand 85, 106, 196
Todaro 212, 226, 233
TOEFL 177
TOI 189
Tokyo 160, 161, 226, 385
TOMCOM 138, 158, 204
Toronto 38, 42, 85
TQR 342–44
Tribes 278, 372
Trump 224
Tukey 383, 385

UAE 9, 11, 43–56, 140, 152, 159, 248, 249, 256, 258, 259, 321, 325, 379, 388, 393
UHC 121, 211

UHH 266
UK 25, 26, 33–35, 38, 74, 89, 95, 100, 116, 123, 124, 132, 137, 138, 140, 142, 152, 153, 159, 160, 162, 164, 165, 177, 179, 180, 189, 206, 215, 225, 230, 241, 288
ULB 317
UN 127, 209, 210, 241, 260
UNDESA 209
undocumented 224
UNDP 240
unemployment 52, 53, 226, 267, 268, 308, 320, 331, 334, 386, 389, 401
UNESCO 209, 228, 309, 319
UNHCR 209, 228
unique 87, 103, 222, 246, 388, 391, 392
Universal 121, 211
unorganized 307
unpaid 44, 51, 88, 254–57, 260, 265, 284, 285, 300
unskilled 20, 54, 219, 323, 324, 346, 380, 389, 393, 401
untouchables 86
UNU-WIDER 386
upgradation 153
UPR 347
upskilling 53
USA 52, 138, 164, 210, 215
utopian 166, 191
Uttarakhand 18, 289, 303, 336, 337
Uttaranchal 345, 346
Uttar Pradesh 206, 345

vaccines 210, 223, 227
Vande 245, 255, 262, 324
vendor 323
ventilator 179
Vietnam 131, 147, 154, 288
violators 388
virus 223, 254, 306, 308, 309
visa 10, 14, 23, 48–51, 54, 92, 138, 140, 141, 198, 203, 206, 208, 216, 250, 252, 254, 259, 323
vulnerabilities 198, 256, 308, 322

WA 160
wage-theft 261, 262
Walton-Roberts 1, 8, 11, 49, 56, 58, 81, 82, 86, 87, 89, 106, 112, 114, 117, 119, 120, 158, 161, 165, 190, 196, 198–202, 206, 208, 212, 213, 215, 216, 228
wave 202, 244, 262, 320, 376

WCMS 331
wealth 228, 230, 231, 233, 268, 271,
  334, 336, 338–43, 347, 401
WEF 214, 229
welfare 122, 130, 141, 142, 144, 150,
  151, 153, 155, 160, 203, 216, 247,
  252, 262, 264, 307, 308, 313, 315,
  317, 347, 371, 383–85, 394
well-being 58, 152, 211, 213, 255, 334,
  335, 338, 340, 346, 371, 386
WFMI 162
WIAD 42
workforce 13, 16, 23, 26–28, 30, 31,
  35, 36, 39, 41–43, 45, 48, 58, 82,
  85–90, 92, 93, 96–104, 121–28, 130,
  132, 135, 137, 139, 155, 161, 162,
  164, 165, 188, 192, 196, 197, 200,
  201, 205–8, 210, 215, 224, 229, 310,
  312, 321–23
World Bank 158, 286, 288
WPS 286
WRI 289

yearbook 370
yoga 147, 152, 200, 224
Yojana 152, 307, 308, 313

Zachariah 246, 248, 249, 262, 263,
  293, 303, 333, 371, 378, 380,
  386–89, 402, 403
Zealand 12–24, 26, 52, 53, 124, 131,
  137, 165, 194, 201

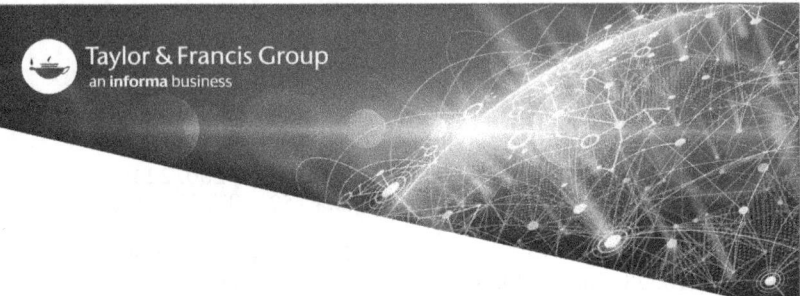
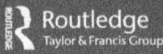
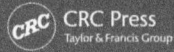